BREAST CANCER: BIOLOGICAL AND CLINICAL PROGRESS

Developments in Oncology

49. K.H. Hollmann and J.M. Verley (eds.): *New Frontiers in Mammary Pathology.* 1986 ISBN 0-89838-852-X
50. D.J. Ruiter, G.J. Fleuren and S.O. Warnaar (eds.): *Application of Monoclonal Antibodies in Tumor Pathology.* 1987 ISBN 0-89838-853-8
51. A.H.G. Paterson and A.W. Lees (eds.): *Fundamental Problems in Breast Cancer.* 1987 ISBN 0-89838-863-5
52. M. Chatel, F. Darcel and J. Pecker (eds.): *Brain Oncology.* Biology, Diagnosis and Therapy. 1987 ISBN 0-89838-954-2
53. M.P. Hacker, J.S. Lazo and T.R. Tritton (eds.): *Organ Directed Toxicities of Anticancer Drugs.* 1988. ISBN 0-89838-356-0
54. M. Nicolini (ed.): *Platinum and Other Metal Coordination Compounds in Cancer Chemotherapy.* 1988 ISBN 0-89838-358-7
55. J.R. Ryan and L.O. Baker (eds.): *Recent Concepts in Sarcoma Treatment.* 1988 ISBN 0-89838-376-5
56. M.A. Rich, J.C. Hager and D.M. Lopez (eds.): *Breast Cancer.* Scientific and Clinical Aspects. 1988 ISBN 0-89838-387-0
57. B.A Stoll (ed.): *Women at High Risk to Breast Cancer.* 1989 ISBN 0-89838-416-8
58. M.A. Rich, J.C. Hager and I. Keydar (eds.): *Breast Cancer.* Progress in Biology, Clinical Management and Prevention. 1989 ISBN 0-7923-0507-8
59. P.I. Reed, M. Carboni, B.J. Johnston and S. Guadagni (eds.): *New Trends in Gastric Cancer.* Background and Videosurgery. 1990 ISBN 0-7923-8917-4
60. H.K. Awwad: *Radiation Oncology: Radiobiological and Phsyiological Perspectives.* The Boundary-Zone between Clinical Radiotherapy and Fundamental Radiobiology and Physiology. 1990 ISBN 0-7923-0783-6
61. J.L. Evelhoch, W. Negendank, F.A. Valeriote and L.H. Baker (eds.): *Magnetic Resonance in Experimental and Clinical Oncology.* 1990 ISBN 0-7923-0935-9
62. B.A. Stoll (ed.): *Approaches to Breast Cancer Prevention.* 1991 ISBN 0-7923-0995-2
63. M.J. Hill and A. Giacosa, (eds.): *Causation and Prevention of Human Cancer.* ISBN 0-7923-1084-5
64. J.R.W. Masters (ed.): *Human Cancer in Primary Culture.* A Handbook. 1991 ISBN 0-7923-1088-8
65. N. Kobayashi, T. Akera and S. Mizutani (eds.): *Childhood Leukemia.* Present Problems and Future Prospects. 1991 ISBN 0-7923-1138-8
66. P. Paoletti, K. Takakura, M.D. Walker, G. Butti and S. Pezzotta (eds.): *Neuro-oncology.* 1991 ISBN 0-7923-1215-5
67. K.V. Honn, L.J. Marnett, S. Nigam and T. Walden Jr. (eds.): *Eicosanoids and Other Bioactive Lipids in Cancer and Radiation Injury.* 1991 ISBN 0-7923-1303-8
68. F.A. Valeriote, T.H. Corbett and L.H. Baker (eds.): *Cytotoxic Anticancer Drugs: Models and Concepts for Drug Discovery and Development.* 1992 ISBN 0-7923-1629-0

SPRINGER SCIENCE+BUSINESS MEDIA, LLC

BREAST CANCER: BIOLOGICAL AND CLINICAL PROGRESS

Proceedings of the Conference of the International Association for Breast Cancer Research, St. Vincent, Aosta Valley, Italy, May 26-29, 1991

Edited by:

L. Dogliotti
A. Sapino
G. Bussolati

Springer Science+Business Media, LLC

Library of Congress Cataloging-in-Publication Data

International Association for Breast Cancer Research. Conference
(1991 : Saint-Vincent, Italy)
Breast cancer : biological and clinical progress : proceedings of
the Conference of the International Association for Breast Cancer
Research, St. Vincent Aosta Valley, Italy, May 26–29, 1991 / edited
by L. Dogliotti, A. Sapino, G. Bussolati.
p. cm. — (Developments in oncology ; 69)
ISBN 978-1-4613-6549-5 ISBN 978-1-4615-3494-5 (eBook)
DOI 10.1007/978-1-4615-3494-5
1. Breast—Cancer—Congresses. I. Dogliotti, Luigi. II. Sapino,
A. III. Bussolati, G. IV. Title. V. Series.
[DNLM: 1. Breast Neoplasms—pathology—congresses. 2. Breast
Neoplasms—physiopathology—congresses. 3. Breast Neoplasms-
-therapy—congresses. WI DE998N v. 69 / WP 870 1578b 1991]
RC280.B8I54 1991
616.99'449—dc20
DNLM/DLC
for Library of Congress 92-7660
CIP

Originally published by Kluwer Academic Publishers in 1992
Softcover reprint of the hardcover 1st edition 1992

CONTENTS

CONTRIBUTORS

J. Alexieva-Figusch, Dept. of Medical Oncology, The Dr. Daniel den Hoed, Cancer Center, PO Box 5201, 3008 AE Rotterdam, The Netherlands

M. Bansal, Dept. of Cell Biology, Baylor College of Medicine, Texas Medical Center, Houston, Texas 77030, USA

P.M.J.J. Berns, Dept. of Medical Oncology, The Dr. Daniel den Hoed, Cancer Center, PO Box 5201, 3008 AE Rotterdam, The Netherlands

S. Bettuzzi, Università di Modena, Istituto Chimica Biologica, 41100 Modena, Italy

M. Bontenbal, Dept. of Medical Oncology, The Dr. Daniel den Hoed, Cancer Center, PO Box 5201, 3008 AE Rotterdam, The Netherlands

P. Briand, Lab. of Tumor Endocrinology, The Fibiger Institute, The Danish Center Society, DK- 2100, Conpenhagen, Denmark

G. Bussolati, Dept. of Biomedical Sciences and Human Oncology, University of Turin, Via Santena 7, 10126 Torino, Italy

G. Calaf, Dept. of Pathology, Fox Chase Cancer Center, 7701 Burholme Avenue, Philadelphia, PA 19111, USA

G. Capony, Université de Montpellier, INSERM U 148, 60 rue de Navacelles, 34100 Montpellier Cedex, France

R.D. Cardiff, Department of Pathology, University of California Medical School, Room 3453, Med. Sci. 1-A, Davis, CA 95616, USA

R. Catane, Dept. Radiation and Clinical Oncology, Hadassah University Hospital, Jerusalem, 91120 Israel

P. Comoglio, Dept. Biomedical Sciences, C.so Massimo d'Azeglio 52, 10126 Torino, Italy

T. Crepaldi, Dept. Biomedical Sciences, C.so Massimo d'Azeglio 52, 10126 Torino, Italy

M.F. Di Renzo, Dept. Biomedical Sciences, C.so Massimo d'Azeglio 52, 10126 Torino, Italy

W.D. Dupont, Dept. of Pathol. and Preventive Medicine, Vand erbilt, University Medical Center, C-3321, Nashville, Tennessee 37232, USA

J.A. Foekens, Dept. of Medical Oncology, The Dr. Daniel den Hoed, Cancer Center, PO Box 5201, 3008 AE Rotterdam, The Netherlands

R. Fuchs-Young, The Ben May Lab. for Cancer Research, 950 East 59th Street, Chicago, Illinois 60637, USA

M. Garcia, Université de Montpellier, INSERM U 148, 60 rue de Navacelles, 34100 Montpellier Cedex, France

G. Greene, The Ben May Lab. for Cancer Research, 950 East

59th Street, Chicago, Illinois 60637, USA

P. Gugliotta, Dept. of Biomedical Sciences and Human Oncology, University of Turin, Via Santena 7, 10126 Torino, Italy

W.J. Gullick, Dept. of Oncology, Imperial Cancer Research Fund, Hammersmith Hospital, Ducane Road, London W12 OHS, England

R. Ishai-Michaeli, Dept. Radiation and Clinical Oncology, Hadassah University Hospital, Jerusalem, 91120 Israel

B. Iwasiow, Dept. of Physiology, Univ. of Manitoba, Inst. of Cell Biology, Winnipeg, Manitoba, R3EOW3 Canada

J.G.M. Klijn, Dept. of Medical Oncology, The Dr. Daniel den Hoed, Cancer Center, PO Box 5201, 3008 AE Rotterdam, The Netherlands

U. Koldovsky, Dept. of Gynaecology, Immunological Laboratory, University of Dusseldorf, Moorenstr. 5, 4000 Dusseldorf, FRG

G. Korner, Dept. Radiation and Clinical Oncology, Hadassah University Hospital, Jerusalem, 91120 Israel

C. La Vecchia, Istituto di Ricerche Farmacologiche "Mario Negri2, Via Eritrea 62, 20157 Milano, Italy

I. Laursen, Lab. of Tumor Endocrinology, The Fibiger Institute, The Danish Center Society, DK- 2100, Conpenhagen, Denmark

P. Leder, Dept. of Genetica, Harvard Medical School, Boston, MA 02115, USA

F. Lee, Dept. of Genetica, Harvard Medical School, Boston, MA 02115, USA

I. Lipp, Dept of Statistics and Biometry, Freiburg University, Germany

F.J. Lofts, Dept. of Oncology, Imperial Cancer Research Fund, Hammersmith Hospital, Ducane Road, London W12 OHS, England

A. Lykkesfeldt, Lab. of Tumor Endocrinology, The Fibiger Institute, The Danish Center Society, DK- 2100, Conpenhagen, Denmark

L. Macrì, Dept. of Biomedical Sciences and Human Oncology, University of Turin, Via Santena 7, 10126 Torino, Italy

C. Manini, Dept. of Biomedical Sciences and Human Oncology, University of Turin, Via Santena 7, 10126 Torino, Italy

A. Manni, Dept. of Medicine, Div. of Endocrinology, Box 850, The Milton S. Hershey Medical Center, Hershey, PA 17033, USA

D.L. Manning, Tenovus Institute for Cancer Research, University of Wales, College of Medicine, Heath Park, Cardiff, CF 44 XX, U.K

D. Marx, Dept. of Statistics and Biometry, Freiburg University, Germany

D. Medina, Dept. of Cell Biology, Baylor College of Medicine, Texas Medical Center, Houston, Texas 77030, USA

Y. Myal, Dept. of Physiology, Univ. of Manitoba, Inst. of Cell Biology, Winnipeg, Manitoba, R3EOW3 Canada

W.R. Miller, Imperial Cancer Research Fundation, Medical Oncology Unit, Western General Hospital, Edinburgh EH4 2XU, Scotland

M. Mohsen, Dept. Radiation and Clinical Oncology, Hadassah University Hospital, Jerusalem, 91120 Israel

R. Moreadith, Dept. of Genetica, Harvard Medical School, Boston, MA 02115, USA

R. Mukhopadhyay, Dept. of Cell Biology, Baylor College of Medicine, Texas Medical Center, Houston, Texas 77030, USA

W. Muller, Dept. of Genetica, Harvard Medical School, Boston, MA 02115, USA

R.I. Nicholson, Tenovus Institute for Cancer Research, University of Wales, College of Medicine, Heath Park, Cardiff, CF 44 XX, U.K.

J. Ochieng, Dept. of Pathology, Fox Chase Cancer Center, 7701 Burholme Avenue, Philadelphia, PA 19111, USA

M. Olivero, Dept. Biomedical Sciences, C.so Massimo d'Azeglio 52, 10126 Torino, Italy

D. Ornitz, Dept. of Genetica, Harvard Medical School, Boston,

MA 02115, USA

D.L. Page, Dept. of Pathol. and Preventive Medicine, Vand erbilt, University Medical Center, C-3321, Nashville, Tennessee 37232, USA

K. Plaut, NIH-NCI, Lab. of Tumor Immunology and Biology, Bldg. 10, Room 5B56, 9000 Rockville Pike, Bethesda, MD, 20892, USA

M. Prat, Dept. Biomedical Sciences, C.so Massimo d'Azeglio 52, 10126 Torino, Italy

H. Rauschecker, Dept. of Surgery, Gottingen University, Germany

A. Robinson, The Ben May Lab. for Cancer Research, 950 East 59th Street, Chicago, Illinois 60637, USA

D. Robinson, Dept. of Physiology, Univ. of Manitoba, Inst. of Cell Biology, Winnipeg, Manitoba, R3EOW3 Canada

H. Rochefort, Université de Montpellier, INSERM U 148, 60 rue de Navacelles, 34100 Montpellier Cedex, France

I.H. Russo, Dept. of Pathology, Fox Chase Cancer Center, 7701 Burholme Avenue, Philadelphia, PA 19111, USA

J. Russo, Dept. of Pathology, Fox Chase Cancer Center, 7701 Burholme Avenue, Philadelphia, PA 19111, USA

A. Sapino, Dept. of Biomedical Sciences and Human Oncology,

University of Turin, Via Santena 7, 10126 Torino, Italy

R. Sauer, Dept. of Radiotherapy, Erlangen University, Germany

H. Sauerbrei, Dept. of Surgery, Gottingen University, Germany

A. Schauer, Dept. of Pathology, Georg-August University, Robert-Koch-Strasse 40, D-3400 Gottingen, Germany

M. Schumacher, Dept. of Statistics and Biometry, Freiburg University, Germany

R.P.C. Shiu, Dept. of Physiology, Univ. of Manitoba, Inst. of Cell Biology, Winnipeg, Manitoba, R3EOW3 Canada

R. Silvestrini, Div. Oncologia Sperimentale C, Istituto Nazionale per lo Studio e la Cura dei Tumori, Via G. Venezian 1, 20133 Milan

E. Sinn, Dept. of Genetica, Harvard Medical School, Boston, MA 02115, USA

D.A. Spandidos, University of Heraklioy, Inst. of Virology, Medical School, Crete, Greece

Q. Tahin, Dept. of Pathology, Fox Chase Cancer Center, 7701 Burholme Avenue, Philadelphia, PA 19111, USA

D. Tsuyuki, Dept. of Physiology, Univ. of Manitoba, Inst. of Cell Biology, Winnipeg, Manitoba, R3EOW3 Canada

I. Vlodavsky, Dept. Radiation and Clinical Oncology, Hadassah

University Hospital, Jerusalem, 91120 Israel

B. Vonderhaar, NIH-NCI, Lab. of Tumor Immunology and Biology, Bldg. 10, Room 5B56, 9000 Rockville Pike, Bethesda, MD, 20892, USA

P. Watson, Dept. of Physiology, Univ. of Manitoba, Inst. of Cell Biology, Winnipeg, Manitoba, R3EOW3 Canada

A. Yarmill, Dept. of Physiology, Univ. of Manitoba, Inst. of Cell Biology, Winnipeg, Manitoba, R3EOW3 Canada

P.-L. Zhang, Dept. of Pathology, Fox Chase Cancer Center, 7701 Burholme Avenue, Philadelphia, PA 19111, USA

PREFACE

The fight against breast cancer is expected to be effectively stimulated by interdisciplinary approaches and cross-fertilization between laboratory and clinical research findings. Of major importance are therefore meetings promoting fast transfer to clinical applications of findings by basic scientists.

The present volume, reporting the proceedings of the 1991 Biennial Conference of the International Association for Breast Cancer Research, hopes to achieve this goal by presenting the most recent observations in the laboratory and their possible applications for diagnostic evaluations and clinical treatments.

The sections of the book focus first on the oncogenes more likely involved in mammary tumorigenesis and on the polypeptide factors and steroid hormones affecting proliferation and possibly inducing carcinogenesis in breast epithelium. A section is devoted to the epidemiological studies and to the identification of risk factors, a way to select populations at higher risk and, possibly, to help in preventing the disease.

Special emphasis is given to the establishment of diagnostic criteria and to the selection of prognostic factors, which must support an effective therapeutic planning.

It is our hope that this volume, a timely update of the most recent advances in specific fields presented by basic scientists, pathologists and clinicians will stimulate new insights and progresses leading ultimately to the control of breast cancer.

L. DOGLIOTTI
A. SAPINO
G. BUSSOLATI

The Editors are grateful to the University of Turin, to the Aosta Valley Region and to all the sponsors, which made the Conference possible. Publication of the proceedings has been supported by a special grant by Farmitalia Carlo Erba (Milan).

This book is dedicated to Prof. P.M. Gullino, who greatly contributed for the organization and the success of the Conference.

SECTION I

ACTIVATION OF CELLULAR ONCOGENES

THE ROLE OF ONCOGENES AND ONCO-SUPPRESSOR GENES IN HUMAN BREAST CANCER

DEMETRIOS A. SPANDIDOS [1,2]

[1] Institute of Biological Research and Biotechnology, National Hellenic Research Foundation, 48 Vas. Constantinou Ave., Athens 11635, Greece.
[2] Medical School, University of Crete, Heraklion, Greece.

ABSTRACT

Breast carcinoma is the principle cancer affecting women and has a complex biological behaviour ranging from a non-invasive to a rapidly metastasizing disease. Recent studies have suggested the involvement of certain oncogenes and onco-suppressor genes in the development of this disease. Ras oncogenes in particular are activated in a high proportion of breast tumors and increased levels of ras protein correlates with poor prognosis. Ras signals may be mediated through the nuclear oncoproteins jun and fos as suggested from the in vitro and in vivo cell transformation studies. The co-operation of ras with other onco-proteins such as myc or erbB-2 and the inactivation of onco-suppressor genes such as p53 or Rb may be important for the progression to the malignant phenotype.

INTRODUCTION

The importance of oncogenes in the development of cancer is now generally accepted (reviewed in refs. 1,2). However, the details of their action during the multistage process of carcinogenesis are not known. Some of the proto-oncogenes which have been shown to be activated in a proportion of breast cancer tumors are discussed below.

<u>Ras</u>

The human ras genes encode proteins called ras p21 that are highly conserved between species, are located in the internal part of the cytoplasmic membrane, are homologous in aminoacid sequence to G proteins, possess GTPase activity and are thought to participate in transducing the proliferation signal (3). The expression of the ras gene family in breast cancer has been studied by immunohistochemical techniques (4), RNA hybridization analysis (5) and Western blots (6). The results of these studies indicate that the H-ras oncogene is important in the progression of malignant breast cancer and that K-ras and N-ras may also play a major role. Amplification of ras genes in breast cancer seems to be a rare event (7,8). Loss of one of the H-ras1 alleles on chromosome 11p was detected in 27% of breast cancer patients who were constitutionally heterozygous for this locus (7). The loss of H-ras alleles in these tumor tissue specimens may indicate the existence of a regulatory sequence that is important in the initiation of breast cancer. Alternatively, the normal H-ras1 gene or another gene located near to it may act as an onco-suppressor gene (2).

<u>Myc</u>

The human c-myc gene encodes for a protein of 62 Kd which is located in the cell nucleus where it binds DNA. Its function is not known (9),although it is suspected of being a transcription factor. Amplification of the c-myc gene in malignant breast cancer has been found at varying frequencies by different investigators (10). These frequencies vary from 6% to 50%

(11,12). However, amplification of N-myc or L-myc is rare (13). The absence of consistent results makes it difficult to draw conclusions concerning the relevance of c-myc in breast cancer. However, it appears that elevated c-myc expression observed at the RNA level does correlate with the prognosis of the patients with breast cancer (13). Using monoclonal antibodies to the c-myc protein, it was found that there were high levels of staining intensity in all malignant tumors, and also in the majority of the benign breast lesions analysed, whereas normal breast tissue exhibited very low levels of c-myc protein (14).The expression of c-myc was also studied in fibrocystic disease (15). High levels of c-myc protein were found in mucous metaplastic cells of epitheliosis and multiple papillomas and it was suggested that elevated expression of c-myc in these cells might be involved in an early stage of malignant cell transformation. A sensitive and quantitative ELISA has been developed for the c-myc oncoproteins and it has been used to assess the level of c-myc in tumor tissue and normal tissue from breast cancer patients (16). No correlation was found between the survival of these patients and elevated c-myc expression in the tumor tissue, and this may be due to the fact that the majority of the patients had advanced disease.

c-erbB-2

The human c-erbB-2 gene and the rat equivalent, neu gene, share homology with the epidermal growth factor receptor gene (17). These genes are also homologous to the viral erbB oncogene. The c-erbB-2 gene encodes a 185 Kd receptor-like protein which has tyrosine protein kinase activity, like the EGF receptor (17) but is distinct from it. Amplification of the c-erbB-2 gene has been observed in breast cancer tissues (10). It has been suggested that amplification of the gene is an indicator of poor prognosis in patients with positive lymph nodes at pathology (18). However, other studies (19) argue for the lack of evidence for the prognostic significance of c-erbB-2 amplification in human breast carcinoma. In vitro transfection studies which showed that a 10-fold elevation of the transfected c-erbB-2 gene in NIH3T3 cells gives rise to transformed cells (20) suggesting that overexpression of this gene in breast tissue may have implications for the progression of the disease. c-erbB-2 expression has been evaluated by an immunohistochemical technique in breast cancer (21-25). No correlation was found between c-erbB-2 expression and survival (21-23). However, others have reported that overexpression of this oncogene correlated with earlier relapse and shorter overall survival (24).

Jun

The first example to be demonstrated of a mutant transcription factor inducing cancer is the product of the oncogene jun. (26).Jun was discovered as a cell-derived genetic insert in the genome of the replication defective retrovirus avian sarcoma virus 17 (ASV 17) isolated from a spontaneous chicken sarcoma (27). The jun interacts with the fos protein to form a complex which binds to DNA at a regulatory element known as the AP-1 site (28). AP-1 is a family of related proteins that have similar binding characteristics and sequences (29). The levels of AP-1 activity as determined by gel retardation assays in human breast lesions and adjacent normal tissue were studied. It was found that AP-1 activity was elevated in 100% of the 12 tumors examined (30).

p53

p53 is a nuclear phosphoprotein that was first identified as a host cell protein that bound to the large tumor (T) antigen of the DNA tumor virus SV40 (31,32). It has subsequently been shown that mutant p53 is a dominant oncogene (33). However,the normal protein is probably an onco-suppressor gene since it can revert the tumor phenotype (34). Mutations in p53 often increase the half life of the mutant protein and immunohistochemical staining to detect the appearance of mutant p53 (35).

DISCUSSION

The development of breast cancer is a multistage process (1). Oncogenes have been implicated in every recognizable stage of this process (2). The evidence in support of this conclusion comes from two directions. Firstly, from experimental model systems involving either the malignant transformation of normal breast epithelial cells with carcinogens or oncogenic viruses or transfection studies with cloned cellular or viral oncogenes (36).Secondly, analysis of human breast lesions for alterations in oncogene structure and expression (4,5,8, 37). Several types of experiments have suggested that oncogenes are involved in the tumorigenic conversion of breast epithelial cells in vitro and in vivo. For example human breast tumors express oncogenes such as ras or myc at abnormally high levels as compared to the adjacent normal tissue. Moreover, genetic alterations in oncogenes in breast tumors occur frequently.

In our studies we have employed a variety of techniques including molecular hybridization using DNA and oligonucleotide probes, immunohistochemistry and ELISA to demonstrate quantitative and qualitative changes in oncogene structure and expression in breast lesions compared with normal tissue (4,5,8). These types of studies provide a better understanding of the possible role of oncogenes in generation of mammary carcinogenesis and might be useful in diagnosis and prognosis.

They might also have implications in the treatment of breast cancer as it might be possible to devise oncogene-based treatments. This is suggested by a number of experimental systems where oncogene action can be halted by transfecting recombinant DNA vectors making anti-sense RNA in the cell, oligonucleotides blocking oncogene expression into protein, site directed mutagenesis procedures, monoclonal antibodies or oncoprotein inhibitors (2).

REFERENCES

1. Spandidos D.A. Bioscience Rep. 6, 691-708, 1986.
2. Spandidos D.A. and Anderson M.L.M. J. Pathol. 157, 1-10, 1989.
3. Spandidos, D.A. (Ed.) Ras oncogenes. Plenum Press. New York and London. pp1-323, 1989.
4. Agnantis N.J., Petraki C., Markoulatos P. and Spandidos D.A. Anticancer Res. 6, 1157-1160, 1986.
5. Spandidos D.A. and Agnantis N.J. Anticancer Res. 4, 269-272, 1984.
6. Clair, T., Miller, W.R. and Cho-Chung, Y.S. Cancer Res. 47, 5290-5293, 1987.
7. Theillet, C., Lidereau, R. and Escot, C. Cancer Res. 46, 4776-4781, 1986.
8. Spandidos D.A. Anticancer Res. 7, 991-996, 1987.
9. Alilalo, K., Koskinein, P., Makela, T.P., Saksela, K., Sistonen, L. and Winquist, R. Biochim. Biophys. Acta 907, 1-32, 1987.
10. Guerin, M., Barrois, M., Terrier, M.J., Speilmann, M. and Riou, G. Oncogene Res. 3, 21-31, 1988.
11. Bonilla, M., Ramirez, M., Lopez-Cueto, J. and Gariglio, P. J. Natl. Cancer Inst. 80, 665-671, 1988.
12. Escot, C., Theillet, C., Lidereau, R., Spyratos, F., Campeme, M., Gest, J. and Callahan, R. Proc. Natl. Acad. Sci. USA 83, 4834-4838, 1986.
13. Varley, J.M., Swallow, J.W., Breammar, W.J., Whittaker, J.L. and Walker, R.A. Oncogene 1, 423-430, 1987.
14. Spandidos D.A., Pintzas A., Kakkanas A., Yiagnisis M., Mahera H., Patra E. and Agnantis N.J. Anticancer Res. 7, 1299-1304, 1987.
15. Papamichalis, G., Francia, K., Karachaliou, F.F.,

Anastassiades, O.Th. and Spandidos, D.A. Anticancer Res. 8, 1223-1228, 1989.

16. Spandidos D.A., Field J.K., Agnantis N.J., Evan G.I. and Moore J.P. Anticancer Res. 9, 821-826, 1989.
17. Semba, K., Kamata, N., Toyoshima, K. and Yamamoto, T.A. Proc. Natl. Acad. Sci. USA 64, 6497-6501, 1985.
18. Slamon, D.J., Clark, G.M., Wong, S.G., Levin, W.J., Ullrich, A. and McGuire W.K.L. Science 235, 177-182, 1987.
19. Ali, I.V., Campbell, G., Liderau, R. and Callahan, R. Oncogene Res. 3, 139-144, 1988.
20. DiFiore, D.P., Pierce, J.H., Kraus, M.H., Segato, O., Richter-King, C. and Aaronson, S.A. Science 237, 178-182, 1987.
21. Gusterson, B.A., Machin, L.G., Gullick, W.J., Gibbs, N.M., Powles, T.J., Price, P., McKinna, A. and Harrison, S. Int. J. Cancer 42, 842-845, 1988.
22. Van de Vijver, M., Peterse, J.L., Mooi, W.J., Wiseman, P., Lomans, J., Dalesio, O. and Nusse, R. New Engl. J. Med. 319, 1239-1234, 1988.
23. Barnes, D.M., Lammie, G.A., Millis, R.R., Gullick, W.L., Allen, D.S. and Altman, D.G. Br. J. Cancer 58, 448-452, 1988.
24. Wright, C., Angus, B., Nicholson, S., Richard, J., Sainsbury, C., Cairns, J., Gullick, W.J., Kelly, P., Harris, A.L. and Wilson-Horne, C.H. Cancer Res. 49, 2087-2090, 1989.
25. Spandidos, D.A., Yiagnisis, M., Papadimitriou, K. and Field, J.K. Anticancer Res. 9, 1385-1394, 1989.
26. Vogt, P.K. and Bos, T.J. TIBS 14, 172-175, 1989.
27. Maki, Y., Bos, T.J., Davis, C., Starbuck, M. and Vogt, P.K. Proc. Natl. Acad. Sci. USA 84, 2848-2852, 1987.
28. Abate, C. and Curran, T. Sem. Cancer Biol. 1, 19-26, 1990.
29. Rauscer III, F.J., Cohen, D.R., Curran, T., Bos, T.J., Vogt, P.K., Bohmann, D., Tjian, R. and Franza, B.R.Jr. Science 240, 1010-1016, 1988.
30. Linardopoulos, S., Malliri, A., Pintzas, A., Vassilaros, S., Tsikkinis, A. and Spandidos, D.A. Anticancer Res. 10, 1711-1714, 1990.
31. Lane, D.P. and Benchimol, S. Genes Development 4, 1-8, 1990.
32. Levine, A.J. and Momand, J. Biochem. Biophys. Acta 1032, 119-136, 1990.
33. Finlay, C.A., Hinds, P.W. and Levine, A.J. Cell 57, 1083-1093.

34. Chen, P.-L., Chen, Y.,Bookstein, R. and Lee, W.-H. Science 250, 1576-1580, 1990.
35. Harris, A.L. J. Pathol. 162, 5-6, 1990.
36. Spandidos D.A. and Anderson M.L.M. Mutation Res . 185, 271-291, 1987.
37. Agnantis N.J., Parissi P., Anagnostakis D. and Spandidos D.A. Oncology 43, 366-369, 1986.

EXPRESSION OF THE *MET* ONCOGENE IN HUMAN TUMORS

M.F. Di Renzo, M. Prat, M. Olivero, T. Crepaldi and P.M.Comoglio

Department of Biomedical Sciences and Oncology, University of Torino Medical School, Torino, Italy.

In human tumorigenesis oncogene over-expression appears to be a frequent event. Oncogenes encoding tyrosine kinases are amplified and/or overexpressed in many human cancers. The *ERBB-1* gene was found to be overexpressed in squamous carcinomas (1-3), in renal cell carcinomas (4) and in glioblastomas (5-6); the *ERBB-2* gene in carcinomas of the breast (7), ovary (8), stomach (9), colon (10) and salivary glands (10). In most cases *ERBB-2* gene overexpression has been associated with poor prognosis (7, 11-12). *FLG* and *BEK*, both encoding tyrosine kinase receptors, were found to be amplified in breast cancers (13).

In human cancer, oncogene activation by structural alteration has also been reported (for a review see 14). Two oncogenes encoding tyrosine kinase receptors (*TRK* and *RET*) were found to be activated by rearrangement at high frequency in human thyroid carcinomas (15-16), suggesting that the activation of this class of oncogenes has a role in the development and/or the progression of human tumors.

The *MET* oncogene encodes the receptor for Hepatocyte Growth Factor/Scatter Factor.

We showed that the protein encoded by the *MET* proto-oncogene is the prototype of a new class of tyrosine kinase receptor by virtue of having a heterodimeric subunit structure (17). A truncated form of the *MET* oncogene was originally identified by transfection assay from a chemically treated human tumor cell line (18). Structural analysis of the *MET* gene product in a cell line where the gene is amplified and overexpressed (17), revealed that it is a 190kDa protein ($p190^{MET}$) composed of two disulphide-linked chains: an extracellular 50kDa α subunit ($p50^{MET}$) and a 145kDa transmembrane β chain ($p145^{MET}$), that contains the tyrosine kinase domain (19-21) and phosphorylation sites involved in the regulation of its activity (22). The kinase activity, in fact, is positively regulated by autophosphorylation on tyrosine (23), and it is negatively regulated by protein kinase-C activation (24) or transient increases of intracellular Ca^{2+} concentrations (25). The aminoacid sequence deduced for the human cloned gene is consistent with this structure (26-27). The molecule is synthesized as a single-chain 170 kDa precursor, which undergoes co-translational glycosylation. Disulphide rearrangements and proteolytic cleavage lead to the mature two-chain 190kDa heterodimer (28).

By using monoclonal antibodies specific for the extracellular domain of the *MET* receptor, two additional *MET* protein of 140 kDa and 130 kDa were identified (29). The former is membrane bound whereas the latter is released from the cell membrane; both have lost the intracellular kinase domain and are likely to be generated by proteolytic processing of $p190^{MET}$. $P140^{MET}$ and $p130^{MET}$ are consistently detected *in vivo*, together with $p190^{MET}$, in different cell lines or their culture supernatants. The generation of the the C-terminal truncated *Met* forms may have a physiological role in modulating the *Met* receptor function.

Recently, Hepatocyte Growth Factor/Scatter Factor (HGF/SF) has been identified as the ligand for the *MET*-encoded receptor (30,31). Hepatocyte Growth Factor (HGF; 32) is a powerful mitogen for hepatocytes in primary cultures and a major mediator of liver regeneration *in vivo* (for a review see 33). HGF was also shown to stimulate the growth of other epithelial tissues, such as kidney tubular epithelium and keratinocytes (34), endothelial cells and melanocytes (35). Scatter Factor (SF) is a protein secreted by fibroblasts which promotes motility and matrix invasion of epithelial cells (36-38). It was reported to be chemotactic and not mitogenic for target cells (39). SF might be involved in the progression of carcinoma cells to a more malignant invasive phenotype (37). While the biological activities of SF and HGF are apparently unrelated, purification of the molecules revealed a surprising degree of structural similarity. Both HGF and SF are disulphide-linked heterodimers consisting of a heavy (α) subunit of 55-65 kDa and a light (β) subunit of 32 or 36 kDa. The coding sequences of SF and HGF genes were shown to be identical (40-42). SF and HGF were also shown to be interchangeable and equally effective in assays for cell growth, motility and invasion (41). Both bind with identical affinities to the same sites in target cells. The formal proof that the receptor for SF/HGF was the product of the *MET* oncogene was given by Naldini et al. (41).

Expression of the *MET* oncogene in normal tissues

In order to gain additional information about the physiological role of the *MET* encoded receptor, its expression was examined in a variety of human tissues at both RNA and protein levels. RNAs of the thyroid, uterus, ovary, adrenal glands, spleen and organs of the gastrointestinal tract were prepared from fresh samples harvested from organ donors. Samples of other organs were harvested from surgical specimens. Northern blot analysis was performed on total RNA using a cDNA probe encompassing the entire *MET* coding sequence. In normal tissues, a 9kb mRNA was the only *MET* transcript detectable. It showed the same size as the major transcript described in cultured cell lines (17). High levels of specific mRNA were found in the liver and thyroid. The transcript was also found in tissues of the gastrointestinal tract, including stomach, ileum, colon and rectum, and in kidney, prostate, seminal vesicles and breast. In lung, uterus, ovary, skin and skeletal muscles specific mRNA was barely detectable while other organs, such as adrenal glands, bone marrow and spleen, were negative.

For Western blot analysis, total proteins of specimens were solubilized in the presence of SDS and separated on PAGE. The $p190^{MET}$ was labelled by an antiserum raised against a synthetic peptide corresponding to the C-terminal tail of the human *Met* protein. High levels of $p190^{MET}$ were found in liver, kidney, ovary, in endometrium and in tissues of the gastrointestinal tract including stomach, ileum, caecum, colon, sigma and rectum (43). In these samples also the 170kDa *Met* precursor (28) was revealed by the antiserum. Lower levels of p190^{MET} were found in the lung, prostate, seminal vesicles, skin and breast. The *Met* protein was barely detectable in the thyroid and in samples of skeletal and smooth muscle. It was undetectable in other tissues, such as bone marrow, lymphoid tissues and adrenal glands. Samples of nervous tissues were taken from fragments of encephalic lobes or spinal cords surgically removed from patients with deeply localized tumors. The *Met* protein was expressed at high levels in the brain, whereas it was barely detectable in the sample of spinal cord and undetectable in the *dura mater* (43).

The cellular localization of the *Met* protein was studied with indirect immunofluorescence on frozen sections of a wide panel of normal adult human organs, using a monoclomal antibody directed against the extracellular domain of the p190^{MET} (44). The results show that immunoreactive *Met* protein is expressed at detectable levels only in restricted cell types (Table 1). The antibody reacted with the epithelial cells of the parenchymal liver, of the major biliary ducts, of the stomach, and of the small and the large intestine. The epithelium of the endometrium and the epithelial component of the ovary were also positive. Basal keratinocytes of the skin and of the oesophagus were stained as well. In hepatocytes and endometrial cells antibody reactivity was preferentially localized at the level of the plasma membrane, with a homogeneous pattern. Basal keratinocytes of the skin and of the oesophagus and major biliary ducts were heterogeneously decorated. In the case of coelomic epithelium of the ovary a diffuse cytoplasmic staining was observed. An identical pattern of reactivity was observed also when specimens were decorated with the immunoperoxidase method. In other normal tissues immunoreactive *Met* protein was undetectable or barely detectable. Surprisingly, the tissues scoring negative by immunofluorescence include thyroid, and placenta, where specific *MET* transcripts were detectable. Since also in Western blot the *Met* protein was barely detectable in thyroid, we concluded that in this tissue either the messenger is not efficiently translated or the protein is particularly unstable.

Table 1. Expression of immunoreactive *Met* protein in normal adult tissues

positive tissues	cell type
Liver	Hepatocytes, major biliary ducts
Oesophagus	Basal keratinocytes
Stomach	Surface and neck glandular epithelium
Jejunum	Cryptal epithelium
Colon-rectum	Basal and middle mucosal gland epithelium
Skin	Basal keratinocytes
Ovary	Coelomic epithelium
Endometrium	Superficial and deep glandular epithelium, endocervical glands
Bronchus	epithelium

Altogether these data suggest that the *Met* receptor plays physiological roles other than the control of hepatocyte proliferations and is implicated in sustaining the growth of a variety of epithelial cells.

Expression of *MET* oncogene in human tumors

The expression of the *Met* receptor was also analyzed in samples of spontaneously occurring human tumors, to investigate its possible involvement in pathological processes.

The *MET* gene is expressed in tumors derived from the epithelial component of different organs (43,44). The expression in gastrointestinal tumors was analyzed at both RNA and protein levels. The level of specific mRNA of stomach and large intestine carcinomas was compared to that of the neighbouring normal tissue. In all tumors the level of *MET* expression was increased. In the whole series of samples, a 9kb transcript was detected. In some stomach carcinoma samples 7.0 and 5.2kb *MET* transcripts were also found. Surgical specimens were also analyzed by Western blotting. The results are summarized in

Table 2. The *Met* protein was expressed in all the tumors of the gastrointestinal tract examined. In a third of the cases of carcinomas of the stomach and colon, it was possible to compare the normal and neoplastic tissues of the same patient; in the whole series, the amount of $p190^{MET}$ was found to be increased in the neoplastic tissue. In most samples also the p170 *Met* precursor was revealed by the antiserum. Similar results were obtained examining carcinomas of the sigma and rectum. Southern blot analysis of carcinoma samples revealed that the increased expression was not accompanied by gene amplification. In a hepatoma the level of *Met* protein was comparable to that of the normal liver. $P190^{MET}$ was undetectable in a gastric lymphoma. By immunofluorecence microscopy, the monoclonal anti-*Met* antibodies stained a high percentage of liver (11/14) and colon-rectal (19/21) carcinomas. A significant percentage of carcinomas of the stomach (11/22) were also positive. The level of *Met* proteins in carcinomas of the liver and of the gastro-intestinal tract was always higher than that observed in their normal counterparts. In the majority of tumors all the cells were stained and the reactivity was restricted to the plasma membrane. Expression of immunoreactive *Met* proteins did not appear to correlate with the degree of differentiation or the histotype of the tumor.

In a sample of colon mucosa, a protein of the approximate mol. wt. of 200kDa was labelled in Western blots in addition to $p190^{MET}$. This protein was recognized by the antiserum directed against the C terminus of the human *Met* protein, but it was not recognized by monoclonal antibodies directed against the *Met* extracellular domain. The structure of the *MET* gene in this patient was studied by Southern analysis of DNA from peripheral blood lymphocytes. Using a combination of different restriction enzymes and probes, unique restriction fragments were found. Together these data suggest that the novel *Met* protein may be the result of a germ-line rearrangement of the 5' portion of the *MET* gene.

Thyroid carcinomas were compared with normal glands and non-neoplastic thyroid diseases. In normal thyroids, as well as in thyroids affected by non neoplastic diseases, only trace amounts of *Met* protein were detectable.

Table 2. Expression of the *Met*/HGF receptor: comparison of normal and neoplastic tissues

Tissue samples	No. positive / No. tested	*Met* protein[1] (relative amounts)
Stomach	16/16	+
Gastric ca.	21/21	++
Gastric lymphoma	0/1	-
Small intestine	4/4	+
Ileal carcinoma	1/1	++
Large intestine	32/32	+
Colorectal ca.	52/52	+++
Liver	3/3	+
Hepatocarcinoma	1/1	+
Thyroid	0/7	-
Thyroid adenoma	1/9	-
Goiter	0/10	-
Thyroid anaplastic ca.	0/1	-
Thyroid papillary ca.	9/15	+++
Thyroid follicular ca.	1/7	++
Thyroid medullary ca.	0/5	-
Breast (mammary gland)	2/2	+
Breast cancer	0/15	-

[1]The relative amount scores are as follows: ± trace amounts; + detectable level; ++ or +++ increased level with respect to the normal counterpart

MET overexpression at protein level was found in 9 out of the 15 papillary carcinomas examined, in 1 out of 7 follicular carcinomas and in 1 out of 9 adenomas. Five medullary carcinomas, as well as the unique sample of anaplastic carcinoma, were negative. The protein expressed in thyroid papillary carcinomas was indistinguishable from the *Met* protein detected in normal human tissues and in epithelial cell lines, as shown by their immunoreactivity with monoclonal antibodies directed against both the C terminal tail and the extracellular domain of the *Met* protein. In addition to the $p190^{MET}$, in thyroid samples it was also possible to detect the truncated p140^{MET}, that is generated from the p190^{MET} by proteolytic cleavage of the intracellular domain and is detectable in all the cell lines expressing the *Met* protein (29). Southern blot analysis revealed that *MET* gene overexpression was not accompanied by *MET* gene amplification and confirmed that also at DNA level the *MET* gene did not show detectable rearrangements. In fact, similar restriction fragments were detected using two different restriction enzymes and a probe encompassing the entire *MET* sequence. By immunofluorescence microscopy the expression of the p190^{MET} was confirmed in 11 out of 13 carcinoma derived from the follicular epithelium.

Unlike normal breast, among the few breast carcinomas examined (15 cases) by Western blot analysis, none showed detectable *Met* protein. As a control, a polyclonal antiserum specific for the *Her-2/neu* protein showed *HER-2* expression in all the breast cancers.

Conclusion and perspectives

By different evidences, many of the known oncogenes have been implicated in the genesis of human cancers. It is likely that multiple genetic abnormalities must develop in order for a cell to become neoplastic, in keeping with the classic multistep theories. Indeed, in many tumors and cell lines more than one oncogene has been implicated. Thus, the discovery that an oncogene, such as the *MET* gene, is overexpressed in a high percentage of carcinomas of the gastro-intestinal and of the thyroid, points to the possible involvement of this oncogene in tumorigenesis affecting these organs.

Whatever the functional consequence of the *MET* gene overexpression is, *Met* protein does accumulate, becoming marker of transformation and target for therapy. Monoclonal antibodies have proved to be a valuable tool for diagnostic and prognostic studies. The discovery of the ligand for the *Met* encoded receptor will be exploited in pharmacology and therapy.

REFERENCES

1. Lu, S.H., Hsieh, L.L., Luo, F.C. and Wienstein, I.B. Int. J. Cancer 42: 502-505, 1988.
2. Hendler, F.J. and Ozanne, B.W. J. Clin. Invest. 74: 647-651, 1984.
3. Yamamoto, T., Kamata, N., Kawano, H., Shimizu, S., Kuroki, T., Toyoshima, K., Rikimaru, K., Nomura, N., Ishizaki, R., Pastan, I., Gamou, S. and Shimizu, N. Cancer Res. 46: 414-416, 1986.
4. Weidner, U., Peter, S., Strohmeyer, T., Hussnatter, R., Ackermann, R. and Sies, H. Cancer Res. 50: 4504-4509, 1990.
5. Libermann, T.A., Nusbaum, H.R., Razon, N., Kris, R., Lax, I., Soreq, H., Whittle, N., Waterfield, M.D., Ullrich, A. and Schlessinger, J. Nature 313: 144-147, 1985.
6. Wong, A.J., Bigner, S.H., Bigner, D., Kinzler, K.W., Hamilton S.R. and Vogelstein, B. Proc. Natl. Acad. Sci USA 84: 6899-6903, 1987.
7. Slamon, D.J., Clark, J.M., Wong, S.C., Levin, W.J., Ullrich, A. and McGuire, L. Science 235: 177-182, 1987.
8. Slamon, D.J., Godolphin, W., Jones, L.A., Holt, J.A., Wong, S.C., Keith, D.E., Levin, W.J., Stuart, S.G., Udove, J., Ullrich, A. and Press, F.M. Science 244: 707-712, 1989.
9. Park J. Bae., Rhim, J.S., Park. S.C., Kimm S.W. and Kraus M.H. Cancer Res. 49: 6605-6609, 1989.
10. Cohen J.A., Weiner, D.B., More K.F., Kokai, Y., Williams, W.V., Maguire, H.C., LiVolsi, V. and Greene M. Oncogene 4: 81-88, 1989.
11. Berchuck, A., Kamel, A., Whitaker, R., Kerns, B., Olt, G., Kinney, R., Soper, J.T., Dodge, R., Clarke-Pearson, D.L., Marks, P., McKenzie, S., Yin, S. and Bast, R.C. Jr. Cancer Res. 50: 4087-4091, 1990.
12. Yonemura, Y., Ninomiya I., Yamaguchi, A., Fushida, S., Kimura, H., Ohoyama, S., Miyazaki, I., Endou, Y., Tanaka, M. and Sasaki, T. Cancer Res. 51: 1034-1038, 1991.
13. Adnane, J., Gaudray, P., Dionne, C.A., Crumley, G., Jaye, M., Schlessinger, J., Jeanteur, P., Birnbaum, D. and Theillet, C. Oncogene 6: 659-663, 1991.
14. Bishop, M. In Weinberg W. "Oncogenes and the Molecular Origins of Cancer, pp. 327-359, Cold Spring Harbor Laboratory Press, 1989.
15. Bongarzone, I., Pierotti, M.A., Monzini, N., Mondellini, P., Manenti, G., Donghi, R., Pilotti, S., Grieco, M., Santoro, M., Fusco, A., Vecchio, G. and Della Porta, G. Oncogene 4: 1457-1462, 1989
16. Grieco, M., Santoro, M., Berlingeri, M.T., Melillo, R.M., Donghi, R., Bongarzone, I., Pierotti, M., Della Porta, G., Fusco, A. and Vecchio, G. Cell, 60: 557-563, 1990.
17. Giordano, S., Ponzetto, C., Di Renzo, M.F., Cooper, C.S. and Comoglio, P.M. Nature 339: 155-156, 1989
18. Cooper, C.S., Park, M., Blair, D., Tainsky, M.A., Huebner, K., Croce, C.M. and Vande Woude, G.F. Nature 311: 29-33, 1984.

19. Dean, M., Park, M., Le Beau, M.M., Robins, T.S., Diaz, M.O., Rowley, J.D., Blair, D.G. and Vande Woude, G.F. Nature 318: 385-388, 1985.
20. Tempest, P.R., Cooper, C.S. and Major, G.N. FEBS Lett. 209: 357-361, 1986.
21. Gonzatti-Haces, M., Seth, A., Park, M., Copeland, T., Oroszlan, S. and Vande Woude, G.F. Proc. Natl. Acad. Sci. USA 85: 21-25, 1988.
22. Ferracini, R., Longati, P., Naldini, L., Vigna, E. and Comoglio, P.M. J. Biol. Chem. 266: 000-000, 1991.
23. Naldini, L., Vigna, E., Ferracini, R., Longati, P., Gandino, L., Prat, M. and Comoglio, P.M. Mol. Cell. Biol. 11: 1793-1803, 1991.
24. Gandino, L., Di Renzo, M.F., Giordano, S., Bussolino, F. and Comoglio, P.M. Oncogene 5: 721-725, 1990
25. Gandino, L., Munaron, L.M., Naldini, L., Ferracini, R., Magni, M. and Comoglio P.M. J. Biol. Chem. 266: 16098-16104, 1991.
26. Park, M., Dean, M., Kaul, K., Braun, M.J., Gonda, M.A. and Vande Woude, G. Proc. Natl. Acad. Sci. USA 84: 6379-6383, 1987.
27. Ponzetto, C., Giordano, S., Peverali, F., Della Valle, G., Abate, M., Vaula, G. and Comoglio, P.M. Oncogene 6: 553-559, 1991.
28. Giordano, S., Di Renzo, M.F., Narsimhan, R.P., Cooper, C.S., Rosa, C. and Comoglio, P.M. Oncogene 4: 1383-1388, 1989.
29. Prat, M., Crepaldi, T., Gandino, L., Giordano, S., Longati, P. and Comoglio, P.M. Mol. Cell. Biol., in press.
30. Naldini, L., Vigna, E., Narshiman, R.P., Gaudino, G., Zarnegar, R., Michalopoulos, G. and Comoglio, P.M. Oncogene 6: 501-504, 1991.
31. Bottaro, D.P., Rubin, J.S., Faletto, D.L., Chan, A.M.L., Kmiecick, T.E., Vande Woude, G.F. and Aaronson, S.A. Science 251: 802-804, 1991.
32. Nakamura, T., Teramoto, H. and Ichihara, A. Proc. Natl. Acad. Sci. USA 86: 6489-6493, 1986.
33. Michalopoulos, G.K. FASEB J. 4: 176-187, 1990.
34. Kan, M., Zhang, G.H., Zarnegar, R., Michalopoulos, G., Myoken, Y., Mckeehan, W.L. and Stevens, J.L. Biochem. Biophys. Res. Commun. 174: 331-337, 1991.
35. Rubin, J.S., Chan, A.M.L., Bottaro, D.P., Burgess, W.H., Taylor, W.G., Cech, A.C., Hirschfield, D.W., Wong, J., Miki, T., Finch, P.W. and Aaronson, S.A. Proc. Natl. Acad. Sci. U.S.A. 88: 415-419, 1991
36. Stoker, M., Gherardi, E., Perryman, M. and Gray, J. Nature, 327: 239-242, 1987.
37. Weidner, K.M., Behrens, J., Vandekerckove, J. and Birchmeier, W. J. Cell Biol. 111: 2097-2108, 1990.
38. Rosen, E.M., Meromsky, L., Setter, E., Vinter, D.W. and Golberd, I.D. Metastasis 10: 49-64, 1990.
39. Gherardi, E., Gray, J., Stoker, M., Perryman, M. and Furlong, R. Proc. Natl. Acad. Sci. USA 86: 5844-5848, 1989.
40. Weidner, K.M., Arakaki, N., Vandekerchove, J., Weingart, S., Hartmann, G., Rieder, H., Fonatsch, C., Tsubouchi, H., Hishida, T., Daikuhara, Y. and Birchmeier, W. Proc. Natl. Acad. Sci. USA, in press.

41. Naldini, L., Weidner, K.M., Vigna, E., Gaudino, G., Bardelli, A., Ponzetto, C., Narsimhan, R.P., Hartmann, G., Zarnegar, R., Michalopoulos, G., Birchmeier, W. and Comoglio, P.M. EMBO J. 10: 000-000, 1991.
42. Gherardi, E. and Stoker, M. Nature 346: 228, 1990
43. Di Renzo, M.F., Narsimhan, R.P., Olivero, M., Bretti, S., Giordano, S., Medico, E., Gaglia, P., Zara, P. and Comoglio, P.M. Oncogene 6: 000-000, 1991.
44. Prat, M., Narsimhan R.P., Crepaldi, T., Nicotra, M.R., Natali, P.G. and Comoglio, P.M. Int. J. Cancer, in press.

ACKNOWLEDGEMENTS

The original papers quoted in this article have been supported by grants from the Italian Association for Cancer Research (A.I.R.C.) and the Italian C.N.R. (PF Biotecnologie and PF A.C.R.O.).

c-*erb*B-2, a Tyrosine Kinase Growth Factor Receptor and its Role in Breast Cancer

F.J. LOFTS and W.J. GULLICK

I.C.R.F. Molecular Oncology Group, 3rd Floor Cyclotron Building, Hammersmith Hospital, Du Cane Road, London W12 OHS.

INTRODUCTION

The tyrosine kinase growth factor receptors form a group of transmembrane glycoproteins with intracellular tyrosine kinase activity and extracellular ligand binding domain. The group is subdivided into four subgroups based on differences in predicted structure (1). The type I subgroup includes the epidermal growth factor receptor (EGFR), encoded by the c-*erb*B-1 gene, c-*erb*B-2 and c-*erb*B-3, which have two cysteine rich domains within the extracellular region and a single tyrosine kinase domain intracellularly. Subgroup II consists of the insulin receptor family, which differ in forming heterotetrameric structures covalently linked by disulphide bonds. Members of subgroup III, e.g. platelet derived growth factor receptor (PDGFR) and colony stimulating growth factor receptor (CSF-1R) have five immunoglobulin-like domains in the extracellular region instead of the cysteine rich domains of subgroups I and II and the tyrosine kinase region is divided by a kinase insert. Subgroup IV, which includes the fibroblast growth factor receptors, is essentially very similar to subgroup III but the extracellular domain has only three immunoglobulin-like structures. The kinase insert of group III and IV contains a tyrosine which can be phosphorylated and has been shown to be involved in substrate binding (2); similarly variable numbers of tyrosine residues in the C-terminus of these receptors, the so called autophosphorylation sites are thought to be involved in either substrate binding and specificity or regulation of receptor kinase activity (3). All the subgroups have a single transmembrane domain across which the mitogenic signal heralded by ligand binding must be propagated. Two theories to explain this process have been proposed.

Firstly, the intramolecular theory proposes that monomeric receptors undergo conformational change on addition of ligand which would be transduced across the membrane. There are theoretical objections to this model with regard to the energy changes required for such a conformational change and in addition incorporation of unrelated sequence in the juxtamembrane region of the CSF.1R are without effect on signal transduction (4), implying no conformational structural constraints on this area. Evidence for the second or intermolecular theory is increasing and includes the following. Kinase negative mutant receptors can be transphosphorylated when coexpressed with a wild type receptor (5); coexpression of insulin and EGF chimeric receptors allows for intermolecular cross phosphorylation by the corresponding ligand (6); dimerisation and activation of EGFR by bivalent monoclonal antibodies but not by their Fab fragments (7) and ligand induced oligomerisation of receptors detected either in living cells, membrane preparations or with purified receptors (8,9,10). It is now generally accepted that growth factors induce dimerisation of their receptors and it is the close association of two intracellular tyrosine kinase domains so derived that results in a conformational change causing activation of kinase activity with binding of ATP and phosphorylation of substrate or the receptor itself on tyrosine residues.

In this chapter we will describe the proposed mode of action of these receptors, with respect to c-*erb*B-2, the evidence for its acting as an oncogene *in vitro* and in human cancer, and lastly possible strategies for inhibiting c-*erb*B-2 in those cancers where it is thought to be over-expressed as in breast cancer.

c-*erb*B-2 OR HER/*neu* FUNCTION AS PROTOONCOGENE AND ONCOGENE

The greatest homology within the type I subgroup is observed in the tyrosine kinase domain, at over 60%. The degree of homology falls to around 40% for the extracellular presumed ligand binding domain (11). Ligands known to activate EGFr include epidermal growth factor (EGF) itself, transforming growth factor alpha (TGFalpha), amphiregulin (12), heparin binding EGF (13), cripto (14) and schwannoma derived growth factor (15). However as yet no ligand for c-*erb*B-2 with full mitogenic activity has been described. Those proteins that have been isolated and shown to have affinity for c-*erb*B-2 - gp30 (16) and another protein of 34 KDaltons (17) when added to cells expressing the c-*erb*B-2 protein will cause increased tyrosine kinase activity but will not cause a proliferative effect on these cells. When EGF is added to EGFr, either solubilized or contained within the cell membrane, it induces dimerization of the receptor (8,9). Using receptors which have been mutated to lack tyrosine kinase activity it has been shown that wild type receptor can be induced to dimerise on addition of EGF to the mutated receptor and cross phosphorylate the C-terminal tyrosine residues as well as intracellular substrates (5).

Thus a model for receptor activation has been proposed whereby EGF binding to the extracellular domain induces a conformational change that allows for dimerization of two receptors which is associated with the increase in tyrosine kinase activity. In the absence of ligand the dimerisation state of c-*erb*B-2 can not be stimulated. However, when cells expressing the rat homologous gene c-*neu* are labelled with ^{32}P orthophosphate and subjected to crosslinkage analysis, 30% of *neu* protein is found to be dimeric (18). Yarden (19) developed monoclonal antibodies to the extracellular domain of *neu* which could stimulate tyrosine kinase activity if bivalent, Fab fragments were ineffective, suggesting a role for dimerization in signal transduction.

This equivalent gene in the rat, *neu*, is known to be a proto-oncogene that can be activated by a point mutation within the predicted transmembrane region. This sequence is composed of approximately 28 hydrophobic amino acids which are thought to form an alpha helix within the environment of the plasma membrane. The mutated *neu* protein, p185*neu*, has a glutamic acid substituted for a valine at position 664 (20). Similar substitutions with aspartic acid and glycine which like glutamic acid would be protonated in the lipid bilayer have been shown to be activating (21), but not other residues. It has been proposed that these specific mutations may explain the observed increase in tyrosine kinase activity of oncogenic p185*neu* by stabilising the receptor in the dimeric state. The presence of an additional hydrogen atom on the substituted residues could form an hydrogen bond between that residue and the carbonyl oxygen of the alanine residue at position 661, thus decreasing the energy state of the dimeric mutant protein compared to the wild type (22,23). Indeed the mutant receptor has been to shown to be 70% dimeric as opposed to only 30% for the wild type, in crosslinkage studies on cell lines transfected with each of the two genes (18). As already stated the oncogenic *neu* has increased tyrosine kinase activity (24) which is essential for its transforming activity (25). In addition Yarden's antibodies were unable to stimulate the kinase activity of oncogenic *neu* implying that it is constitutively active (19).

The activation of rat c-*neu* was first detected in a neuroblastoma cell line derived from tumours that developed in the offspring of rats treated with ethylnitrosourea during pregnancy (26). Attempts have been made to find similar activating mutations in human tumours. So far no such transmembrane mutations have been found in specimens examined by differential hybridization of DNA amplified from primary tumours by the polymerase chain reaction (27-31). However this does not rule out other as yet unidentified activating mutations in the human p185 encoded by c-*erb*B-2. Experimentally engineered glutamic acid for valine substitutions within the transmembrane region of c-*erb*B-2 are found to be activating and the resulting oncogene will transform mouse fibroblasts *in vitro* (32).

However, p185c-*erb*B-2 is capable of acting as a transforming oncogene in the absence of mutation. Overexpression of the human protooncogene in mouse fibroblasts will induce transformation as assessed by focus formation, colony growth in soft agar and growth of tumours in nude mice (33,34). Similarly expression of c-*erb*B-2 in transgenic mice leads to tumours in those tissues in which it is expressed (35). Many human tumours have been investigated for evidence of overexpression of c-*erb*B-2, either due to gene amplification assessed by increased signal on Southern blot, or increased expression by either Northern blot, for RNA transcription, or by immunocytochemistry for protein synthesis. The latter has the advantage of localizing the expression of c-*erb*B-2 to the tumour cells and to the membrane. The significance of staining in the cytoplasm is not known and positive tumours are classified as those with increased membrane staining which has been shown to be associated with gene amplification. In addition immunocytochemistry will detect those tumours which have overexpression in the absence of gene amplification.

c-*erb*B-2 IN HUMAN BREAST CANCER

The relevance of c-*erb*B-2 overexpression in human cancer, particularly in breast adenocarcinoma, has been investigated extensively, helped by the availability of antibodies that can stain paraffin blocks of archival tissue sections. Thus large series have been relatively quickly assessed by immunocytochemical techniques and the association between c-*erb*B-2 positivity and various recognised prognostic indicators established. Within the whole range of breast cancer pathology c-*erb*B-2 membrane overexpression is mainly found in ductal carcinomas. Benign tumours very rarely stain for c-*erb*B-2 (36). Malignant tumours vary in the extent of staining. Ductal carcinoma *in situ* of comedo type has positive staining in 90% of tumours whereas the other histological subtypes such as cribriform, solid or papillary *in situ* carcinomas are predominantly negative (37). Paget's disease of the nipple which is often associated with an intraductal carcinoma also exhibits membrane staining in approximately 90% of cases, whereas extra mammary Paget's is much less likely to express p185 (38,39). Positive staining invasive carcinomas are almost exclusively ductal in origin, lobular carcinoma is not found to have increased c-*erb*B-2 membrane staining (40). Confining oneself to the invasive ductal carcinomas the overall prevalence of c-*erb*B-2 amplification and/or overexpression is approximately 21%, a figure derived from the published data between 1987 and early 1991 and including over nine thousand primary breast cancers examined (41).

This 21% of invasive ductal carcinomas with overexpression of p185 c-*erb*B-2 is found to correlate with poor prognostic indicators. Slamon et al (42) originally described the association of c-*erb*B-2 amplification with poor overall survival and disease free interval in patients with breast cancer. The association was limited to node positive patients who already fell into a poor prognosis group, but c-*erb*B-2 was found to be an additional independent predictor of limited survival of similar power to nodal status. Since this report in 1987 there have been many breast cancer series published looking at c-*erb*B-2 as a prognostic factor. McGuire recently listed a set of guidelines for assessing proposed prognostic factors (43) which included the following, a) a biological hypothesis, and c-*erb*B-2 could indeed be involved in malignant change or progression as it is a known oncogene; b) a pilot study as provided by Slamon et al.(42); and c) definitive studies to determine reproducibility of assays for the factor, optimized cut off values, large multicentre patient populations to avoid bias and methodological validation. Unfortunately, many of the subsequent studies have added little as the numbers of primary tumours examined are too small or the follow-up period to short to allow for any meaningful conclusions on prognosis. Similarly different histological methods and different antibodies used in immunocytochemical studies may give rise to varying sensitivities in detecting p185 membrane staining. Some groups include cytoplasmic staining as positive although the significance of this is not understood and it is not associated with c-*erb*B-2 amplification.

Taking these factors into consideration the balance of evidence is for c-*erb*B-2 amplification and/or overexpression being an independent and significant predictor of poor outcome, be that disease free survival or overall survival. Fig. 1 depicts the published data as a histogram showing the larger the number of primary tumours examined the more often the association with poor outcome was found to be significant.

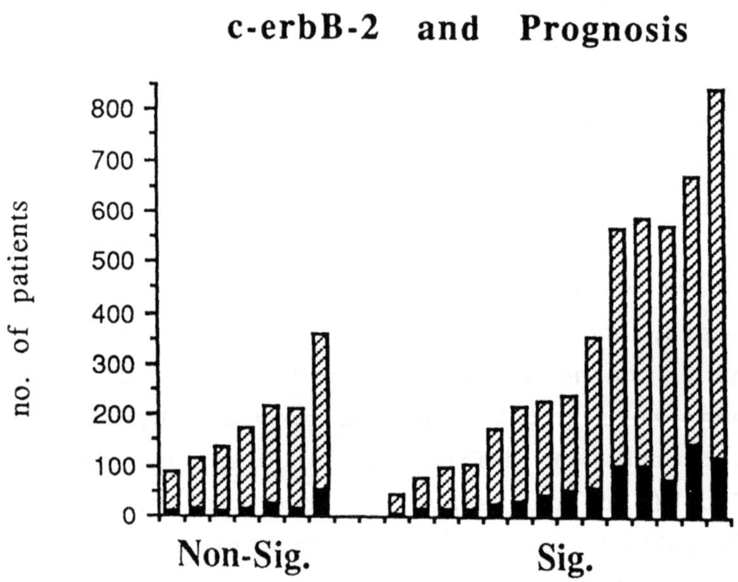

FIGURE 1: Histogram of primary tumours examined for c-*erb*B-2 overexpression in increasing order and separated into those studies finding non-significant or significant prognostic power. Solid bars represent proportion of tumours found to be positive for c-*erb*B-2 and the hatched bar the total number examined in

each series.

As well as c-*erb*B-2 being found to be independently predictive of shortened survival it has been found to be associated with other classical poor prognostic factors. Overexpression is inversely correlated with oestrogen receptor and progesterone receptor (44), positively correlated with histological grade (45), tumour size (37), mitotic index (46) and inflammatory tumours (47).

In spite of all this evidence supportive of c-*erb*B-2 overexpression as a prognostic indicator in human cancer there remains controversy as to its role in the node negative group. Node positive patients already carry a worse prognosis and benefit from adjuvant therapy (48). It is the node negative group, a proportion of whom will also progress, that need to be investigated to try and determine those characteristics associated with and possibly responsible for the aggressive nature of their disease. Hence the importance of determining if c-*erb*B-2 overexpression is truely independently predictive of relapse in this subgroup. Slamon's original report in 1987 (42) did not find evidence for c-*erb*B-2 as a prognostic indicator in the node negative group, but the numbers were small. Node negative patients have a lower probability of relapsing than node positive patients, thus to investigate prognostic markers in this group requires large patient numbers and long term follow-up to accrue sufficient events to correlate with the prognostic indicator of interest.

Studies which have each looked at approximately five hundred primary cancers or more have failed to fully resolve this issue. One study failed to find an independent predictive role in node negative patients (49) whereas another found the opposite with c-*erb*B-2 being of prognostic value only in the node negative group (50). Others have found c-*erb*B-2 to be predictive of a reduced survival or more rapid relapse independently of tumour stage or nodal status (51-54). Figure 2 summarises in histogram form the studies looking at node negative patients specifically and the association between c-*erb*B-2 overexpression and its value as a significant or non-significant prognostic indicator. As can be seen there is not the clear distinction seen on the general histogram and the debate remains open.

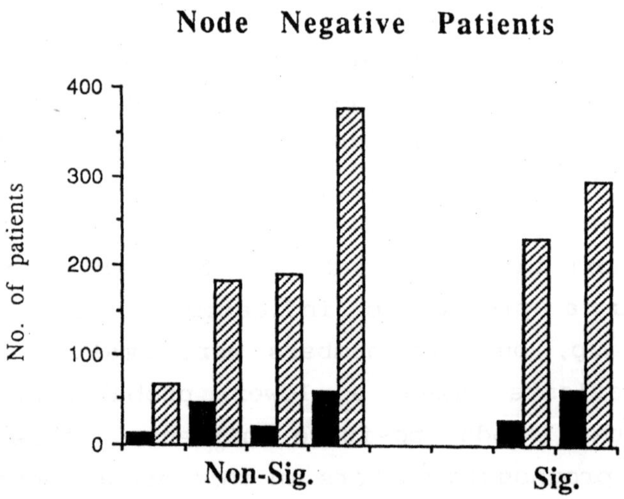

Figure 2: Histogram of number of node negative patients examined (hatched bars) and proportion positive for c-*erb*B-2 overexpression (solid bars) in a series of studies divided into those finding a significant (SIG) or a non-significant (NON-SIG) role for c-*erb*B-2 as a prognostic indicator.

INHIBITION OF c-*erb*B-2

Accepting that c-*erb*B-2 is an oncogene when overexpressed in fibroblasts and that it is found to be overexpressed in various human adenocarcinomas as well as breast it could have a role in the development of these tumours. In addition to breast cancer c-*erb*B-2 is amplified and/or overexpressed in ovarian cancer (55), gastric cancer (56), bladder cancer (57) and non-small cell lung cancers (58). Thus if one could inhibit the function of c-*erb*B-2 one could potentially limit the progression of disease, particularly in breast cancer where it confers a worse prognosis with increased probability of relapse. There are various theoretical approaches to inhibiting growth factor receptor function and some have been utilized experimentally and we will briefly review the data available so far.

Ligand antagonists

As described above a ligand for c-*erb*B-2 or *neu* with full mitogenic activity has not yet been recognised. However when such information is available no doubt it will attract similar interest as has the EGF peptide. The sequence of EGF is known and its three dimensional structure has been determined by NMR spectroscopy. By altering residues within the sequence that are thought to be involved in binding to receptor one can attempt to generate antagonists to EGF which maintain binding activity but have no ability to stimulate kinase. Such peptides have been made but although they lack stimulatory activity they also lack affinity for the receptor compared to EGF (59). The three dimensional structure of the binding pocket has not yet been determined and until this is known it is unlikely that more specific antagonistic analogues of EGF will be synthesised.

Monoclonal antibodies

Antibodies directed against the extracellular domain could have the capacity to either stimulate the receptor, compete for the ligand binding site or induce down-regulation without phosphorylation. An antibody with the latter characteristics against *neu*, 7.16.4, has been shown to reduce the ability of *neu* transformed fibroblasts to grow as colonies in soft agar or tumours in nude mice (60). Similarly an antibody to human c-*erb*B-2 has been generated and shown to inhibit the growth of human breast cancer cell lines *in vitro* (61). Although there are problems in administering monoclonal antibodies to humans with poor accessability of a large macromolecule to the site of the tumour and anti mouse antibody responses, such antibodies are now being considered for use in Phase I clinical trials.

Extracellular domains

There are two approaches to the use of extracellular domains. One group has reported on the use of secreted extracellular domains of p185 c-*erb*B-2 as a source of immunogen. Experimental animals immunised with this protein developed cellular immunity against c-*erb*B-2 expressing cells and antibodies that were inhibitory to growth of breast cancer cell lines (62). Unfortunately, within the human situation the species differences exploited by this method cannot be utilised. Basu et al. (63) used the external domain of EGFR secreted from A431 cells to show that this soluble form of the receptor could form heterodimers with the membrane bound form of the receptor and thus inhibit tyrosine kinase activity, it was not found to be due to competition for EGF binding (although the soluble extracellular domains can bind EGF) as the effect was still seen in saturating concentrations of EGF. In the PDGFR system addition of soluble extracellular domain was found to inhibit the binding of PDGF to the whole receptor and thus blocked the mitogenic response (64).

Dimerisation Inhibitors

Just as the extracellular domain of EGFR can form heterodimers which inhibit kinase activity any form of truncated receptor which lacks a kinase domain may have the ability of forming inactive complexes with whole wild type receptor thus competitively blocking mitogenic signal transduction. This has been shown to be the case for EGFR when the whole receptor is expressed with a receptor lacking only the intracellular domain but still anchored in the membrane (65) and for the PDGFR with similar deletions (66). In this laboratory we are taking a similar approach but trying to determine the minimal length of receptor that can still dimerise with whole receptor to inhibit homodimers and thus form inactive heterodimers.

Tyrosine Kinase Inhibitors

The tyrosine kinase region could be considered as the effector for these receptors, thus the enzyme's function could be inhibited either by inhibition of ATP or substrate binding. The ATP binding site has considerable homology between kinases with the sequence Gly-X-Gly-x-x-Gly followed at a variable distance by Val-Ala-X-Lys determining the site. Thus although effective antagonists to ATP binding have been found e.g. genistein which inhibit tyrosine kinases, but not serine and threonine kinases, it lacks specificity and would act on all tyrosine kinase receptors as well as the intracellular tyrosine kinases (67). Erbstatin is a naturally occurring compound with tyrosine kinase inhibitory properties due to its ability to compete with substrate for binding to the substrate binding pocket of tyrosine kinases. An analogue of erbstatin has been shown to be growth inhibitory to EGF treated A431 cells (68). The structure of these substrate antagonists is related to tyrosine and chemical synthesis of similar tyrosine based inhibitory analogues has allowed development of compounds which appear to have greater affinity for EGFR kinase domain than that of the insulin receptor, by three orders of magnitude, assessed in purified receptor kinase assays. These compounds blocked EGF induced proliferation but not EGF independent proliferation of A431 cells (69). Thus exploiting the differences in substrate specificity between receptors may allow the development of specific tyrosine kinase inhibitors.

Antisense oligonucleotides

The aim of antisense oligonucleotides is to block the translation of the mRNA specific to the protein of interest by administering a sequence of DNA complementary to the message which will thus hybridise to it and either interrupt translation or lead to destruction of the message. The technology of designing nuclease resistant oligonucleotides and administration to the cell is developing rapidly, inspite of technical problems with such a strategy antisense oligonucleotides can be effective in blocking expression of some proteins (70,71). No published data on inhibition of c-*erb*B-2 or *neu* translation is available.

CONCLUSIONS

c-*erb*B-2 is an oncogene that is activated by amplification and/or overexpression. It is found to be amplified and overexpressed in approximately 20% of some human adenocarcinomas. In breast cancer it's expression is associated with a poor prognosis and thus it is a potential therapeutic target. Various approaches towards inhibiting c-*erb*B-2 or other tyrosine kinase growth factor receptor function have been discussed.

REFERENCES

1. Yarden Y. and Ullrich A., Ann. Rev. Biochem. 57:443-478, 1988.
2. Cantley L.C., Auger K.R., Carpenter C., Duckworth B., Graziani A., Kapeller R. and Soltoff S. Cell 64:281-302, 1991.
3. Ullrich A. and Schlessinger J. Cell 61:203-212, 1990.
4. Lee A.W-H. and Nienhuis A.W. Proc. Natl. Acad. Sci. USA 87:7270-7274, 1991.
5. Honegger A.M., Schmidt A., Ullrich A. and Schlessinger J. Mol. Cell. Biol. 10:4035-4044, 1990.
6. Ballotti R., Lammers R., Scimeca I-C., Dull T., Schlessinger J., Ullrich A. and van Obberghen E. EMBO J. 8:3303-3309, 1989.
7. Spaargaren M., Defize L.H.K., Boonstra J. and de Laat S.W. J. Biol. Chem. 266:1733-1739, 1991.
8. Yarden Y. and Schlessinger J. Biochemistry 26:1434-1442, 1987.
9. Yarden Y. and Schlessinger J. Biochemistry 26:1443-1451, 1987.
10. Schlessinger J. Biochem. Sci. 13:443-447, 1988.
11. Yamamoto T., Ikawa S., Akiyama T., Semba K., Nomura N., Miyajima N., Saito T. and Toyoshima K. Nature 319:230-234,1986.
12. Plowman G.D., Green J.M., McDonald V.L., Neubauer M.G., Disteche C.M., Todaro G.J. and Shoyab M. Mol. Cell. Biol. 10: 1969-1981, 1990.
13. Higashiyama S., Abraham J.A., Miller J., Fiddes J.C. and Klugsbrun M. Science 251:936-939, 1991.
14. Ciardiello F., Dono R., Kim N., Persico G. and Salomon D.S. Cancer Res. 51:1051-1054, 1991.
15. Kimura H., Fischer W.H. and Schubert D. Nature 348:257-260, 1990.
16. Lupu R., Colomer R., Zugmaier G., Sarup, J., Shepard M., Slamon D. and Lippman M.E. Science 249:1552-1555, 1990.
17. Yarden Y. and Peles E. Biochemistry 30:3543-3550, 1991.
18. Weiner D.B., Liu J., Cohen J.A., Williams W.V. and Greene M.I. Nature 339:230-231, 1989.
19. Yarden Y. Proc. Natl. Acad. Sci. USA 87:2569-2573, 1990.
20. Bargmann C.I., Hung M-C. and Weinberg R.A. Cell 45:649-657, 1986.

21. Bargmann C.I. and Weinberg R.A. EMBO J. 7:2043-2052, 1988.
22. Sternberg M.J.E. and Gullick W.J. Nature 339:587, 1989.
23. Sternberg M.J.E. and Gullick W.J. Protein Engineering 3:245-248, 1990.
24. Bargmann C.I. and Weinberg R.A. Proc. Natl. Acad. Sci. USA 85:5394-5398, 1988.
25. Weiner D.B., Kokai Y., Wada T., Cohen J.A., Williams W.V. and Greene M.I. Oncogene 4:1175-1183, 1989.
26. Shih C., Padhy L.C., Murray M. and Weinberg R.A. Nature 290:261-264, 1981.
27. Lemoine N.R., Staddon S.L., Dickson C., Barnes D.M. and Gullick W.J. Oncogene 5:237-239, 1990.
28. Lemoine N.R., Wyllie F.S., Lillehaug J.R., Staddon S.L., Hughes C.M., Aasland R., Shaw J., Varhaug J.E., Brown C.L., Gullick W. J. and Wynford-Thomas D. Eur. J. Cancer 26:777-779,1990.
29. Hall P.A., Hughes C.M., Staddon S.L., Richman P.I., Gullick W.J. and Lemoine N.R. J. Pathology 161:195-200, 1990.
30. Tuzi N.L., Venter D.J., Kumar S., Staddon S.L., Lemoine N.R. and Gullick W.J. Br. J. Cancer 63:227-233, 1991.
31. Lemoine N.L., Jain S., Silvestre F., Lopes C., Hughes C.M., McLelland E., Gullick W.J. and Filipe M.I. Br. J. Cancer 64:79-83, 1991.
32. Segatto O., King C.R., Pierce J.H., Di Fiore P.P. and Aaronson S.A. Mol. Cell. Biol. 8:5570-5574, 1988.
33. Di Fiore P.P., Pierce J.H., Kraus M.H. Segatto O., King C.R. and Aaronson S.A. Science 237:178-182, 1987.
34. Hudziak R.M., Schlessinger J. and Ullrich A. Proc. Natl. Acad. Sci. USA 84:7159-7163, 1987.
35. Suda Y., Aizawa S., Furuta Y., Yagi T., Ikawa Y., Saitoh K., Yamada Y., Toyoshima K. and Yamamoto T. EMBO J. 9:181-190, 1990.
36. Gusterson B.A., Machin L.G., Gullick W.J., Gibbs N.M., Powles T.J., Elliott C., Ashley S., Monaghan P. and Harrison S. Br. J. Cancer 58:453-457, 1988.
37. van de Vijver M.J., Peterse J.L., Mooi W.J., Wisman P., Lomans J., Dalesio O. and Nusse R. N.E.J.M. 319:1239-1245, 1988.
38. Lammie G.A., Barnes D.M., Millis R.R. and Gullick W.J. Histopathology 15:505-514, 1989.
39. Meissner K., Riviere A., Haupt G. and Loning T. Am. J. Path. 137:1305-1309, 1990.
40. Ramachandra S., Machin L., Ashley S., Monaghan P. and Gusterson B.A. J. Path. 161:7-14, 1990.
41. Lofts F.J. and Gullick W.J. In:Breast

Cancer:Cellular and Molecular Biology III(Eds. Dickson R.B. and Lippman M.E.) Kluwer Acad. Publishers, Norwell, 1991.
42. Slamon D.J., Clarke G.M., Wong S.G., Levin W.J., Ullrich A. and McGuire W.L. Science 235:177-182, 1987.
43. McGuire W.L. J.N.C.I. 83:154-155, 1991.
44. Zeillingar R., Kury F., Czerwenka K., Kubista E., Sliutz G., Knogler W., Huber J., Zielinski C., Reiner G., Jakezz R., Staffen A., Reiner A., Wrba F. and Spona J. Oncogene 4:109-114, 1989.
45. Parkes H.C., Lillycrop K., Howell A. and Craig R.K. Br. J. Cancer 61:39-45, 1990.
46. Marx D., Schauer A., Reiche C., May A., Ummenhofer L., Roles A., Rauschecher H., Sauer R. and Schumacher M. J. Cancer Res. Clin. Oncol. 116:15-20, 1990.
47. Guerin M., Gabillot M., Mathieu M-C., Travagli J-P., Spielmann M., Andrieu N. and Riou G. Int. J. Cancer 43:201-208, 1989.
48. Early Breast Cancer Trialists Collaborative Group. Treatment of Early Breast Cancer vol. 1, Oxford University Press, 1990.
49. Clark G.M. and McGuire W.L. Cancer Res. 51:944 - 948, 1991.
50. Dykins R., Corbett I.P., Henry J.A., Wright C., Yuan J., Hennessy C., Lennard T.J.W., Angus B. and Home C.H.W. J. Path. 163:105-110, 1991.
51. Paterson M.C., Dietrich K.D., Danyluk J., Paterson A.H.G., Lees A.W., Jamil N., Hanson J., Jenkins H., Krause B.E., McBlain W.A., Slamon D.J. and Fourney R.H. Cancer Res. 51:556-567, 1991.
52. Gullick W.J., Love S.B., Wright C., Barnes D.M., Gusterson, B., Harris A.L. and Altman D.G. Br. J. Cancer 63:434-438, 1991.
53. Lovekin C., Ellis I.O., Locker A., Robertson J.F.R., Bell J., Nicholson R., Gullick W.J., Elston C.W. and Blamey R.W. Br. J. Cancer 63: 439-443, 1991.
54. Winstanley J., Cooke T., Murray G.D., Platt-Higgins A., George W.D., Holt S., Myskov M., Spedding A., Barraclough B.R. and Rudland P.S. Br. J. Cancer 63:447-450, 1991.
55. Slamon D.J., Godolphin W., Jones L.A., Holt J.A., Wong S.G., Keith D.E., Levin W.J., Stuart S.G., Udove J., Ullrich A. and Press M.F. Science 244:707-712, 1989.
56. Falck V.G. and Gullick W.J. J. Path 159:107- 111, 1989.
57. Moriyama M., Akiyama T., Yamamoto T., Kawamoto T., Kato T., Sato K., Watanuki T., Hikage T., Katsuta N. and Mori S. J. Urology 145:423-427, 1991.

58. Kern J.A., Schwartz D.A., Nordberg J.E., Weiner D.B., Greene M.I., Torney L. and Robinson R.A. Cancer Res. 50:5184-5191, 1990.
59. Matsunami R.K., Campion S.R., Niyogi S.K. and Stevens A. FEBS Letters 264:105-108, 1990.
60. Drebin J.A., Link V.C., Stern D.F., Weinberg R.A. and Greene M.I. Cell 41:695-706, 1985.
61. Hudziak R.M., Lewis G.D., Winget M., Fendly B.M., Shepard H.M. and Ullrich A. Mol. Cell. Biol. 9:1165-1172, 1989.
62. Fendly B.M., Kotts C., Vetterlein D., Lewis G.D., Winget M., Carver M.E., Watson S.R., Sarup J., Saks S., Ullrich A. and Shepard H.M. J. Biol. Response Modifiers 9:449-455, 1990.
63. Basu A., Raghunath M., Bishayee S. and Das M. Mol. Cell. Biol. 9:671-677, 1989.
64. Duan D-S.R., Pazin M.J., Fretto L.J. and Williams L.T. J. Biol. Chem. 266:413-418, 1991.
65. Kashles O., Yarden Y., Fischer R., Ullrich A. and Schlessinger J. Mol. Cell. Biol. 11:1454-1463, 1991.
66. Ueno H., Colbert H., Escobedo J.A. and Williams L.T. Science 252:844-848, 1991.
67. Gullick W.J. In:Genes and Cancer (Eds Carney D. and Sikora K.) J. Wiley & Sons Ltd.,263-273, 1990.
68. Yaish P., Gazit A., Gilon C. and Levitzki A. Science 242:933-935, 1988.
69. Umezawa K., Hori T., Tajima H., Imoto M., Isshiki K. and Takeuchi T. FEBS Letters 260:198-200, 1990.
70. Tidd D.M. Br. J. Cancer 63:6-8, 1991.
71. Stein C.A. and Cohen J.S. Cancer Res. 48:2659-2668, 1988.

ACKNOWLEDGEMENTS

We would like to thank Miss Zoe Redley for invaluable help in the preparation of this manuscript.

MAMMARY MORPHOGENESIS AND ONCOGENES

Robert D. Cardiff[1], David Ornitz[2], Frederick Lee[2], Randall Moreadith[2], Eric Sinn[2], William Muller[2], and Philip Leder[2]

[1]Department of Pathology, School of Medicine, University of California, Davis CA, 95616; [2]Department of Genetics, Harvard Medical School, Boston MA, 02115 .

INTRODUCTION

The effects of specific oncogenes on the differentiation of the mammary epithelium can now be studied using transgenic animals and glands (1). Many studies have now appeared describing the use of different transgenes and several different promotor systems to produce mammary tumors (1,2). The use of binary systems for tissue-specific promotion of oncogenes and the production of bigenic and trigenic animals through hybrid crosses promise to expand the analysis of different oncogenes in mammary epithelium (3). Some investigators have recognized the presence of various types of mammary hyperplasia and mammary dysplasia in these animals (4,5). However, there has been very little discussion of the growth and development of the mammary gland in these animals and there have been no comparative studies of the effects of different oncogenes on the morphogenesis of the mammary gland. In the following review, we will summarize our collective experience with mammary growth and development and with mammary tumorigenesis in one set of transgenic animals.

GROWTH AND DEVELOPMENT

Control

The growth and development of the FVB mouse mammary tree was followed using the whole mount technique and histological sections of the FVB mouse from the age of three weeks through pregnancy and into retirement from a breeding colony. In general, the FVB mammary gland showed the normal growth and development expected of laboratory strains of mice. At three weeks of age the mammary tree extended into less than 10% of the mammary fat pad. By 9 weeks, the gland frequently filled 100% of the fat pad and consisted of ducts with very little lobulo-alveolar development. The virgin animal maintained this configuration throughout its lifetime.

The mammary gland of the pregnant animal proliferated to form lobulo-alveolar units as expected. The most unusual aspect of the physiology of the FVB mammary gland was the very long period for the gland to regress after weaning. Some animals examined three months after weaning had strikingly persistent lobulo-alveolar hyperplasia. However, no focal lesions and no mammary tumors were found in the FVB mammary gland.

Transgenic

Growth and development in the transgenic mammary gland appears to be influenced by the type of oncogene, quantity of the transgene expressed and the hormonal milieu. Most of the transgenic animals examined exhibited normal growth and development of the mammary gland. None of the animals with ras, myc, mos, fos, or jun transgenes demonstrated abnormal mammary development in virgin animals. Only one of many monogenic int-2 animals examined by the whole mount technique had a focal cystic lesion in a virgin mammary tree.

The most striking abnormalities of the virgin mammary gland were found in the binary int-2 animals, created by using a dual mammary promoter system, which were expressing very high levels of the mRNA (3). These animals had extensive cystic ductal dysplasia and stunted mammary growth. Transplantation of these abnormal structures resulted in abnormal outgrowths of binary int-2 mammary tissue into the stroma of the normal FVB fat pad.

RESPONSE TO HORMONES

Mammary epithelium is very responsive to a variety of hormones. The LTR of the mouse mammary tumor virus contains hormone response elements and increases the hormone responsiveness of mammary tissue (2,3). Murine and human mammary cancer are both effected by hormones. Some transgenic animals respond to lactogenic hormones with massive hyperplasia and others with little or no morphological abnormalities.

Under the influence of lactogenic hormones or dexamethasone stimulation, the mammary tree of most transgenic animals was within normal limits. The most dramatic exception to this rule has been the mammary trees of the non-binary int-2 and neu transgenics which developed a massive mammary hyperplasia under the influence of pregnancy (3,6). However, some strains develop more subtle changes in their mammary trees that are intermediate between the two extremes. For example, the myc transgenics did not develop gross abnormalities when stimulated by hormones but did have greater lobulo-alveolar development relative to control wild type liter mates when stimulated with dexamethasone. This suggests that the physiological effect of some transgenes may be overlooked if the development of the mammary tree is not studied in its entirety.

PERSISTENT HYPERPLASIAS

The mammary trees of multiparous animals were of particular interest since focal precursors to the neoplasms can usually be detected in retired breeding stock (7). Based on the study of mammary tumorigenesis in the laboratory mouse, one expects that the number and type of hyperplastic lesions found in the regressed mammary gland will correlate with tumor incidence (7). As with other aspects of this comparative study, different oncogenes were associated with different patterns of persistent lesions following hormone stimulation.

In a series of over 100 whole mounts from myc and ras transgenics, only 10% had focal hyperplasias. These hyperplasias were typically hyperplastic alveolar nodules (HAN) closely resembling those found in the laboratory mouse. Since a large proportion of these animals develop mammary tumors, the number of focal hyperplasias should have been greater. The most striking dysplasias were observed in the whole mounts of a group of myc bearing transgenic animals which also contained exogenous MuMTV. In this select population, all of the retired breeders had multiple focal dysplasias with not only alveolar hyperplasia but many lesions also had extensive stromal proliferation.

The diffuse mammary hyperplasias associated with int-2 and neu resulted in quite a different pattern. They did not completely regress but persisted throughout the animal's lifetime (3,6). However, careful histological examination of the mammary fat pad did reveal partial regression. Focal areas of persistent glandular and stromal hyperplasia stood out from the general regressing background. It should also be noted that the abnormal growth pattern of the int-2 mammary epithelium persisted when transplanted into virgin FVB mammary fat pads, indicating that the abnormality is not related to an abnormal hormonal milieu in the transgenic animal.

INT-2 HISTOLOGY

The hyperplastic lesions of the pregnant and postpartum int-2 transgenic females exhibited a remarkable glandular and stromal hyperplasia under the influence of hormones (3). Even more remarkable was the similarity between these mammary hyperplasias and the pregnancy-dependent tumors or plaques of the GR/A mouse. The GR plaque differs from the int-2 transgenic hyperplasia only in the focal nature of the lesion in the GR as opposed to the diffuse involvement of the transgenic mammary gland. However, the severity of the hyperplasia in the transgenic mammary gland is variable, leading to focal lesions that stand out from the background. These persistent foci may represent local transformation and warrant further study.

The analogy is extended into the molecular biology of the two lesions in that most of the GR plaques have MuMTV induced clonal rearrangement of the int-2 locus (8). Thus, the "spontaneous" lesion of domestic mice and the engineered lesion of transgenic mice are molecularly and histologically identical.

MAMMARY TUMORIGENESIS

The introduction of activated oncogenes/transgenes into the mouse genome with the appropriate tissue specific promotor leads to increased mammary tumor incidence (9-11). The tumors arise in a stochastic manner in most situations (10). However, some of the tumors seem to arise with kinetics predicted for one hit kinetics (6). The stochastic production of tumors suggest that other genes are important in the production of mammary tumors even in the these transgenic animals.

The data comparing the mammary tumor latency periods and tumor incidence proved difficult to interpret. It is clear that the transgene will be associated with different effects in different circumstances. For example, the comparison of two transgenic colonies with the <u>neu</u> gene revealed vastly different tumor incidences and latency periods. For example, the TG.NK and TG.NF strains both carry <u>neu</u> as a transgene. The TG.NF strain has a 96% mammary tumor incidence and a mean latency of 97 days. The TG.NK tumor incidence is 50% with a mean latency of 202 days (2). This suggests that positional and/or gene dosage effects will influence tumorigenesis (2). These observations make comparisons across strains very difficult and limits the generalizations that can be made about the tumor potential of a single oncogene.

However, the study of the interactions of oncogenes can be enhanced by the production of hybrid animals on a single, uniform background. Most remarkably, the hybrid animals resulting from the mating of two dissimilar transgenic parents also resulted in the stochastic production of mammary tumors (10,11). This observation was expanded to include the production of trigenic animals by crossing bigenic animals with monogenic animals (Table 1). Once again, the tumor kinetics suggested stochastic production (10). Thus, even the presence of more than one activated oncogene is not sufficient for mammary tumorigenesis.

MAMMARY TUMOR PHENOTYPE

One of the central assertions of this review is that each activated oncogene is associated with a distinctive histological and cytological pattern or tumor phenotype. As a result, at least in murine tumors, the pathologist can predict which oncogenes are activated in a tumor by studying the tumor phenotype.

Most spontaneous mammary tumors of domestic mice are induced by the mouse mammary tumor virus (7). These tumors are associated with the insertion activation of either int-1 or int-2 depending upon the mouse strain and the origin of the virus (7,8). These tumors have been classified alphabetically in the classical work of Thelma Dunn (12). In our experience, over 95% of these

MuMTV-induced tumors can be readily classified as either type A or type B. It is essential to recognize that only 20-30% of the tumors from transgenic mice are of the types described by Dunn.

Our comparison showed that 76% of mammary tumors from transgenic mice were not the types described by Dunn as generally found in the laboratory mouse. Although we have examined mammary tumors from a variety of sources, the most comprehensive study comes from a retrospective analysis of transgenic animals with neu, ras and/or myc oncogenes. This study of 607 tumors from 407 animals provided statistical support for the hypothesis that the activated oncogene is reflected in the morphological pattern of the tumor (2).

Tumors from the ras animals tend to have a papillary pattern with the tumor cells aligned around blood vessels (2). The cells tend to have small oval uniform nuclei and eosinophilic cytoplasm and are referred to as small cell tumors (SC). In contrast, tumors associated with myc transgene expression are large cell tumors and have a glandular differentiation (LC). The nuclei are large and pleomorphic. The chromatin pattern is coarse with prominent nuclei. The cytoplasm tends to be basophilic. The tumors characteristic of neu associated tumors have an intermediate cell and nodular patterns (IC). The nuclei are larger than those found in the ras tumors and have a more open chromatin but the cytoplasm tends to stain a light pink.

The tumor phenotype could be correlated with the tumor genotype with 90% accuracy (2). The large cell tumor was found in association with the myc transgene. The intermediate cell tumor associated exclusively with the neu transgene. However, the papillary small cell phenotype was associated with both the ras and the neu transgene. The latter observation reduced the sensitivity of detection for the neu to 47%.

TABLE 1.
TRIGENIC ANIMALS
TG.NKMSH

Genes	SLIDES # Tu	# Mice	HISTOLOGICAL MAMMARY TUMOR TYPES SC	LC	IC	DUNN	TOTAL COLONY %Tu (#MICE)	Mean Days
myc/ras/neu	24	17	3	18	2	1	100(17)	72
myc/ras	7	5	2	5	0	0	100(10)	89
myc/neu	25	19	1	16	0	8	91(22)	141
neu	10	10	10	0	0	0	73(28)	228
ras	2	2	2	0	0	0	67(6)	263
neu/ras	6	5	4	1	0	1	38(16)	180
myc	1	1	0	0	0	1	20(10)	299
wild type	-	-	-	-	-	-	0(64)	-
TOTALS=	75	59	22	40	2	11	46(173)	

The more intriguing part of this extensive retrospective study involved the trigenic strain whose tumors were classified without knowledge of the animals actual genotype (Table 1). Since the parents were all heterozygous animals, the genotype of the offspring could contain combinations of different oncogenes.

The offspring that did not inherit any of the

transgenes (wild type) did not develop a single mammary tumor. The other animals developed tumors at different rates depending on the combination of oncogenes present in the genome. All of the animals with all three oncogenes developed tumors with a mean latency of 72 days (Table 1.). Bigenic myc and ras animals all developed tumors with a mean latency of 89 days. While only 50% of the neu and ras bigenics developed tumors with a mean of 180 days. The monogenic animals developed proportionately fewer tumors with prolonged latency periods.

Most remarkably, the tumors that emerged from these hybrid animals accurately reflected the presence of the oncogene. The large cell, basophilic tumors (LC) occurred exclusively in animals with at least one myc The papillary small cell tumors (SC) appeared only in animals with neu or ras.

We have also studied tumors from other transgenic mice. Although this experience is more limited than those described above, some patterns seem to emerge which suggest other associations between oncogenes and tumor phenotype.

While our experience with malignant tumors of the int-2 mouse is relatively meager, these tumors seem to be emerging from the binary strains at a high frequency. These tumors tend to be lobulo-alveolar adenocarcinomas with a prominent papillary component. Their pattern of development deviates from the pattern observed in the hyperplasias of these animals. Although they do resemble the type A tumor described by Dunn, these tumors are not identical to the types of tumors generally found in the GR mouse. However, the sample of these transgenic tumors is scant and generalizations may not be justified.

SUMMARY AND DISCUSSION

The comparative studies summarized above provide data concerning the effect of selected transgenes on the mammary epithelium and their potential role in the origin and evolution of mammary tumors. From these observations, it is apparent that normal mammary growth and differentiation is possible even though one or two activated oncogenes are expressed in the tissue. The oncogenes which disturb normal development appear to be the exception and to act only when expressed at very high levels.

On the other hand, epithelium containing some forms of transgenic oncogenes will respond to hormone stimuli with either accentuation of normal physiological processes, such as with myc, or development of massive dysplastic hyperplasias, such as with int-2. The hyperplastic tissue may exhibit retarded regression once the hormone stimulus is withdrawn or demonstrate persistent dysplastic focal lesions. In either case, relatively few candidate preneoplastic lesions appear in the mammary glands of transgenic mice.

Since most of the neoplasms from this genetic background arise in a stochastic pattern, a number of other oncogenes must be involved in the development of mammary tumors. However, at least some of the oncogenes studied here have such a remarkable association with certain unique histological patterns that the transgene must have a dominant effect on the structure and function of the neoplastic cell.

At the present time, little attempt has been made to draw attention to oncogene specific patterns, or phenotypes, in human breast pathology. Moreover, relatively little data concerning the molecular events leading to human breast cancer is available (13-19). The most thoroughly documented relationship between tumor type and human breast oncogenes involve the her-2 and ras genes which are associated with poor prognosis and comedocarcinomas (14-19). Since the rodent homolog, neu, was found to be a transgenic oncogene whose phenotype was readily overshadowed by ras or myc, it is conceivable that the human counterpart of the phenomena observed here will emerge as we learn more about the molecular basis of human breast cancer. We believe that the phenomena observed in our comparative studies of the transgenic mouse mammary gland will lead to a definition of similar events in the human.

The biological significance of the histological and cytological patterns associated with each of the transgenes is not understood. Oncogenes may be expressed without leading to disturbances of mammary growth, suggesting that the transgene does not lead directly to transformation but that it acts in concert with other genes. The specific pathway of transformation may be related to the time at which the transgene is expressed or the state of differentiation of the target cell when the transgene is expressed. The second generation of study with the transgenic mammary systems should be designed to study these phenomena.

ACKNOWLEDGEMENTS

This work has been supported by grants from the Howard Hughes Foundation, American Cancer Society grant #MV-428C and partially supported by a grant from E.I. Dupont de Nemours Company, Inc. We appreciate the technical support of Mr. Robert Munn and Ms. Judy Walls.

REFERENCES

1. Strange, R. and R.D. Cardiff. In: Breast Cancer: Progress in Biology, Clinical Management and Prevention. (M.A. Rich, J.C. Hager and I. Keydar, eds.) Kluwer Academic Publishers. Boston, Dordecht, London. pgs 1-14, 1989.
2. Cardiff,R.D., E. Sinn, W.J. Muller, and P. Leder. Am. J. Path.(In Press)
3. Ornitz, D.M., Moreadith, R.S., and Leder, P. Proc. Natl. Acad. Sci. (USA) 88:698-702, 1991.
4. Bouchard, L., Lamarre, L. Tremblay,P.J. and

Joliceour, P. Cell, 57:1455-931-961, 1989.
5. Matsui, Y., Halter, S.A., Holt, J.T., Hogan, B.L., and Coffey A.J. Cell 61:1147-1155, 1990.
6. Muller, W.J., Sinn, E., Pattengale, P.K., Wallace, R., Leder, P. Cell 54:105-115,1988.
7. Cardiff, R.D. European J.Cancer and Clin.Onc. 24:15-20, 1988.
8. D.W. Morris, P.A. Barry, H.D. Bradshaw, and R.D. Cardiff. J. Virology 64:1794-1802, 1990.
9. Stewart, T.A., Pattengale, P.K., Leder, P. Cell 38:627-637, 1984.
10. Pattengale, P.K., Stewart, T.A., Leder, A., Sinn, E., Muller, W., Tepler, I., Schmidt, E., Leder, P. Am.J. Path. 135:39-61, 1989.
11. Sinn, E., Muller, W., Pattengale, P.K., Tepler, I., Wallace, R., Leder, P. Cell 49:465-475, 1987.
12. Dunn, T.B. "Morphology of mammary tumors in mice." In: F. Homburger(ed.), Physiopathology of Cancer, A.J. Phiebig, Inc., White Plains NY, pp. 38-82, 1959.
13. Varley, J.M., Brammar, W.J., Lane, D.P., Swallow, J.E., Dolan, C. and Walker, R.A. Oncogene 6:413-421, 1991.
14. Callahan, R. and Campbell, G. J. Natl. Cancer Inst. 81:1780-1786, 1989.
15. Slamon D.J., Goldolphin, W., Jones L.A., Holt, J.A., Wong, S.G., Keith, D.E., Levin, W.J., Stuart, S.G., Udove, J., Ullrich, A., Press, M.F. Science 244:707-712, 1989.
16. Barnes, D.M. Brit. Med. J. 299:1061, 1989.
17. Borg, A., Linell, F., Idvall, I., Johansson, S., Sigurolsson, H., Ferno, M., Killander, D. Lancet, i:1268-1269, 1989.
18. van de Vijver, M.J., Peterse, M.D., Mooi, W.J., Wisman,P., Lomans, J., Dalesio, O., Nusse, R.J.: N.Engl. J. Med. 319:1239-1245,1988.
19. Querzoli, P., Marchetti, E., Bagni, A., Marzola, A., Fabris, G, Nenci, I: Breast. Ca. Res. and Treat., 12:23-30, 1988.

SECTION II

POLYPEPTIDES
AND
GROWTH FACTORS EXPRESSION

INTERDEPENDENCE OF HORMONES AND GROWTH FACTORS IN LOBULO-ALVEOLAR DEVELOPMENT OF THE MAMMARY GLAND AND IN TUMORIGENESIS

BARBARA K. VONDERHAAR AND KAREN PLAUT

Laboratory of Tumor Immunology and Biology National Cancer Institute National Institutes of Health Bethesda, MD 20892, USA.

INTRODUCTION

In normal breast development, two major pathways for cell growth regulation act in parallel. One is the positive pathway, generally believed to involve growth factors such as epidermal growth factor (EGF), transforming growth factor alpha (TGF-a), insulin-like growth factors (IGF-I and IGF-II), fibroblast growth factors (FGF) [1], and possibly platelet derived growth factor (PDGF) [2]. The other is the negative pathway involving agents such as members of the transforming growth factor beta family (TGF-b1, -b2, and -b3) [3], a putative c-erbB2 ligand [4], mammostatin [5], and products of the retinoblastoma (Rb) [6] and p53 antioncogenes [7]. Both of these pathways are influenced both positively and negatively by the classical hormones such as estrogen (E), progesterone (P), and prolactin (Prl). These same hormones and growth factors are also intertwined in their action in the development and promotion of breast cancer (Fig 1). Increased response to, or overexpression of, positive factors and/or loss of response to, or decreased expression of, negative factors contribute to tumor development.

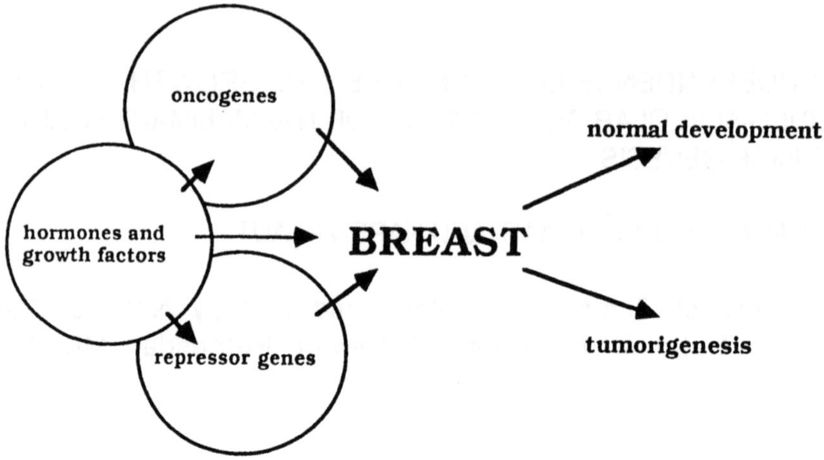

Fig. 1. Schematic of the hormonal and growth factor influences on oncogenes and repressor genes involved in normal mammary development and tumorigenesis.

A good in vitro model for studying human breast development is not yet available. Some "normal" human breast cells can be grown in primary culture but to date they appear to be estrogen receptor negative, a characteristic which is not common to the majority of mammary epithelial cells. These cells can only be grown for finite periods of time or after being immortalized with oncogenes or an infective agent such as SV40 [8, 9]. While we await the development of a good, reliable, and accurate human model system, studies in the mouse can afford us many insights into the complex array of hormones and growth factors involved in breast development. The results in the mouse do not always translate readily to the human condition. However, the rodent systems do allow us to gain some insights into the roles of the various hormones and growth factors in breast cancer. Armed with this knowledge, potential sites for therapeutic intervention may be identified.

Estrogen and Progesterone

The importance of estrogen and progesterone in the induction and progression of mammary tumors in rodents is clearly established [10]. Estrogen administration effectively induces breast tumors, and treatment with antiestrogens, such as tamoxifen, can reduce or even prevent the occurrence of tumors. Tamoxifen treatment has also been shown to result in remission of established cancer in rodents [11]. In humans a parallel situation occurs. By destroying ovarian function through oophorectomy or radiation-induced menopause for reasons other than breast cancer, a reduction by up to 75% in the incidence of subsequent breast cancer can be achieved [12, 13].

Differences in hormonal responsiveness to the ovarian steroids may reflect the stage of development of the mammary gland. Estrogen (E) stimulates ductal growth and increases progesterone (P) receptors in the mammary gland of mature mice [14]. Supplementation with E increases DNA synthesis in the duct end epithelium [15, 16] and P stimulates DNA synthesis by increasing ductal side branching in the mammary gland from ovariectomized mice [17]. Supplementation with E and P causes a synergistic increase in DNA synthesis and epithelial cell proliferation. This is coupled with a large increase in P receptors [15]. It is likely that induction of the P receptor in the mammary gland by E accounts for some of the synergistic increase in mammary proliferation in the presence of E and P [18].

Prior to sexual maturity, E does not induce the P receptor in the mammary gland of ovariectomized mice. Stimulation by E still increases DNA synthesis in mammary end buds and ducts but the response is not altered when both E and P are administered [15]. In addition, P alone has little effect on mammary development.

Insulin

Recently, Papa et al. [19] showed that the insulin receptor content in human breast cancer tumors is more than six-fold higher than in normal breast tissues. Receptors were localized in malignant epithelial cells and not in stromal and inflammatory tissues [19]. In addition, Giorgino et. al. [20] showed that overexpression of normal insulin receptors transfected into fibroblasts and CHO cells induces a ligand-dependent transformed phenotype.

It has been postulated that many of the effects of insulin on mammary development are due to interaction of insulin with the receptor for insulin-like growth factor I (IGF-I). While some mammary functions may be mediated through IGF-I, it is apparent that insulin is responsible for some aspects of epithelial cell maintenance. Insulin is necessary for maintaining ductal parenchyma and cell survival in whole organ culture of mouse mammary glands [21, 22]. The effects of IGF-I in whole organ culture have not been previously examined.

Prosser et al. [23] compared the effect of insulin and IGF-I in mouse mammary explants from pregnant and lactating mice. Insulin is capable of inducing accumulation of b-casein mRNA and synthesis at ten-fold lower concentrations than IGF-I. This is in line with previous findings by Bolander et al. [24] which indicate that insulin is essential for accumulation of casein mRNA in mouse mammary epithelial cells. Insulin and IGF-I are additive in stimulating glucose transport activity in pregnant or lactating mouse mammary glands [23, 25]. Therefore, the relative efficacy of insulin and IGF-I can vary with the developmental state and functional activity of the mammary gland.

Prolactin

The role of Prl in normal development and tumorigenesis in the rodent is well accepted [26]. The role of this hormone in normal development of human breast is less clear; its role in breast cancer remains controversial [27]. While some studies in humans show that serum levels of lactogenic hormones are elevated in some women at risk for familial breast cancer [28, 29] and in breast cancer patients [30], other studies fail to find such increases or correlations with prognostic factors [31, 32]. In contrast to the rodent models where CB154 treatment can dramatically alter the course of the disease [33], only limited success in humans is achieved by attempts to lower serum Prl by a variety of means [34, 35, 36]. By immunocytochemistry, Prl is localized in up to 85% of human breast cancer biopsies [37]. Over 70% of human breast cancers contain Prl receptor [38] although no consistent correlation is reported between Prl receptors and age, weight, menopausal status, or pathological features such as differentiation, histoprognostic grading, and cellular density [39, 40]. However, better differentiated (grade I) carcinomas appear to lack Prl receptors [40].

In normal rodent development, the minimal hormonal requirement for lobulo-alveolar development in vivo is estrogen, progesterone, and Prl [41]. The effects of Prl on mammary development are both direct and indirect through its luteotropic action. During pregnancy, however, hypophysectomy does not affect mammary cell number or lobulo-alveolar development, suggesting that the structurally similar placental lactogen is an important lactogen at this time [42]. In vitro, primary cultures of human [43], as well as rodent mammary epithelial cells [44, 45], display an absolute requirement for Prl for growth and passage on tissue culture plastic or inside of collagen gels. The essential role of Prl in lobulo-alveolar development in vitro in rodents has been firmly established using whole organ cultures and hormonally supplemented, chemically defined medium [22, 46, 47].

Growth Hormone

The role of growth hormone in inducing mammary development has been debated for many years. Early researchers reported that growth hormone causes mammogenesis in mice [41], however these studies were dismissed since early pituitary preparations were contaminated with Prl. Recent studies have brought the role of growth hormone in mammary development back to the forefront. Kleinberg et al. [48] implanted pellets of either human growth hormone (hGH), rat growth hormone (rGH), human prolactin (hPrl) or rat prolactin (rPrl) locally into the mammary gland of hypophysectomized, castrated male rats that had been treated with E. A 10 to 100 fold increase in mammary development and IGF-I mRNA level is achieved in response to hGH versus hPrl. This is not entirely surprising since hGH is known to have both lactogenic and somatogenic properties [49].

This concept is further supported by a recent study reporting that transgenic mice containing sequences of the hGH gene display morphological development and functional differentiation of the mammary gland by 8 weeks of age. Development is comparable to that normally observed after 14 to 15 days of gestation [50]. Precocious development is related to mammary specific expression of hGH mRNA [50]. Although IGF-I is elevated in response to hGH gene constructs, elevated IGF-I alone does not stimulate mammary epithelial development in transgenic mice [50]. Gunzburg et al. [51] micro-injected the hGH gene coupled to the WAP promoter into mice embryos.

While glands from virgin, transgenic, female animals express low levels of the transgene, it is unclear whether hGH protein is expressed. Many animals become pregnant and lactate normally although expression of the transgene is unregulated [51].

Unlike hGH which has somatogenic and lactogenic properties, Kleinberg et al. [48] observed that rGH is more potent than either rPrl or hPrl in stimulating mammary development in altered male rats. This is contrary to previous studies which suggest that rGH is not lactogenic [52]. Recently it has also been reported that GH receptors line the ductal epithelium of the proliferating rat mammary gland [53]. In addition, transgenic mice containing a metallothionein-ovine-GH fusion gene have increased mRNA for both Prl and GH receptors in liver in response to expression of the gene [54].

Therefore, there are a number of possibilities that could account for the actions of GH. Growth hormone increases IGF-I which may act directly on the mammary gland [23, 25]. It is also possible that GH alters the responsiveness of the mammary gland to Prl. Prolactin receptor numbers in the liver increases in response to oGH in transgenic mice [54]. A third possibility is that GH acts directly on the mammary gland. GH receptors or receptor mRNA have been identified in the ductal epithelium of rat, bovine, and rabbit mammary glands [53, 55, 56 57] lending support to the concept that GH may act directly on the mammary gland during development.

Transforming growth factor-a and epidermal growth factor

Transforming growth factor alpha (TGF-a) is structurally and functionally similar to epidermal growth factor [58]. Responses to TGF-a or EGF are probably mediated through a common receptor, the epidermal growth factor receptor. It appears that TGF-a is capable of inducing neoplastic transformation in mouse mammary epithelial cells [59, 60].

Recently, a number of investigators have developed transgenic mice models that express human TGF-a in the mammary gland. Expression of TGF-a increases DNA synthesis by the gland and in many cases causes abnormalities ranging from hyperplasia through adenocarcinoma [61, 62, 63]. Abnormalities are predominantly observed in adult animals [62, 63]. This coincides with the increase in EGF receptors in response to ovarian steroids. However, in one study increased DNA synthesis was observed in immature mice expressing the transgene [61].

Responses to EGF or TGF-a in the normal gland may vary with stage of mammary development. Expression of mRNA for TGF-a and EGF occurs in mammary tissue from virgin and pregnant mice whereas only EGF mRNA is found during lactation [64]. TGF-a mRNA has been detected in mammary glands from lactating rats [65]. Both EGF and TGF-a are secreted into milk [66]. Both are localized in different layers of the mammary epithelium but are able to elicit local ductal development of the mammary gland in ovariectomized mice [64].

EGF plays a role in mitogenesis and morphological development of the mouse mammary gland [67, 68]. However, in some circumstances, EGF inhibits mammary ductal development [69]. EGF can also promote proliferation of cultured mammary epithelial cells from pregnant and lactating mice [70, 71] and can regulate synthesis and secretion of some milk proteins [72]. Furthermore, in whole organ culture of the mouse mammary gland, EGF is an absolute requirement for a second round of lobulo-alveolar development after a full cycle of mammary development, milk protein secretion and involution has occurred [73].

Transforming growth factor b-1

Diffusible negative growth regulators play key roles in normal growth control and differentiation not only during embryogenesis but also in the adult state. The most studied of the known negative regulators are probably the highly ubiquitous and potent members of the transforming growth factor-b (TGF-b) family. The TGF-bs are believed to play a major role in the genesis of cancer as evidenced by studies in a variety of systems [74]. Their mechanisms of action at the molecular level appear to implicate a variety of oncogenes and tumor suppressor genes [75]. Several human breast cancer cell lines secrete TGF-b into the medium [76, 77]. The expression of mRNA for TGF-b1, -b2 or -b3 varies with the different cell lines studied [78]. In estrogen receptor positive cells, decreased mRNA levels for TGF-b2 and -b3 are observed after 48hr. treatment with estradiol; the levels of TGF-b1 mRNA are not affected [78]. Tamoxifen causes a five fold increase in production of TGF-b by MCF-7 cells probably through a posttranscriptional mechanism [76]. In estrogen receptor negative cells no effect of either estradiol or tamoxifen occurs on expression of mRNA for any member of the TGF-b family [78].

The role of TGF-bs in normal development of the human breast is unknown, but it is becoming increasingly clear that they play an important role in normal rodent mammary development. Rat mammary epithelial cells in primary culture secrete a latent form of TGF-b, some of which is activated in situ and contributes to the growth potential of these cells in an autocrine manner [79]. TGF-b1 inhibits mouse mammary ductal development when implanted locally in the mammary gland of virgin mice [80, 81]. Furthermore, it appears that TGF-b1 stimulates the extracellular matrix indicating that it may play a role in mediating epithelial-stromal interactions [82]. When TGF-b1 is implanted locally in the glands of steroid hormone-primed or pregnant mice, lobulo-alveolar development is not altered [80]. This further supports the concept that TGF-b1 is important for mammary development prior to puberty. Hence it was hypothesized that once the glands are exposed to the ovarian steroids and the animal achieves sexual maturity, TGF-b1 can no longer inhibit lobulo-alveolar development [80].

Whole organ culture

Due to the complexity of the interrelationships among the hormones and growth factors involved in mammary development, a culture system has been developed which allows one to mimic, in vitro, natural cycles of mammogenesis, milk protein synthesis and secretion, and regression. Administration of E and P to 3-4 week old mice primes the mammary gland for in vitro culture. Subsequently, complete lobulo-alveolar development can be achieved in vitro by culturing whole mouse mammary glands in a hormonally supplemented, serum-free medium. The required hormones are I, Prl, aldosterone(A) and hydrocortisone(H) [22, 46]. I, H and Prl are necessary for milk protein synthesis and regression can be obtained by withdrawal of all hormones except I [83]. A second round of development can then be achieved by addition of the four hormones and EGF [73].

The whole organ culture system is uniquely suited to examine the effect of hormones and growth factors on normal morphogenesis. This culture system allows epithelial-mesenchymal interactions, which are important to mammogenesis, to remain intact [84, 85]. Isolation of the mammary gland in culture allows for observation of the effects of specific factors alone, or in combination, on lobulo-alveolar development. Elucidation of the mechanism underlying normal mammary development will provide keys to understanding the uncontrolled regulation that occurs in tumorigenesis.

Whole organ cultures were initially performed using the thoracic #2 mammary gland of mice since this was reported to be the most active gland [47]. However, through comparison of lobulo-alveolar development in abdominal vs thoracic glands we determined that the abdominal #4 gland is equally, if not more, active in whole organ culture than the thoracic gland of E/P primed mice (Fig. 2).

Initially, mammary glands were incubated at 37 C in an atmosphere of 95% O2 with 5% CO2 [46]. We have determined that an atmosphere consisting of 50% oxygen with 5% CO2 is sufficient for complete lobulo-alveolar development [86]. Although development will occur in the absence of oxygen (i.e. 5% CO2 in air), responses tend to be delayed and less pronounced [87].

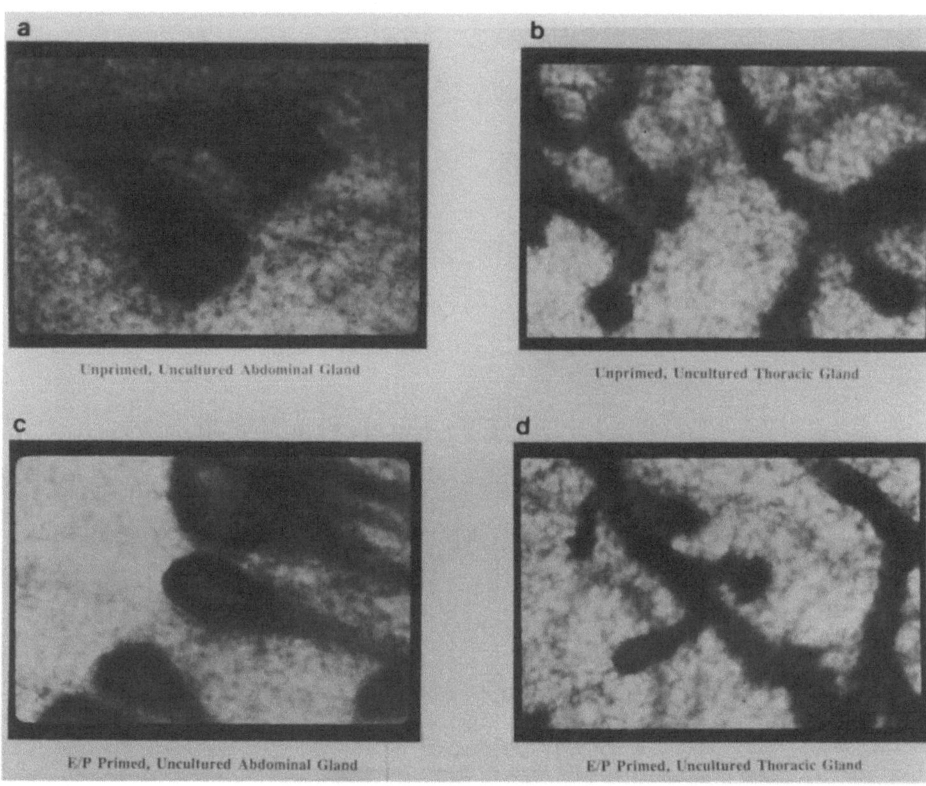

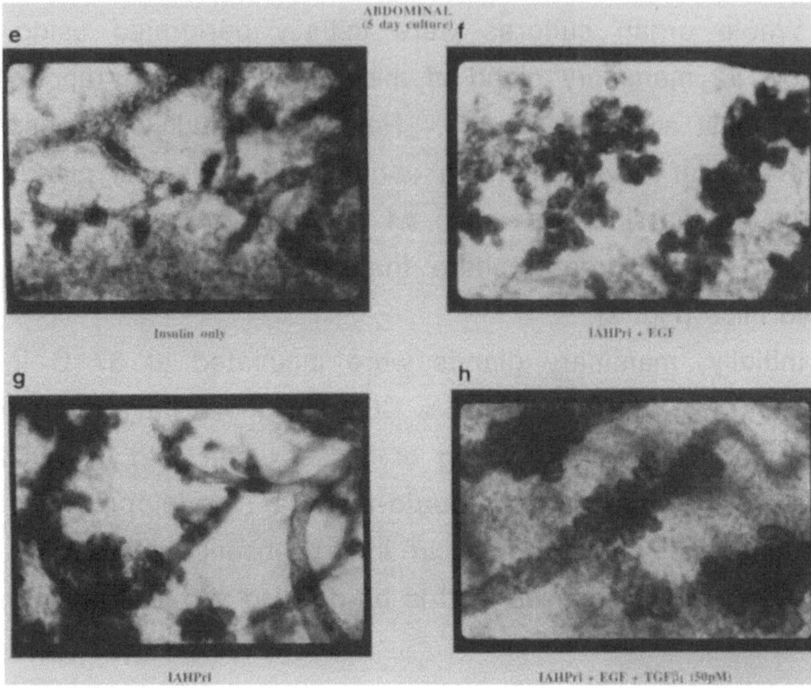
ABDOMINAL
(5 day culture)
e
f
Insulin only
IAHPri + EGF
g
h
IAHPri
IAHPri + EGF + TGFβ1 (50pM)

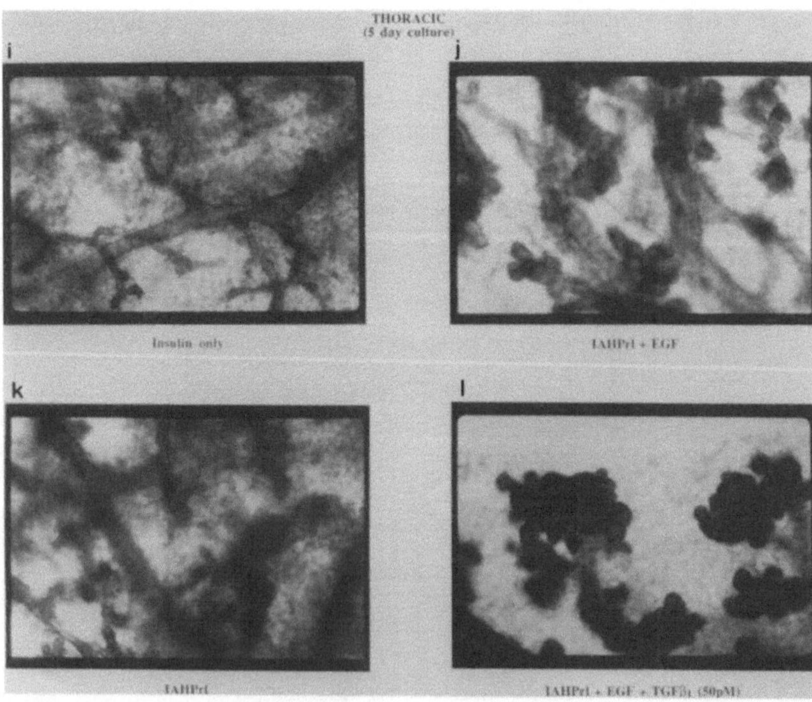
THORACIC
(5 day culture)
i
j
Insulin only
IAHPri + EGF
k
l
IAHPri
IAHPri + EGF + TGFβ1 (50pM)

Fig. 2. Whole mounts of mammary glands from sub-adult mice: a) Unprimed, uncultured, abdominal gland b) E/P primed, uncultured, abdominal gland c) Unprimed, uncultured, thoracic gland d) E/P primed, uncultured, thoracic gland e) cultured with I, abdominal gland f) cultured with IAHPrl, abdominal gland g) cultured with IAHPrl + EGF, abdominal gland h) cultured with IAHPrl + EGF + b-TGF (50pM), abdominal gland i) cultured with I, thoracic gland j) cultured with IAHPrl, thoracic gland k) cultured with IAHPrl + EGF, thoracic gland l) cultured with IAHPrl + EGF + b-TGF (50pM), thoracic gland.

Effects of estrogen and progesterone priming

It is still unclear why E and P priming is necessary to obtain lobulo-alveolar development in vitro. Elucidation of the response to E and P at the biochemical and molecular levels is currently being pursued. E/P priming of 4 week old ovary-intact mice for 9 days increases DNA synthesis in the mammary gland by about 50%. When each hormone is given individually to these mice, P increases DNA synthesis while E does not (Plaut, Ginsburg, and Vonderhaar, unpublished). Unlike the study performed by Haslam [84], the treatment period is for 9 days rather than 24hr. following a single injection of steroid. It is hypothesized that either extended treatment periods or the continued presence of very low levels of E in the mice are required to allow P to exert its effects on DNA synthesis in the mammary glands of these sub-adult mice.

Supplementation of mice with E and P increases binding of EGF to receptors in the epithelial-rich region of the mammary gland [87]. That this is a localized effect which occurs specifically in the nipple region where extensive ductal and end bud development has occurred has been confirmed by Western blot analysis (Ikeda and Vonderhaar, unpublished). We do not know which cell type has the induced, active EGF receptors since both epithelial cells and the surrounding fibroblasts have been shown to bind EGF during early development [68]. The development of these receptors under the influence of the steroidal hormones may allow the mammary gland to respond to TGF-a or EGF under normal physiological conditions.

It appears that EGF decreases the time needed to obtain lobulo-alveolar development. When E/P priming is shortened from 9 to 6 days, full lobulo-alveolar development in whole organ culture occurs only if the medium is supplemented with EGF along with the four hormones [87]. When EGF is added to the medium in place of Prl, only a few aveolar buds develop, pointing out the essential requirement for Prl.

Priming with E/P results in an increase in the content of EGF in the submaxillary gland of mice [88]. However, blood concentrations of EGF are not altered. In addition, testosterone, which causes large increases in submaxillary EGF, cannot mimic the priming effects of E and P [88]. Alteration in the concentration of EGF is not likely to be the only change occurring during E/P priming since infusion of EGF into the mouse via an Alzet minipump does not mimic the effects of E/P priming on lobulo-alveolar development in whole organ culture [88].

The steroid hormones do cause an increase in a local mammary-derived growth factor that is detectable in the mammary gland of primed animals. Like EGF and TGF-a, the factor can induce lobulo-alveolar development after 6 days in whole organ culture with I,A,H, and Prl. The cultured mammary glands are about 20 times more sensitive to the mammary derived growth factor than to EGF [87, 88]. Acid-alcohol extracts of the mammary glands containing the derived growth factor do not contain immunologically detectable EGF; the extract does, however, compete in an assay for EGF binding activity [87]. Based on these data, it would not be unreasonable to speculate that the mammary-derived growth factor is in fact TGF-a. Liscia has detected, by in situ hybridization, the presence of TGF-a mRNA in the mammary glands of virgin mice (D. S. Liscia, personal communication) and lactating rats [65]. Furthermore, preliminary evidence from our laboratory indicates that mammary derived growth factor is immunologically indistinct from TGF-a.

The hypothesis that TGF-a may be a physiological regulator of mammary development is further supported by data obtained using locally implanted pellets. The mouse mammary gland is more sensitive to the effects of TGF-a than to the effects of EGF in vivo [67] and in vitro [87, 88]. In addition, TGF-a stimulates local lobulo-alveolar development without administration of exogenous steroid hormones to the sub-adult animals [67].

It also appears that E/P releases the inhibition of mammary development caused by TGF-b1. When mammary glands from mice primed with E/P are incubated in whole organ culture with 50 pM TGF-b1, lobulo-alveolar development is not altered. This is consistent with the observation of Daniel et al. [80] who reported no local effects of implants of TGF-b on fully developed mammary glands of pregnant mice. These data suggest that E/P priming may play an important role in altering the responsiveness of the mammary gland to TGF-b1. It is hypothesized that E/P decreases expression of the mRNA for TGF-b1. Preliminary evidence from our laboratory suggests that this is indeed the case as the level of TGF-b1 mRNA in mammary glands decreases significantly with E/P priming (Plaut, Ikeda, and Vonderhaar, unpublished).

<u>Effect of other hormones during whole organ culture</u>

It appears that I is necessary for maintenance of the basal ductal structure in whole organ culture. Replacement of I by

0.1ug/ml of IGF-I does not maintain the mammary epithelium. The concentration of IGF-I used is that which elicits responses in glucose transport and casein gene expression after 3 days in mammary explant culture [23].

Recent studies in our laboratory show that when lower concentrations of bovine GH (250ng/ml) are used in place of Prl in the cultures, lobulo-alveolar development does not occur. Higher concentrations of bGH (1ug/ml) substitute for Prl in the presence of I, A, and H, and fully developed glands are obtained in the presence of IAH-GH and EGF. These observations are consistent with the findings of Kleinberg [48] and suggest that results obtained with GH in vivo [41] were not due solely to contaminating Prl.

CONCLUSION

A working hypothesis emerges from these studies suggesting that it is through the priming effects of estrogen and progesterone, that the mammary epithelial cells begin their path to full development. E/P priming results in suppression of production of TGF-b1 by the mammary cells, induction of the EGF receptor and production of TGF-a (Fig 3). These key events set into play a variety of subsequent steps resulting in cells able to fully respond to the further influences of I, A, H, and Prl as well as EGF or TGF-a and culminating in full lobulo-alveolar development of the mammary gland.

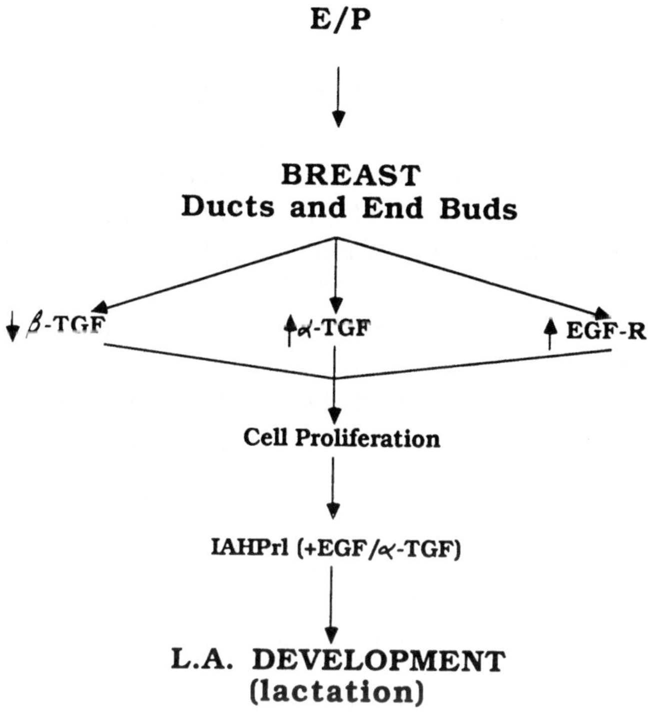

Fig 3. Hypothesis for the role of estrogen and progesterone in the priming process prior to lobulo-alveolar development in vitro. To whom all correspondence should be sent at: Laboratory of Tumor Immunology and Biology, National Cancer Institute, National Institutes of Health, Bld 10 Rm 5B56, Bethesda, MD 20892.

Current address: Department of Animal Science University of Vermont Burlington, VT 05405

REFERENCES

1. Lippman, M.E. and Dickson, R.B. Recent Prog. Hormone Res. 45: 383 - 440, 1986.
2. Ginsburg, E. and Vonderhaar, B.K. Cancer Letters in press, 1991.
3. Moses, H.L., Bascom, C.C., Coffey, R.J., Keski-Oja, J., Lyons, R.M. and Sipes, N.J. In: Progress in Cancer Research and Therapy (Eds. F. Bresciani, R.J.B. King, M.E. Lippmanand J.P. Raynaud), Raven Press, Ltd, New York, 1988, pp. 197 - 202.
4. Lupu, R., Colomer, R., Zugmaier, G., Slamon, D. and Lippman, M.E. Science 249: 1552 - 1554, 1990.
5. Ervin, P.R., Kaminski, R.C., Cody, R.C. and Wicha, M.S. Science 244: 1585 - 1587, 1989.
6. Lee, E., Bookstein, R. and Lee, W.H. In: Regulation of Breast Cancer (Eds. M.E. Lippmanand R.B. Dickson), Kluwer Press, Boston, 1990, pp. 23 - 44.
7. Nigro, J.M., et al. Nature 232: 705 - 708, 1989.
8. Stampfer, M.R. and Bartley, J. In: Cellular and Molecular Biology of Mammary Cancer (Eds. D. Medina, W. Kidwell, G. Heppnerand E. Anderson), Plenum Press, New York, 1987, pp. 419 - 436.
9. Chang, S.E., Keen, J., Lane, E.B. and Taylor-Papadimetriou, J. Cancer Res. 42: 2040 - 2053, 1982.
10. Wang, D.Y. and Bulbrook, R.D. In: Principles of Surgical Oncology (Eds. R.W. Raven), Plenum Medical Book Co., New York, 1977, pp. 227 - 261.
11. Heel, R.C., Brogden, R.N., Speight, T.M. and Avery, G.S. Drugs 16: 1 - 24, 1978.
12. MacMahon, B. and Feinlieb, M. J. Natl. Cancer Institute 24: 733 - 753, 1960.
13. Hirayama, T. and Wynder, E.L. Cancer 15: 28 - 38, 1962.
14. Leung, B.S. In: Hormonal Regulation of Mammary Tumors (Eds. B.S. Leung), Eden press, Vermont, 1982, pp. 118 - 154.
15. Haslam, S.Z. Endocrinology 122: 860 - 867, 1988.
16. Bresciani, F. Cell Tissue Kinet. 1: 51 - 63, 1968.
17. Haslam, S.Z. Endocrinology 122: 464 - 470, 1988.
18. Haslam, S.Z. and Shyamala, G. Endocrinology 108: 825 - 830, 1981.
19. Papa, V., et al. J. Clin. Invest. 86: 1503 - 1510, 1990.

20. Giorgino, F., Belfiore, A., Milazzo, G., Constantina, A., Maddux, B., Whittaker, J., Goldfine, I. and Vigneri, R. Mol. Endocrinol. 5: 452 - 459, 1991.
21. Wood, B.G., Washburn, L.L., Mukherjee, A.S. and Banerjee, M.R. J. Endocr. 65: 1 - 6, 1975.
22. Ichinose, R.R. and Nandi, S. J. Endocrin. 35: 331 - 340, 1966.
23. Prosser, C.G., Sankaran, L., Hennighausen, L. and Topper, Y.J. Endocrinology 120: 1411 - 1416, 1987.
24. Bolander, F.F.J., Nicholas, K.R., Van Wyk, J.J. and Topper, Y.J. Proc. Natl. Acad. Sci. USA 78: 5682 - 5684, 1981.
25. Prosser, C.G. and Topper, Y.J. Endocrinology 119: 91 - 96, 1986.
26. Welsch, C.W. and Nagasawa, H. Cancer Res. 37: 951 - 963, 1977.
27. Vonderhaar, B.K. and Biswas, R. In: Cellular and Molecular Biology of Mammary Cancer (Eds. D. Medina, W. Kidwell, G. Heppnerand E. Anderson), Plenum Publishing Corp., New York, 1987, pp. 205 - 219.
28. Love, R.R. and Rose, D.P. Eur. J. Cancer Clin. Oncol. 21: 1553 - 1554, 1985.
29. Henderson, B.E., Gerkins, V., Rosario, I., Casagrande, J. and Pike, M.C. N. Engl. J. Med. 293: 790 - 795, 1975.
30. Hill, P., Wynder, E.L., Kumar, H., Helman, P., Rona, G. and Kuno, K. Cancer Res. 36: 4102 - 4106, 1976.
31. Cole, E.N., England, P.C., Sellwood, R.A. and Griffiths, K. Eur. J. Cancer 13: 677 - 684, 1977.
32. Sheth, N.A., Ranadive, K.J., Suraiya, J.N. and Sheth, A.R. Br. J. Cancer 32: 160 - 167, 1975.
33. Welsch, C.W. and Gribler, C. Cancer Res. 33: 2939 - 2946, 1973.
34. Klijn, J.G.M., deJong, F.H., Lamberts, S.W.J. and Blankenstein, M.A. J. Steroid Biochem. 23: 867 - 873, 1985.
35. Henson, J.C., Coune, A. and Staquet, M. Eur. J. Cancer 8: 155 - 156, 1972.
36. Murray, R.M.L., Mozaffarian, G. and Pearson, O.H. In: Prolactin and Carcinogenesis (Eds. A.R. Boynesand K. Griffiths), Alpha Omega Publishing, Cardiff, Wales, 1972, pp. 158 - 161.
37. Agarwal, P.K., Tandon, S., Agrawal, A.K. and Kumar, S.

Indian J. Exper. Biol. 27: 1035 - 1038, 1989.

38. Peyrat, J.P., Dewailley, D., Djiane, J., Kelly, P.A., Vandewalle, B., Bonneterre, J. and Lefebvre, J. Breast Cancer Res. Treat. 1: 369 - 373, 1981.
39. Bonneterre, J., Peyrat, J.P., Vandewalle, B., Beuscart, R., Vie, M.C. and Cappelaere, P. Eur. J. Cancer Clin. Oncol. 18: 1157 - 1162, 1982.
40. Codegone, M.L., DiCarlo, R., Muccioli, G. and Bussolati, G. Tumori 67: 549 - 552, 1981.
41. Nandi, S. J. Natl. Cancer Inst. 21: 1039 - 1063, 1958.
42. Ray, E.W., Anerill, S.C., Lyons, W.R. and Johnson, R.E. Endocrinology 56: 359 - 373, 1955.
43. Malarkey, W.B., Kennedy, M., Allred, L.E. and Milo, G. J. Clin. Endocrinol. Metab. 56: 673 - 677, 1983.
44. Ceriani, R.L. Developmental Biology 21: 530 - 546, 1970.
45. Flynn, D., Yang, J. and Nandi, S. Differentiation 22: 191 - 194, 1982.
46. Ichinose, R.R. and Nandi, S. Science 145: 496 - 497, 1964.
47. Banerjee, M.R., Wood, B.G. and Kinder, D.L. In Vitro 9: 129 - 133, 1973.
48. Kleinberg, D.L., Ruan, W., Catanese, V., Newman, C.B. and Feldman, M. Endocrinology 126: 3274 - 3276, 1990.
49. Forsyth, I.A., Folley, S.J. and Chadwick, A. J. Endocrinol. 31: 115 - 126, 1965.
50. Bchini, O., Andres, A.C., Schubaur, B., Mehtali, M., LeMeur, M., Lathe, M. and Gerlinger, P. Endocrinology 128: 539 - 546, 1991.
51. Gunzburg, W.H., Salmons, B., Zimmerman, B., Muller, M., Arfle, V. and Brem, G. Mol. Endocrin. 5: 123 - 133, 1991.
52. Newman, C.B., Cosby, H., Friesen, H.G., Feldman, M., Cooper, P., DeCrescito, V., Pilon, M. and Kleinberg, D.L. Proc. Natl. Acad. Sci. USA 84: 8110 - 8114, 1987.
53. Orian, J.M., Snibson, K., Stevenson, J.L., Brandon, M.R. and Herington, A.C. Endocrinology 128: 1238 - 1246, 1991.
54. Krivi, G.G., Hauser, S.D. and McGrath, M.F. Proc. Endocrin. Soc. 72: 247, 1990.
55. Baumbach, W.R., Horner, D.L. and Logan, J.S. In: Biotechnology in Growth Regulation (Eds. R.B. Heap, C.G. Prosserand G.E. Lamming), Butterworth, London, 1989, pp. 221 - 228.

56. Jammes, H., Gaye, P., Belair, L. and Djiane, J. Proc. Endocrin. Soc. 72: 91, 1990.
57. Lincoln, D.T., Waters, M.J., Breipohl, W., Sinowatz, F. and Lobie, P.E. Acta Histochemica Band 40 (Suppl): S47 - S49, 1990.
58. Salomon, D.S., Kim, N., Saeki, T. and Ciardiello, F. Cancer Cells 2: 389 - 397, 1990.
59. Shankar, V., et al. Mol. Carcinogen. 2: 1 - 11, 1989.
60. McGeady, M.L., Kerby, S., Shankar, V., Ciardiello, F., Salomon, D.S. and Seidman, M. Oncogene 4: 1375 - 1382, 1989.
61. Jhappan, C., Stahle, C., Harkins, R.N., Fausto, N., Smith, G.H. and Merlino, G.T. Cell 61: 1137 - 1146, 1990.
62. Matsui, Y., Halter, S.A., Holt, J.T., Hogan, B.L.M. and Coffey, R.J. Cell 61: 1147 - 1155, 1990.
63. Sandgren, E.P., Luetteke, N.C., Palmiter, R.D., Brinster, R.L. and Lee, D.C. Cell 61: 1121 - 1135, 1990.
64. Snedeker, S.M., Brown, C.F. and DiAugustine, R.P. Proc. Natl. Acad. Sci. USA 88: 276 - 280, 1991.
65. Liscia, D.S., Merlo, G., Ciardiello, F., Kim, N., Smith, G.H., Callahan, R. and Salomon, D.S. Dev. Biol. 140: 123 - 131, 1990.
66. Salomon, D.S. and Kidwell, W.R. In: Breast Cancer: Cellular and Molecular Biology (Eds. M.E. Lippmanand R.B. Dickson), Kluwer Press, Boston, 1988, pp. 363 - 390.
67. Vonderhaar, B.K. J. Cell. Phys. 132: 581 - 584, 1987.
68. Coleman, S., Silberstein, G.B. and Daniel, C.W. Dev. Biol. 127: 304 - 315, 1988.
69. Coleman, S. and Daniel, C.W. Dev. Biol. 137: 425 - 433, 1990.
70. Taketani, Y. and Oka, T. FEBS Lett. 152: 256 - 260, 1983.
71. Taketani, Y. and Oka, T. Endocrinology 113: 871 - 877, 1983.
72. Vonderhaar, B.K. and Nakhasi, H.L. Endocrinology 119: 1178 - 1184, 1986.
73. Tonelli, Q.J. and Sorof, S. Nature 285: 250 - 252, 1980.
74. Barnard, J.A., Lyons, R.M. and Moses, H.L. Biochim. Biophys. Acta 1032: 79 - 87, 1990.
75. Pietenpol, J.A., et al. Cell 61: 777 - 785, 1990.
76. Knabbe, C., Lippman, M.E., Wakefield, L.M., Flanders, K.C., Kasid, A., Derynk, R. and Dickson, R.B. Cell 48: 417 - 428, 1987.

77. Arteaga, C.L., Tandon, A.K., VonHoff, D.D. and Osborne, C.K. Cancer Res. 48: 3898 - 3904, 1988.
78. Arrick, B.A., Korc, M. and Derynck, R. Cancer Res. 50: 299 - 303, 1990.
79. Ethier, S.P. and Van de Velde, R.M. J. Cell. Phys. 142: 15 - 20, 1990.
80. Daniel, C.W., Silberstein, G.B., Van Horn, K., Strickland, P. and Robinson, S. Dev. Biol. 135: 20 - 30, 1989.
81. Silberstein, G.B. and Daniel, C.W. Science 237: 291 - 293, 1987.
82. Silberstein, G.B., Strickland, P., Coleman, S. and Daniel, C.W. J. Cell. Biol. 110: 2209 - 2219, 1990.
83. Terry, P.M., Ganguli, R., Ball, E.M. and Banerjee, M.R. Cell Differ. 4: 113 - 122, 1975.
84. Haslam, S.Z. J. Dairy Sci. 71: 2843 - 2854, 1988.
85. Wiens, D., Park, C.S. and Stockdale, F.E. Dev. Biol. 120: 245 - 258, 1987.
86. Plaut, K. and Vonderhaar, B.K. Proc. Endocrin. Soc. 72: 182, 1990.
87. Vonderhaar, B.K. In: Control of Cell Growth and Proliferation (Eds. C.M. Veneziale), Van Nostrand Reinhold Co., New York, 1984, pp. 11 - 33.
88. Vonderhaar, B.K. In: Breast Cancer: Cellular and Molecular Biology (Eds. M.E. Lippmanand R.B. Dickson), Kluwer Academic Publishers, Boston, 1988, pp. 251 - 266.

THE ROLE OF ESTROGEN REGULATED SECRETED PROTEINS FOR GROWTH REGULATION OF HUMAN BREAST CANCER

Anne E. Lykkesfeldt, Inga Laursen and Per Briand

Laboratory of Tumor Endocrinology, The Fibiger Institute, The Danish Cancer Society, DK-2100 Copenhagen, Denmark.

INTRODUCTION

Breast cancer is the most common cancer disease among women in the western countries. The female sex hormone estradiol plays an important role in the etiology of the disease as a promoter for the growth of initiated cells and as a promotor for growth of the established tumor cells. A prerequisite for estrogen stimulated cell proliferation is presence of estrogen receptors in the tumor cells, and about 60% of the primary breast tumors contain estrogen receptors. About 33% of the breast cancer patients with advanced disease respond to endocrine treatments as antiestrogen or estrogen ablation treatments, indicating the very important role of estrogens even in the metastatic disease (1,2,3,4). The mechanisms by which estrogen stimulates cell proliferation of breast cancer cells have been extensively studied and autocrine or paracrine mechanisms have been indicated in several studies (5,6,7,8). Regulation of cell proliferation by autocrine factors with a negative growth effect has also been shown (9,10); and estradiol (E2) stimulation of human breast cancer cell lines has been suggested to arise from upregulation of positive factors as well as down regulation of negative factors (11,12). Examples of factors shown to have a growth stimulatory effect on breast cancer cells are insulin, IGF-I, IGF-II, EGF and TGF-α (11,13,14,15), whereas TGF-ß has been found to have a negative effect on cell proliferation (9). At present much information is available on factors involved in E2-regulated growth of breast cancer cells, but the regulation seems to be complex and more information is still required to be able to develop new strategies in the treatment of E2-dependent breast tumor growth.

MODEL SYSTEMS FOR THE STUDY OF ESTROGEN STIMULATED GROWTH

We have used the estrogen receptor positive human breast cancer cell line MCF-7 (16) to study E2-regulated cell proliferation. We propagate the cells in phenol red free DME/F12 medium with 1% fetal calf serum (FCS), and in this medium we observe a small increase in cell number in cultures grown with added E2 (12). When we grow the cells in medium with 1% FCS plus 10% newborn calf serum (NCS) we observe a decrease in cell proliferation compared to 1% FCS (17). MCF-7 cells grown with 1% FCS and 10% NCS respond to addition of E2 with an increase in growth rate (doubling time decreases from 65 hours to 36 hours), and after 6 days cell numbers in the E2-treated cultures are 4 times higher than in cultures without E2. MCF-7 cells growing in presence of E2 have a characteristic malignant phenotype with small cells able to grown in multilayers, whereas the MCF-7 cells growing with suboptimal E2 amount tend to stop cell proliferation when they reach a monolayer (18). MCF-7 cells grow in nude mice supplemented with E2, whereas no tumors will grow up in animals without estrogen supplementation. The absolute requirement of E2 to develop tumors in the nude mice can not alone be ascribed to a decrease in cell doubling time, since our observation time of 4 months should be sufficient to observe slow growing tumors. Furthermore we also find this E2-requirement with a MCF-7 subline which grows with a doubling time of 38 hours in chemically defined medium without E2 (15). E2 has been shown to inhibit natural killer (NK) cell activity in nude mice (19), and the requirement for E2 could therefore also be due to the demand for suppression of the NK cell activity in order to obtain a net increase in proliferation of the MCF-7 cells. In our experiments we have, however, not found any indications for suppression of NK cell activity with the doses of estrogens used (P. Briand and M. Madsen, personal communication). We therefore find it more likely that the MCF-7 cells may require estrogens in order to produce factors, which promote growth and also protect the tumor cells against NK cell attack.

PROTEINS SECRETED FROM MCF-7 CELLS

MCF-7 cells grown in tissue culture secrete various proteins to the medium. We have labelled MCF-7 cells grown for 6 days in medium with and without E2 with ^{35}S-methionine for 6 hours in serum free medium to be able to analyse these proteins. The proteins in the conditioned media have been separated by SDS-PAGE under reducing conditions. The autoradiograms show three major protein bands at mol.wt 66 kDa, 61 kDa and 52 kDa, which are present in significantly higher amounts in medium from the E2-treated cultures and one protein band at mol.wt 42 kDa, which is present in significantly lower amount in the conditioned medium from E2-treated cultures (12). SDS-PAGE analysis performed under non-reducing conditions revealed that the 42 kDa protein formed a dimer of a mol.wt about 80 kDa, whereas the E2-stimulated proteins showed identical profiles under reducing and non-reducing conditions.

IDENTIFICATION OF SECRETED PROTEINS FROM MCF-7 CELLS

Immunoprecipitation experiments have shown that monoclonal antibodies to 52 kDa cathepsin D precipitate the 52 kDa protein secreted from our MCF-7 cells, thereby indicating that this protein is identical to the lysosomal protease 52 kDa procathepsin D first described to be secreted from MCF-7 cells by Westley and Rochefort (20). The 61 kDa protein is precipitated by polyclonal rabbit antibodies to serum α_1-antitrypsin indicating a homology with this serum antiprotease. Purification of the 61 kDa protein from conditioned medium from MCF-7 cells is in progress and it will be investigated whether the 61 kDa protein secreted from the breast cancer cells differs from the serum α_1-antitrypsin. Our preliminary experiments have revealed small differences between the two proteins. The 66 kDa protein is precipitated by polyclonal rabbit antibodies to serum α_1-antichymotrypsin. The 66 kDa protein has been purified to homogeneity from conditioned medium from E2-stimulated MCF-7 cells and the comparison between this protein and the serum α_1-antichymotrypsin showed small but distinct differences between these proteins (Inga Laursen, manuscript in preparation). Immunocytochemical analysis with use of polyclonal antibodies to α_1-antichymotrypsin or monoclonal antibodies raised against the 66 kDa secreted protein showed a granular cytoplasmic appearance of the antigen in the E2-stimulated cultures. The 42 kDa protein, the synthesis of which is inhibited by E2, has so far not been recognized by any of the commercially available antibodies tested. It may be of interest to mention that polyclonal rabbit antibodies to mature TGF-ß1 do not react with our 42 kDa protein neither in immunoprecipitation experiments nor in Western Blotting, and neutralizing antibodies to TGF-ß1 have not been able to abrogate the reduced cell proliferation of E2-deprived MCF-7 cells secreting 42 kDa protein (21). We have not yet tested whether the 42 kDa protein is homologous to TGF-ß2, which has been shown to be down regulated by E2 in the hormone responsive breast cancer cell line T47D (22).

THE FUNCTION OF E2-REGULATED PROTEINS

The 52 kDa protein is an acid protease normally located

in the lysosomes in the cells (23). 52 kDa protein purified from conditioned medium from MCF-7 cells has been shown to stimulate the growth of estrogen deprived MCF-7 cells (24). In our model system we find that the number of MCF-7 cells grown with 1% FCS and 10% NCS can be increased with about 30% when we add 52 kDa protein (concentration 12 nM), which we have purified from medium conditioned by E2-stimulated cells, supporting a mitogenic activity of the secreted 52 kDa protein. In a retrospective study the level of 52 kDa protein in cytosols of primary breast cancer biopsies was found to be an independent prognostic factor in predicting relapses in breast cancer patients (25). Transfection of cathepsin D cDNA into tumor cells increases the metastatic potential of these cells in athymic mice (26), indicating that this protease may be involved in metastasis.

The 61 kDa protein is found by us to be homologous to the serum antiprotease α_1-antitrypsin, which inhibits the proteases trypsin and elastase (present in neutrophil leukocytes). We have not yet demonstrated whether our 61 kDa protein is active as an antiprotease, but a recent publication has shown that MCF-7 cells secrete α_1-antitrypsin and α_1-antichymotrypsin and that these protease inhibitors present in medium from MCF-7 cells are active as antiproteases (27). We find that purified α_1-antitrypsin from human serum has no direct growth stimulatory effect when added to estrogen deprived MCF-7 cells. However, polyclonal antibodies to serum α_1-antitrypsin partially inhibit E2-stimulated cell proliferation of our MCF-7 subline, which is propagated in chemically defined medium. This MCF-7 subline adapted to grow in phenol red free chemically defined medium has a high secretion of 61 kDa protein (12), and the inhibitory activity of added antibodies to α_1-antitrypsin on E2-stimulation indicates to us, that the 61 kDa protein is involved in the E2-stimulation in a manner which involves other factors than 61 kDa protein. We suggest that the 61 kDa protein via the antiprotease activity could protect growth factors or growth factor receptors against proteolysis and may be also inhibit proteolytic activation of latent forms of proteins with a negative growth regulatory function.

The 66 kDa protein is homologous to serum α_1-antichymotrypsin, which inhibit the proteases chymotrypsin, chymase (present in mast cells) and cathepsin G (present in neutrophil leukocytes). We find that the protein purified to homogeneity from medium conditioned by E2-stimulated MCF-7 cells is active as an antiprotease shown by its ability to form SDS-stable complexes with chymotrypsin. Presence of active antichymotrypsin in medium from MCF-7 cells has previously been described by others (28,29). Partially purified preparations of the 66 kDa protein had a growth stimulatory effect on MCF-7 cells, but the 66 kDa protein purified to homogeneity exerted no significant effect on cell proliferation. This purified protein might have lost its biological activity during the last purification steps, but this is not very likely since the purified protein as mentioned above was found to be an active antiprotease. Experiments with addition of polyclonal antibodies to serum α_1-antichymotrypsin to E2- stimulated cultures had a growth inhibitory effect, indicating that the function of the 66 kDa protein is essential in the processes resulting in growth stimulation. Mechanisms by which an antiprotease could be involved in stimulation of cell proliferation are mentioned above in the discussion of the effect of the 61 kDa protein.

The 42 kDa protein, which is the monomer of a protein with mol.wt about 80 kDa, is present in very small amounts in E2-stimulated cultures, whereas this protein is the major protein secreted from growth inhibited cells (cells grown in estrogen poor medium (12) and in medium with antiestrogens (Lykkesfeldt, unpublished)). We find that serum free conditioned medium harvested from cells propagated with 1% FCS and 10% NCS has a growth inhibitory effect on our MCF-7 cells growing with 1% FCS. Fractionation of the conditioned medium by gel filtration at neutral pH, revealed that growth inhibitory activity was present in the fractions eluting in the mol.wt area around 100 kDa. SDS-PAGE analysis at non-reducing conditions of the fractions with growth inhibitory activity showed that these fractions contained a 80 kDa protein band and this protein band appeared as a 42 kDa band under reducing conditions, strongly indicating that this protein is identical to the one we find to be inhibited in E2-stimulated cultures. All our experiments have so far indicated that the 42 kDa protein have a negative growth regulatory function (12,21), and it will be interesting to purify this protein to homogeneity and discover the identity and the function of the purified protein.

POSSIBLE FUNCTION OF THE 61 kDa AND THE 66 kDa PROTEIN IN VIVO

Plasma protease inhibitors have been described to modulate the immune responses in vivo (30,31,32,33), and both α_1-antitrypsin and α_1-antichymotrypsin have been found to decrease antibody-dependent cell mediated cytotoxicity and natural killing in a dose-responsive pattern (31,32). α_1-Antichymotrypsin appears to be the most potent antiprotease in inhibiting the NK-cell activity (33) and in inactivating cathepsin G released from neutrophil leucocytes. We find it of great interest that the estrogen dependent breast tumor cells produce and secrete these antiproteases and suggest that they may play an important role for the survival of the tumor cells against attack from the cells of the immune system. Such a defence mechanism could be needed both in the early life of the tumor cells and might be a prerequisite for the survival in the blood circulation and to form metastases in distant organs.

EXPERIMENTS IN PROGRESS

We have set up an NK assay to measure the cytolysis of adherent MCF-7 cells by ^{51}Cr release (33). We have used MCF-7 cells grown with and without E2, but we have not been able to find a significant difference in cytolysis of E2-treated and non-treated cells in our preliminary experiments. The methods need further optimerization before we will be able to draw any conclusions.

We have planned to start another set of experiments to investigate whether the antiproteases are essential for tumor formation in nude mice. We inoculate the nude mice with 10^7 MCF-7 cells subcutaneously in the fourth mammary gland and supplement the mice with estrogen either as estrone given in the drinking water or by an intramuscular injection of a depot of estradiol (Progynone, Schering) (34). Mice supplemented with estrogen will be treated with antibodies to α_1-antitrypsin and/or α_1-antichymotrypsin in order to see whether the antibodies can prevent or reduce the growth of the tumor cells. Alzet osmotic pumps placed subcutaneously in the viscinity of the tumor cells will be used for administration of the antibodies.

Immunohistochemical analyses for presence and distribution of α_1-antitrypsin and α_1-antichymotrypsin in breast tumor biopsies are in progress and the importance of these antiproteases as a marker for the potential to metastasize will be investigated. It has been shown in several papers that many different types of tumors stain positive for these antiproteases, but no specificity of the antiproteases as tumor markers has yet been found (35,36,37).

CONCLUSION

Estrogen stimulation of cell proliferation of MCF-7 cells has been studied, and we have found that growth stimulation is concomitant with an increased synthesis and secretion of three proteins with mol.wt. 52 kDa, 61 kDa and 66 kDa and a decreased synthesis and secretion of one protein with mol. wt 42 kDa. The three estrogen stimulated proteins have been identified as the protease 52 kDa procathepsin D, a protein homologous to the antiprotease α_1-antitrypsin and a protein homologous to the antiprotease α_1-antichymotrypsin, respectively. The protein at mol. wt 42 kDa, which is inhibited by E2, has not yet been identified, but the described experiments indicate that this protein has a negative growth regulatory function on the MCF-7 cells. A mitogenic effect of the 52 kDa protein on growth of MCF-7 cells propagated in estrogen depleted medium has been described in the literature (24) and we have confirmed this observation. No direct effect on cell proliferation was found with the purified antiproteases, but antibodies to the antiproteases were able to reduce the E2-stimulated cell proliferation, indicating a role for the antiproteases either by protecting positive growth regulatory proteins or their receptors against proteolytic break down or by inhibiting the proteolytic activation of latent forms of proteins with negative growth regulatory function. Plasma protease inhibitors have been found to modulate the immune responses (30-33), and we will investigate whether production and release of antiproteases from E2-stimulated MCF-7 cells might protect them against attack from cells of the immune system. It will be interesting to elucidate whether production of antiproteases by tumor cells may play an important role both during the formation of the primary tumor and also in the metastatic process.

ACKNOWLEDGEMENTS.

This research was supported by a grant from the Neye Foundation.

REFERENCES

1. Mouridsen, H., Palshof, T., Patterson, J. and Battersby, L. Cancer Treat. Rev. 5:131-141, 1978.
2. Henderson, I.C., Canellos, G.P. N. Engl. J. Med. 302:17-30, 1980.
3. Henderson,I.C., Canellos, G.P. N. Engl. J. Med. 302:78-90, 1980.
4. McGuire, W.L., Pearson, O.H., Segaloff, A. IN: Estrogen receptors in human breast cancer (Eds. W.L., McGuire, P.P. Carbone, E.P. Vollmer. Raven, New York, 1975, pp. 1-7.
5. Sirbasku, D.A. In: Hormones and Breast Cancer (Eds. M.C. Pike, P.K. Siiteri and C.W. Welsh) Banbury Report No.8, 1981, pp. 425-443.
6. Lippman, M.E. et al. J. Cell. Biochem. 35:1-16, 1987.
7. Vignon, F. Growth Factors and Oncogenes 190:75-86, 1989.
8. Osborne, C.K. and Arteaga, C.L. Breast Cancer Res. Treat. 15:3-11, 1990.
9. Knabbe, C. et al. Cell 48:417-428, 1987.
10. Arteaga, C.L. et al. Cancer Res. 48:3898-3904, 1988.
11. Lippman, M.E. et al. J. Cell. Biochem. 35:1-16, 1987.
12. Lykkesfeldt, A.E., Laursen, I. and Briand. P. Mol. Cell. Endocrinol. 62:287-296, 1989.
13. Van der Burg, B. et al. J. Cell. Physiol. 134:101-108, 1988.
14. Karey, K.P. and Sirbasku, D.A. Cancer Res. 48:4083-4092, 1988.
15. Briand. P. and Lykkesfeldt, A.E. Anticancer Res. 6:85-90, 1986.
16. Soule, H.D. et al. J. Natl. Cancer Inst. 51:1409-1416, 1973.
17. Lykkesfeldt, A.E. and Briand, P. Br. J. Cancer 53:29-35, 1986.
18. Lykkesfeldt, A.E. et al. Eur. J. Cancer Clin. Oncol. 22:439-444, 1986.
19. Hanna, N. and Schneider, M. J. Immunol. 130:974-980, 1983.
20. Westley, B. and Rochefort, H. Cell 20:353-362, 1980.
21. Laursen, I., Briand, P. and Lykkesfeldt, A.E. Anticancer Res. 10:343-352, 1990.
22. Arrick, B.A., Korc, M. and Derynck, R. Cancer Res. 50: 299-303, 1990.

23. Morisset, M., Capony, F. and Rochefort, H. Biochem. Biophys. Res. Commun. 138:102-109, 1986.
24. Vignon, F. et al. Endocrinology 118:1537-1545, 1986.
25. Thorpe, S.M. el al. Cancer Res. 49:6008-6014, 1989.
26. Garcia, M. et al. Oncogene 5:1809-1814, 1990.
27. Tamir, S. et al. Endocrinology 127:1319-1328, 1990.
28. Gendler, S.J. and Tökes, Z.A. Biochim. Biophys. Acta 882:242-253, 1986.
29. Massot, O. et al. Mol. Cell. Endocrinol. 42:207-214, 1985.
30. Gravagna, P. et al. Scand. J. Immun. 15:115-118, 1982.
31. Ades, E.W. et al. Scand. J. Immunol. 15:109-113,1982.
32. Gravagna, P. et al. J. Reticuloendothelial Soc. 32:125-130, 1982.
33. Hudig, D. el al. J. Immunol. 126:1569-1574, 1981.
34. Madsen, M.W. and Briand, P. Eur. J. Cancer 26:793-797, 1990.
35. Ordonez, N.G. and Manning, J.T. Am. J. Gastroent. 79:959-963, 1984.
36. Leader, M., Collins, M. and Henry, K. Am. J. Surg. Pathol. 11:133-139, 1987.
37. Soini, Y. and Miettinen, M. Am. J. Clin. Pathol. 89:131-136, 1988.

THE PROLACTIN-INDUCIBLE PROTEIN / GROSS CYSTIC DISEASE FLUID PROTEIN (PIP/GCDFP-15): GENETIC ANALYSIS AND HORMONAL REGULATION OF GENE EXPRESSION

R. SHIU, Y. MYAL, D. TSUYUKI, D. ROBINSON, B. IWASIOW, A. YARMILL & P. WATSON

Department of Physiology, Faculty of Medicine, University of Manitoba, Winnipeg, Manitoba, Canada R3E 0W3

The prolactin-inducible protein (PIP)/gross cystic disease fluid protein (GCDFP-15) was isolated by us (1, 2) as a glycoprotein secreted by the T47D human breast cancer cell line in response to lactogenic peptide hormones (human prolactin and human growth hormone) and androgen, and independently by Haagensen and co-workers (3) as a protein found in abundance in the fluid of gross cystic disease of the breast. Haagensen and colleagues (3, 4) have measured the clinical profiles of this protein by radioimmunoassay and immunohistochemistry in the blood and tissues of patients having abnormal breast pathology. Based on immunohistochemical data, these investigators concluded that GCDFP-15 is the product of apocrine glands, and that the production of this protein by gross cystic disease and malignant breast tumors is the result of apocrine differentiation. Beside Haagensen's group, many clinical laboratories are using the GCDFP-15/PIP as a marker for abnormal breast functions and have observed, for instance, that the contents of GCDFP-15 in gross cystic disease fluid is correlated with that of androgens, prolactin and epidermal growth factor (5). PIP/GCDFP-15 protein is abundant in gross cystic disease and malignant breast carcinomas (2-4, 6). However, little, if any, of this protein is found in normal human mammary tissue (4). Nevertheless, the protein has been detected by immunocytochemistry in normal apocrine tissues such as the serous cells of the salivary gland, Moll's glands of eyelids, ceruminous glands of the ear canal, sweat glands, perineum and some bronchial glands (3,4). We have also employed Western immunoblot to demonstrate the presence of PIP/GCDFP-15 protein in a variety of physiological fluids such as blood, saliva, tear, sweat, amniotic fluid and breast milk (7). While the studies on PIP/GCDFP-15 protein distribution and tissue contents are informative, they have provided little insight into the cellular origin (site of synthesis) and functional significance of this protein. Also, the genetic mechanisms governing the expression of the PIP/GCDFP-15 gene (PIP*) in normal and neoplastic tissues remain to be explored. For these reasons, we have directed our research into the molecular genetics of PIP gene. [**Since PIP is the official name used in the Genome Data Base and in both Genbank Data Bank and the EMBL Data base, the GCDFP-15 designation will not be used. Throughout this article, PIP is used to denote the gene.*]

Our initial effort has resulted in the cloning of the human PIP cDNA (7) which was used for the first time to study the tissue distribution of the expression of *PIP*. For example, we were able to show the presence of authentic PIP mRNA in normal human skin samples, supporting the notion based on immunocytochemical studies that the sweat gland is the site of production of PIP. Since *PIP* is a multihormonally regulated gene in human breast cancer cell lines (see below and 1,2,7-9), our finding of *PIP* gene expression in normal tissues such as the sweat gland suggests that the latter organ may be subjected to the influence of multihormonal signals such as prolactin, growth hormone, androgen and estrogen. Therefore, studies on the regulation of *PIP* gene expression in normal tissues may lead to the identification of novel target sites for the above hormones.

The availability of the PIP cDNA has also enabled us to detect and quantitate the presence of PIP mRNA in human breast tumor biopsy specimens, gross cystic disease tissues and other human tumors (6). Figure 1 shows a Northern hybridization analysis of RNA samples isolated from a number of human tumor tissues. Among many human tumors tested, only breast tumors and gross cystic breast tissues are positive for PIP mRNA; PIP mRNA is undetectable in a sample of normal human breast tissue obtained from reduction mammoplasty, an observation consistent with the lack of immunoreactive PIP/GCDFP-15 protein in normal human breast tissues reported by Haagensen and colleagues (3,4). Also, PIP mRNA was undetectable in carcinomas of the prostate, colon and bladder (6). It is clear from the strengths of the hybridization signals (Fig. 1) that there is a considerable variation of PIP mRNA levels in human breast cancer samples. At present, the mechanism(s) responsible for this variation of *PIP* gene expression has not been elucidated, although parameters such as cellular heterogeneity, tumor-to-stromal cell ratio, or magnitude of gene expression, have to be considered. Nevertheless, when

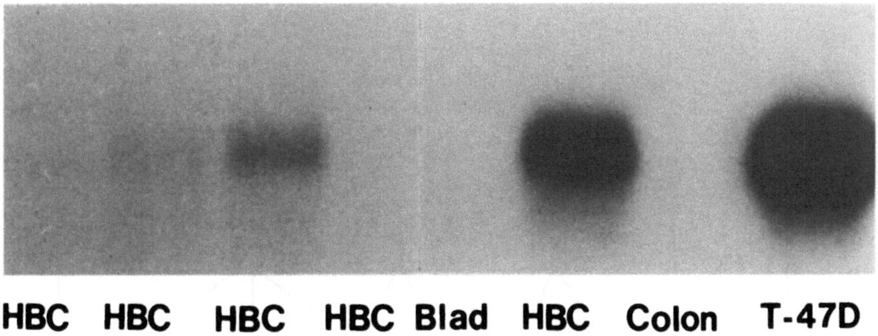

Fig. 1. PIP mRNA in human tumors studied by Northern hybridization. HBC: human breast carcinoma; Blad: bladder carcinoma; Colon: colon carcinoma; T-47D: human breast cancer cell line. (Reprinted with permission from ref. 6).

the levels of PIP mRNA in human breast cancers were compared with that of estrogen receptors (a commonly used diagnostic/prognostic indicator), we found significant correlation ($p < 0.01$) between PIP mRNA and estrogen receptor contents (6), suggesting that PIP gene expression may be a potentially useful marker for a subpopulation of hormone responsive breast cancers. In addition, PIP gene expression may be a useful tool to investigate the potential role of prolactin/growth hormone in human breast cancer.

In order to facilitate studies towards evaluating the potential of the PIP gene as a genetic marker, it was first necessary to isolate and characterize the structure of the gene. The structure of the PIP gene cloned from an EMBL 3 human lymphocyte genomic DNA library is shown in Fig. 2 (10). The PIP gene has many features typical of mammalian genes: the coding region is contained within 7 kb of DNA and is interrupted by 3 introns, and the four exons range in size from 106 bp to 223 bp in length. A fragment of the genomic clone was used for Southern hybridization to DNA isolated from human-hamster somatic cell hybrids, and for *in situ* hybridization to metaphase lymphocyte chromosomes. These studies have allowed the localization of the PIP gene to the long arm of chromosome 7 (7q32-36)(11). Furthermore, a two-allele Taq1 Restriction Fragment Length Polymorphism (RFLP) has been detected at the PIP gene locus (12). Fig. 3 illustrates the Taq1 RFLP pattern of the PIP gene locus in a family of Manitoba Hutterites (a religious sect). Southern hybridization analysis of Taq1

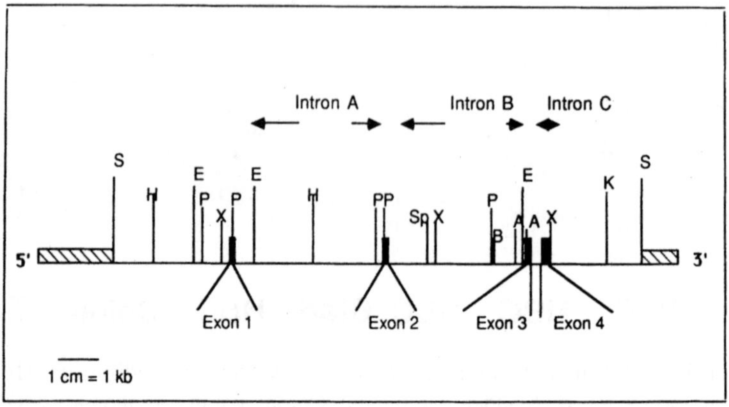

Fig. 2. Restriction map of the recombinant phage clone containing the human PIP gene and flanking sequences. (Reprinted with permission from ref. 10).

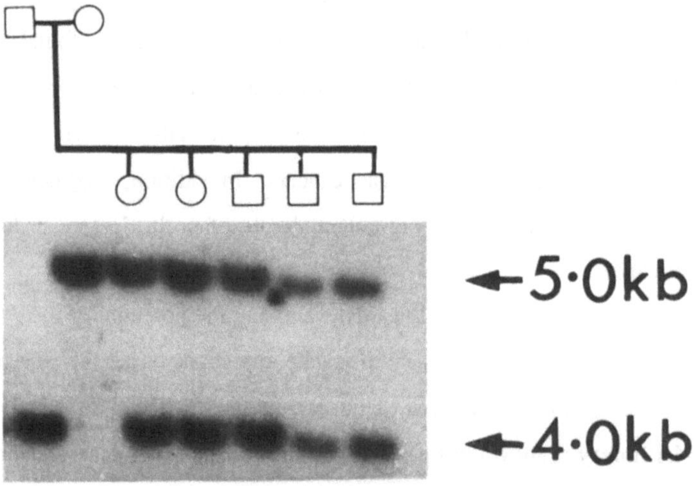

Fig. 3. RFLP profile of the PIP locus in a Manitoba Hutterite family. Allele A is the 5 kb fragment and allele B is the 4 kb fragment.

digested lymphocyte DNA revealed the father is homozygous for the 4.0 kb allele B, whereas the mother is homozygous for the 5.0 kb allele A, and all the children are therefore heterozygotic (AB). This type of analysis was extended to over 100 non-Hutterites, unrelated individuals in the Province of Manitoba (Table 1). When DNA from healthy volunteers was analysed, the majority (17/19) exhibited only the A allele (homozygous A), with the remaining two individuals showing heterozygosity (AB). Included in this study were 101 unrelated breast cancer patients, of which lymphocyte DNA from 1/3, and breast tumor DNA from 2/3, of these patients were analysed (Table 1). Similar to the finding in the normal volunteers, 90% of the breast cancer patients were homozygous for the A allele, and the remaining 10% were heterozygotes. Also, there were no differences in these frequencies between breast tumor DNA and lymphocyte DNA from the patients, indicating that breast tumor development is not associated with the loss of heterozygosity of chromosome 7 containing the PIP gene locus. Finally, it is of interest to note that, of the 101 non-Hutterite individuals, no homozygosity of the B allele was observed. This is in contrast to our observation with the Manitoba Hutterite community where we have detected 2 homozygotes for the B allele in 16 unrelated individuals, in addition to a higher frequency of heterozygotes. The reason for this difference between the Hutterites and the general population is at present unknown.

TABLE 1: ALLELE FREQUENCIES FOR TAQ RFLP AT PIP GENE LOCUS

	# INDIV. (N)	ALLELE A (5 Kb)	ALLELE B (4 Kb)	AB	P
BREAST TUMORS	67	62	0	5	N.S.
PATIENT LYMPHOCYTES	34	29	0	5	N.S.
NORMAL LYMPHOCYTES	19	17	0	2	
HUTTERITE LYMPHOCYTES	16	10	2	4	0.05

Our initial work (1, 2, 7) has indicated that either the lactogens (human prolactin and human growth hormone), or androgens (dihydrotestosterone), or both, effectively increase the level of PIP mRNA in the T47D and ZR-75-1 human breast cancer cell lines. Rochefort and co-workers (8) and Labrie and colleagues (9) subsequently confirmed our observations and in addition, the latter group showed that estradiol antagonizes the effect of androgen on PIP mRNA accumulation (9). As is the case for other eukaryotic genes, hormonal regulation of mRNA levels occurs either transcriptionally or post-transcriptionally, with alterations in mRNA stability being one of the most frequently used mechanisms of post-transcriptional regulation. Since little is known about the molecular events associated with prolactin and androgen actions in gene expression in human cells, a series of experiments were conducted to examine the effects of the two classes of hormones on *PIP* gene expression in the T47D human breast cancer cell line (10). The effects of prolactin and androgen on PIP precursor heteronuclear RNA (hnRNA) and mature messenger RNA (mRNA) stability were first examined. In this study, T47D breast cancer cells were incubated with hormone(s), and the RNA polymerase II inhibitor, 5,6-dichloro-1-ß-D-ribofuranosylbenzimidazole (DRB), was used to block the synthesis of new mRNAs. At various times following DRB treatment, cells were collected and the levels of PIP hnRNA and mRNA were determined by Northern analysis, using both PIP cDNA and genomic DNA intron probes. The results of such a study is summarized in Table 2.

Table 2: Effects of Hormones on PIP RNA stability

HORMONE TREATMENT	HALF LIFE OF PIP	
	hnRNA (min)	mRNA (hour)
NONE	49 ± 15	17 ± 3
PROLACTIN	31 ± 3	18 ± 2
DIHYDROTESTOSTERONE	37 ± 4	14 ± 1
BOTH HORMONES	36 ± 8	22 ± 2

The data presented in Table 2 indicate that the stability of the PIP hnRNA and PIP mRNA is not affected by the hormones, suggesting that neither prolactin nor androgen is involved in post-transcriptional regulation of *PIP* gene expression in human breast cancer cells.

Next, the effects of androgen and human prolactin/growth hormone on the transcriptional activity of the *PIP* gene was studied (10), using the *in vitro* nuclear transcriptional activity of the *PIP* gene was studied (10), using the *in vitro* nuclear run-on assay. To study the transcriptional activities across the *PIP* gene, we hybridized nuclear run-on nascent [^{32}P]-labeled RNA transcripts to a 5' PIP genomic fragment (gPIP1.5 which consists of exon 1 and portions of 5' flanking and intron A sequences), and to a 3' PIP genomic fragment (gPIP0.7 which consists of the last two exons 3 and 4, and intron c)(Fig. 3). Figure 4 shows that the lactogen alone (human growth hormone was used instead of prolactin in this experiment) or androgen alone, stimulates transcription of the *PIP* gene. The lactogen appears to preferentially increase the 3' hybridization signal. However, in subsequent experiments (unpublished) using single-stranded PIP genomic fragments for hybridization to avoid the detection of antisense RNA transcripts, human prolactin/growth hormone or dihydrotestosterone promotes uniform transcription across the *PIP* gene, with the androgen stimulating transcription by approximately 5-fold, and lactogen by 3-fold.

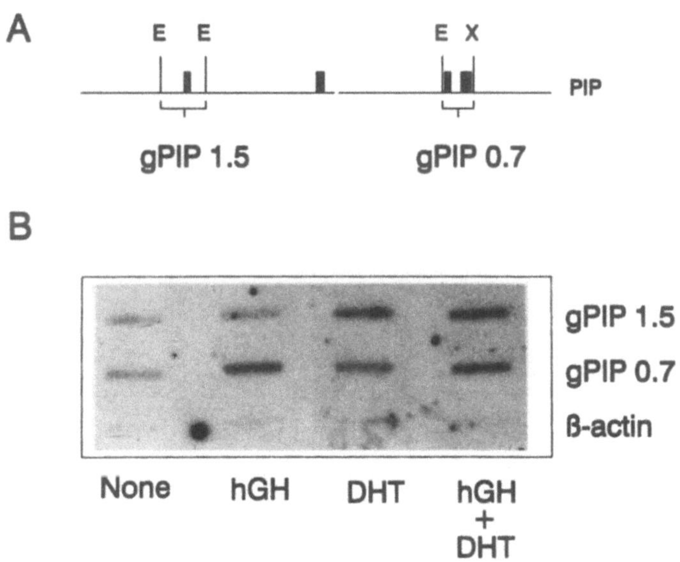

Fig. 4. Effect of hormones on *PIP* gene transcription assessed by the *in vitro* nuclear run-on assays. A) Schematic drawing showing the 5' (gPIP 1.5) and 3' (gPIP 0.7) genoic fragments used for hybridization. B) Hybridization of nuclear run-on transcripts to immobilized DNA. Human growth hormone (hGH), which is equipotent with human prolactin in the induction of *PIP* gene expression, was used as the lactogenic hormone in this experiment. DHT: dihydrotestosterone. (Reprint with permission from ref. 10).

The nucleotide sequences of the 5' flanking region of the human *PIP* gene revealed that the hexanucleotide sequence TGTTCT, which forms the core sequence of the glucocorticoid/androgen cis-acting element of the mouse mammary tumor virus (13), occurs five times within 1.2 kilobases of the 5' flanking region of the *PIP* gene (10). This 1.2 kb 5' flanking sequence containing the promoter region was ligated in front of the chloramphenicol acetyltransferase (CAT) gene. This PIP-CAT chimeric construct was transfected into the hormone responsive ZR-75-1 human breast cancer cells, and the effects of lactogen and androgen on CAT activity was determined. The result of one such experiment is shown in Fig. 5. Dihydrotestosterone but not

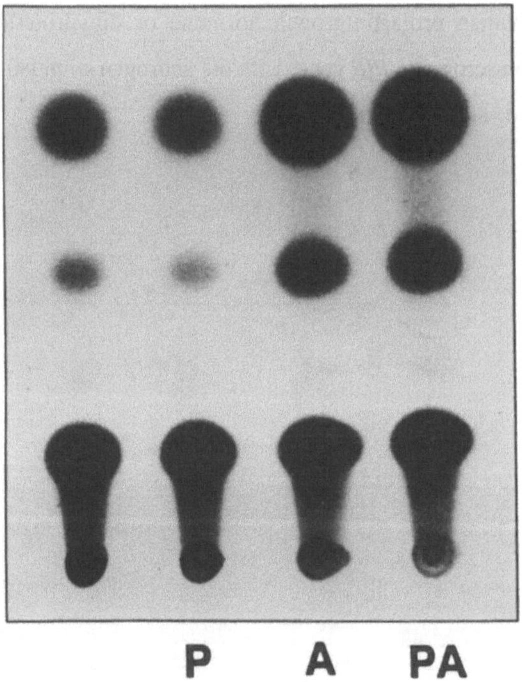

Fig. 5. Transient expression of the PIP-CAT chimeric construct in the ZR-75-1 human breast cancer cell line. P: prolactin; A: androgen (DHT); PA: both hormones.

prolactin was able to stimulate the transient expression of CAT. This finding indicates the presence of androgen response cis-acting elements, possibly containing the hexanucleotide sequence TGTTCT, in the promoter region of the *PIP* gene.

Experiments in progress will define the exact location and sequence of this androgen response element. The observation that prolactin alone failed to induce CAT expression may indicate that the sequence conferring prolactin responsiveness is not contained within this 1.2 kb 5' flanking region, but may lie somewhere else in the *PIP* gene. Additional experiments studying the expression of the full complement of the *PIP* gene are required to gain insight into the molecular basis of prolactin responsiveness in the *PIP* gene.

ACKOWLEDGEMENT

This research is supported by the Medical Research Council of Canada.

REFERENCES

1. Shiu, R.P.C. and Iwasiow, B.M. J. Biol. Chem. 260: 11307-11313, 1985.
2. Shiu, R.P.C., Murphy, L.C., Tsuyuki, D., Myal, Y., Lee-Wing, M. and Iwasiow, B. Rec. Progr. Horm. Res. 43: 277-303, 1987.
3. Haagensen, D.E., Jr. and Mazoujian, G. In: Diseases of the breast (Haagensen, C.D., ed.), W.B. Saunders Co., Philadelphia, 1986, pp. 475-500.
4. Haagensen, D.E., Jr., Dilley, W.G., Mazoujian, G. and Wells, S.A., Jr. Annals N. Y. Acad. Sci. 586: 161-173, 1990.
5. Collette, J., Van Cauwenberge, J-R., Dejardin, L., Carlisi, A., Jaspar, J-M. and Franchimont, P. Annals N. Y. Acad. Sci. 586: 146-157, 1990
6. Murphy, L.C., Lee-Wing, M., Goldenberg, G.J. and Shiu, R.P.C. Cancer Res. 47: 4160-4164, 1987.
7. Murphy, L.C., Tsuyuki, D., Myal, Y., Shiu, R.P.C. J. Biol. Chem. 262: 15263-15241, 1987.
8. Chalbos, D., Haagensen, D., Parish, T. and Rochefort, H. Cancer Res. 47: 2787-2792, 1987.
9. Simard, J., Hatton, A-C., Labrie, C., Dauvois, S., Zhao, H.F., Haagensen, D.E., Jr. and Labrie, F. Mol. Endocrinol. 3: 694-702, 1989.
10. Myal, Y., Robinson, D.B., Iwasiow, B., Tsuyuki, D., Wong, P. and Shiu, R.P.C. Mol. Cell Endocrinol. 80: 165-175, 1991.
11. Myal, Y., Gregory, C., Wang, H., Hamerton, J.L. and Shiu, R.P.C. Somatic Cell Mol. Genet. 15: 265-270, 1989.
12. Myal, Y., Gregory, C.A., Karpan, C., Hamerton, J.L. and Shiu, R.P.C. Nucleic Acids Res. 17: 5879, 1989.
13. Ham, J., Thompson, A., Needham, M., Webb, P. and Parker, M. Nucleic Acids Res. 16: 5263-5277, 1988.

SECTION III

MAMMARY EPITHELIUM AND STROMA IN VIVO AND IN VITRO

ROLE OF RAS ONCOGENE IN HUMAN BREAST CANCER: AN EXPERIMENTAL APPROACH

J. RUSSO, G. CALAF, J. OCHIENG, I.H. RUSSO, Q. TAHIN, P-L. ZHANG

Department of Pathology, Fox Chase Cancer Center, 7701 Burholme Avenue, Philadelphia, PA 19111

INTRODUCTION

There are several reports indicating that oncogenes are associated with breast cancer in humans and animals (1,2). Among the oncogenes, the ras family with their three variants, c-Ha-ras, v-Ha-ras and n-Ha-ras, has been widely studied and reported to be involved in mammary carcinomas induced in experimental animals by chemical carcinogens, in breast cancer cell lines, in primary breast cancers, as rare alleles or as an amplification or expression of the gene product of the ras gene, the p21 protein (3-6). However, whether the ras oncogene is a causative agent of breast cancer has not been proven as yet.

There is experimental evidence that the ras oncogene is able to enhance the tumorigenic phenotype. A mouse mammary epithelial cell line that was not tumorigenic was changed into a tumorigenic line by transfection with c-ras gene, primary rabbit mammary epithelial cells were immortalized after microinjection with simian virus SV40 DNA and became tumorigenic after transfection with an activated human c-Ha-ras gene (7,8), benzo(a)pyrene immortalized human breast epithelial cell were changed into tumorigenic by combination of SV40 antigen and v-Ha-ras transferred into the cells using a retroviral vector (9). In transgenic mice there is evidence that the ras oncogene plays an important role in developing mammary tumors when the mice contain a MMTV-v-ras fusion construct (10).

Collectively the strongest evidence of the initiating role of the ras gene in mammary tumorigenesis comes from the study of mammary tumors induced by chemical carcinogens that selectively induce a point mutation in codon 12 for MNU and a mutation in codon 61 for DMBAs (11,12). In our laboratory we have shown that primary cultures of breast epithelial cells treated with chemical carcinogens are able to produce amplification of the c-Ha-ras gene (13). However, these cells never became tumorigenic in nude mice (14). When newborn rats are treated with a chemical carcinogen, mutation of the c-Ha-ras gene is observed in the mammary gland but not tumorigenesis until the animals reach the puberal age (15). All these data clearly indicate that c-Ha-ras requires a proliferative milieu via immortalization or hormonal stimulation in order to be fully operational (14). However, up to now has been difficult to study the interaction of the oncogenes with normal breast cells due to the lack of a system that allows one to study this process in a systematic approach. Therefore, what is needed is an experimental system in which the process of immortalization can be studied in the realm of physiologic terms and that allows us to clarify the role of the ras gene in relation to the immortalization phenomena and/or in combination to other genes.

NORMAL HUMAN BREAST EPITHELIAL CELLS

The establishment of immortal human mammary epithelial cell lines of nonmalignant origin has been rare (16-22). Normal human mammary epithelial cells can be maintained in vitro for 10-20 passages and then senescence occurs (21). Until recently there has been no report of immortalization occurring in cultures of untreated normal breast epithelium (22). The establishment of an immortal cell line (MCF-10) that arose spontaneously, without viral or chemical intervention, from mortal human diploid mammary epithelial cells of extended life span provided an important tool for understanding how specific genes such as c-Ha-ras, erb/B2 or transforming growth factor alpha (TGF-alpha) are able to induce transformation phenotypes and at the same time provide the basis for understanding the difference between the processes that control senescence, immortalization and malignancy.

MCF-10 cell line is a bonafide human breast epithelial cell in nature (23). These cells express epithelial sialomucins and keratins reported in human breast (22,23). Ultrastructurally the cells are low cuboidal with numerous desmosomes and short microvilli; they grow in plastic as a monolayer forming domes (23). The cells are not tumorigenic in nude mice, grow in culture under the control of hormones and growth factors, they form ductular structures in collagen matrix and they lack anchorage-independent growth (22). Cytogenetic analysis prior to immortalization showed normal diploid cells although later passages after immortalization showed minimal rearrangement and near diploidy (22). Genotypically these cells were clearly demonstrated to be human by DNA hybridization with probes for highly polymorphic sequences such as the hypervariable single copy gene PUM (22). The relationship of MCF-10 to the specific donor was demonstrated by hybridization of identical size HaeIII fragments with a M13 probe that detects multiple hypervariable minisatellites (22). MCF-10 cells do not have amplification of c-erbB2/HER-2-neu, erbA-1, int-2, int-1 or mutated c-Ha-ras-1 gene. In addition they did not contain SV40 antigen (22). These characteristics make this cell line the most near to a normal breast epithelial cell line available.

TRANSFECTION OF MCF-10 WITH MUTATED RAS ONCOGENE

We have used (24) the plasmid Homer 6 (pHomer 6) as a transfection vector as well as a construct containing normal Ha-ras gene or the human T24(T) activated oncogene. In this construct both genes T24 and c-Ha-ras are flanked by enhancers SV40 and MoSV (25). The selection of cells with the integrated foreign DNA was done by growing the cells for three weeks in media containing geneticin. After this time the colonies were counted, measured and replated. After using this selective medium the cells were labelled MCF-10Aneo when they were transfected with pHomer6 only, MCF-10AneoN and MCF-10AneoT when the cells were transfected with the protooncogene or the activated oncogene respectively (24). The transfected mutated c-Ha-ras gene was detected by Southern hybridization analysis of MCF-10Aneo and MCF-10AneoN DNA with ^{32}P labeled EcoR1 411 b.p. fragment of plasmid pKy1. A point mutation in ras gene at codon 12 of exon-1 will result in the abolishment of a MspI.HpaII site which falls in that region of the gene resulting in 411 b.p. fragment instead of the 355 and 56 b.p. fragments expected from a normal ras gene. We detected the 355 b.p. MspI.HpaII fragment corresponding to the normal site at codon 12 as expected in MCF-10A cells transfected with pHo6N carrying the normal ras gene. We detected the 411 b.p. MspI.HpaII fragment in MCF-10A cells transfected with plasmid pHo6T, carrying the mutated ras gene of T24 cell line, indicating the presence of the mutated ras gene in those transfected cells. Restriction mapping with EcoR1 and BamH1 confirmed that no rearrangement of the ras gene was present (26). We also have reported that no amplification of erbB2 or int2 was present in the transfected cells, indicating that we have introduced a mutated ras gene without altering other genes that are known to be associated with breast cancer (24,26). Using two dimensional gel electrophoresis and western blot we have demonstrated that MCF-10AneoT cells also express the mutated p21 protein whereas the other transfectant controls only expressed the normal p21 but not the mutated form (24).

EXPRESSION OF MALIGNANT PHENOTYPES BY THE MUTATED C-HA-RAS GENE

An important and critical question to be answered is whether the mutated ras gene in MCF-10A cells is able to induce all the array of malignant changes observed in breast cancer cells. We have been able to demonstrate that the activated ras gene is able to induce malignant transformation of MCF-10 cells (24). The growth pattern of MCF-10AneoT cells was disorganized, with loss of contact inhibition, the cells forming clumps over the monolayer. In contrast, MCF-10A, MCF-10Aneo and MCF-10AneoN cells did not show alterations in the pattern of growth, forming a single layer of cells with dome formation (Fig. 1). MCF-10AneoT

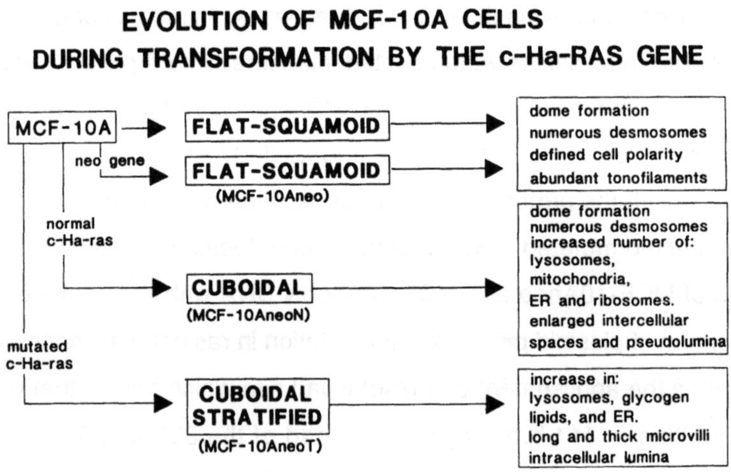

Figure 1: Schematic representation of the pathway of immortalization and transformation of MCF-10A. From: Russo, J., et al. (J. Cell Sci., 1991).

cells were unable to form ductal growth in a collagen matrix, indicating that the mutated gene had altered the ductulogenic properties normally present in these cells (24). The cells transfected with the mutated gene acquired anchorage independent growth and were able to grow in the absence of epidermal growth factor, hydrocortisone and cholera toxin (24). The expression of anchorage independence in these cells was associated with increased motility. This phenomenon was detected using the phagokinetic track assay. For this assay the cells were plated onto a carpet of colloidal gold and incubated with 3F3A, a monoclonal antibody directed to the glycoprotein gp78, which has been identified as a motility receptor (27). After a 24 hour incubation period the phagokinetic tracks were visualized by dark field illumination, photographed and the surface areas cleared of gold were measured utilizing an image analysis sytem. These areas indicated the motility of the cells, expressed in mm^2 (Table 1). The migratoy

Table 1

STIMULATION OF RANDOM MOTILITY
IN RAS-TRANSFECTED MCF-10A CELLS

Cell Line	Mean area cleared of gold particles (mm^2)	
	3F3A	Conditioned medium
MCF-10A-neo	14.7 ± 7.0	4.9 ± 0.2
MCF-10A-neoN	8.0 ± 2.0	7.7 ± 0.7
MCF-10A-neoT	68.0 ± 26.0	13.6 ± 1.6

response of the three cell lines under stimulation of the 3F3A antibody (27) showed that MCF-10AneoT cells had a stimulated random motility higher than MCF-10Aneo and MCF-10AneoN cells (Table 1). None of the three cell lines was able to move or clear the gold particles in the absence of 3F3A, even after a 48-hour incubation period. Addition of MCF-10AneoT conditioned medium to these cells slightly increased motility in MCF-10AneoT cells, indicating that an autocrine loop may be present (27). The high motility observed in MCF-10A cells under the effect of the mutated ras gene also correlated with the invasion assay using the Boyden chamber (Table 2) and with the higher collagenolytic activity observed in transfected cells. Furthermore, the demonstration that MCF-10AneoT cells were tumorigenic in irradiated nude mice (24), clearly indicated that the mutated ras gene was able to induce all the malignant phenotypes during the process of cell transformation (Fig. 2).

Table 2

CHEMOTACTIC AND CHEMOINVASIVE ACTIVITY OF RAS-TRANSFECTED MCF-10A CELLS

Cell Line	Chemotaxis FCM [1]	Chemotaxis SFM [2]	Chemoinvasion MG-25	Chemoinvasion MG-12.5
MCF-10A-neo	28 ± 1	2 ± 1	1 ± 1	1 ± 1
MCF-10A-neoN	11 ± 1	2 ± 1	0 ± 0	1 ± 1
MCF-10A-neoT	44 ± 2 •	2 ± 1	2 ± 1	31 ± 1 •

(1) FCM=fibroblast conditioned media
(2) SFM=serum free media
• ($p < 0.001$)

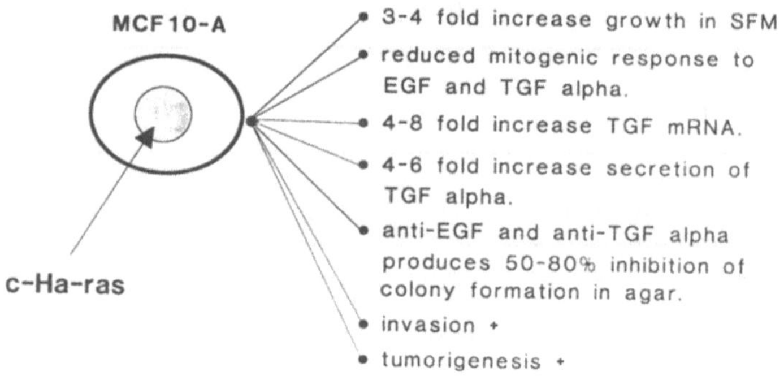

Figure 2: Malignant phentypes induced by the mutated c-Ha-ras in MCF-10A cells.

ROLE OF TGF-ALPHA IN THE NEOPLASTIC TRANSFORMATION OF MCF-10A CELLS

It is well known that in the process of cell proliferation there are negative and positive regulatory factors represented by the TGF-alpha and TGF-beta (28). During the process of transformation the cells are able to secrete their own growth factor, such as TGF-alpha, that occupies the resceptor for epidermal growth factor (EGF) and maintains an autocrine loop of cell proliferation. During the process of cell transformation the cells are unable to respond to TGF-beta, producing a disbalance by the preponderant action of TGF-alpha (29, 30). The ability of the

MCF-10AneoT cells to present anchorage independent growth in the presence or absence of EGF indicated to us that the presence of an autocrine loop may be present. We confirmed this by incubating MCF-10AneoT cells with an antibody against TGF-alpha; this antibody was able to block the growth of these cells in agar methocel. We have determined that MCF-10AneoT and isolated clones of the same produced TGF-alpha in significant amounts, 72-105 ng/ 108 cells during 48 hs (31). It was also demonstrated that the higher expression of TGF-alpha gene was associated with higher expression of the p21 protein of the c-Ha-ras gene (31).

The hypothesis that TGF-alpha is responsible for both the transformation of the cells and the maintenance of the autocrine loop the transformed phenotype was tested by transfecting the TGF-alpha gene to MCF-10A cells in order to determine whether transfected cells would express the same malignant phenotypes induced by the mutated ras gene in MCF-10AneoT cells (24). For that purpose MCF-10A cells were infected with 1522, a replication defective, amphotropic retroviral vector that contains the TGF-alpha cDNA under transcriptional control of an internal mouse MT1 mouse metallothionein-1 promoter. Cadmium chloride induces the expression of TGF-alpha gene through the MT1 promotion. The neomycin resistant gene was used for selection. As depicted in Figure 3, the infected cells

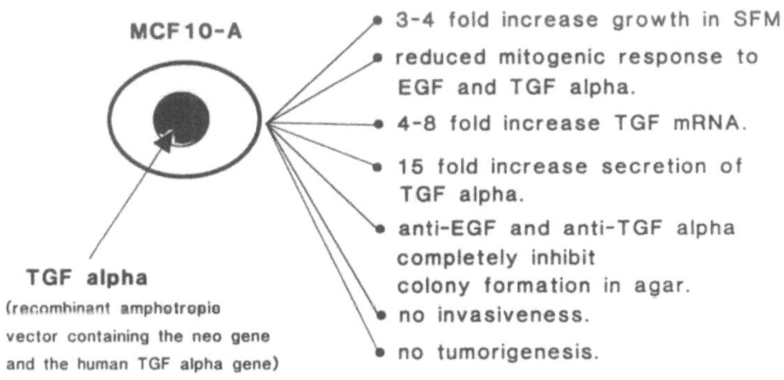

Figure 3: Malignant phenotypes induced by the TGF-alpha gene in MCF-10A cells.

were able to grow in the serum-free medium, and exhibited a 4-8 fold increase in TGF-alpha mRNA, and a 15 fold increase in the secretion of TGF-alpha. Incubation of infected cells with anti-TGF- alpha inhibited colony formation. However, these cells did not express the invasive or the tumorigenic phenotypes. These results indicated that neither the amplification nor the production of TGF-alpha were able to induce certain malignant phenotypes, such as increased motility, invasion and tumorigenesis. Although it is possible that the expression of anchorage independent growth is induced by c-Ha-ras via TGF-alpha secretion, the mutated c-Ha-ras induce other changes that result in the expression of other phenotypes by the transfected cells, such as increases in the expression of mRNA for cathepsin B and L, in the activity in association with plasma membrane/endosomal fractions and in the spontaneous subcellular distribution of cathepsin B activity (32). These findings open new avenues for studying the role of ras gene in the modulation of lysosomal enzymes, proteolytic enzymes and the mobilization of the proton pump in the regulation of the intracellular pH.

ROLE OF THE ERBB-2 GENE IN THE EXPRESSION OF MALIGNANT PHENOTYPES IN MCF-10A CELLS

It has been reported that erbB-2 gene is involved in breast cancer and the amplification of the gene correlates with the clinical aggressive behavior of the disease (33). However its role in the initiation of mammary caricinogenesis is not clear. It is possible to speculate that if erbB2 gene is capable of initiating the process of breast cancer, transfection of MCF-10A cells with this gene will induce the malignant phenotypes observed in MCF-10AneoT cells. For that purpose MCF-10A cells were transfected with an expression vector plasmid pDd-V1J8 containing the full length normal rat c-neu under the transcriptional control of the MSV-LTR and the neomycin gene. C-neu induces increased growth in serum-free medium and colony formation in agar methocel which is inhibited by incubation of transfected cells with anti-erbB2 antibody. Transfected cells, however do not increase the production of TGF-alpha, do not respond to exogenous TGF-alpha or EGF, and they are not invasive or tumorigenic in irradiated nude mice (Fig. 4) (31).

These data indicate that the expression of a malignant phenotype such as anchorage independent growth is induced by different genes such as c-Ha-ras, TGF-alpha or erbB2. Our data also indicate that c-Ha-ras induces anchorage independent growth through a TGF-alpha loop whereas erbB2 induces the same phenotype without the intervention of TGF-alpha. Interestingly enough, other malignant phenotypes, such as invasion and tumorigenesis, are induced only by the mutated ras gene.

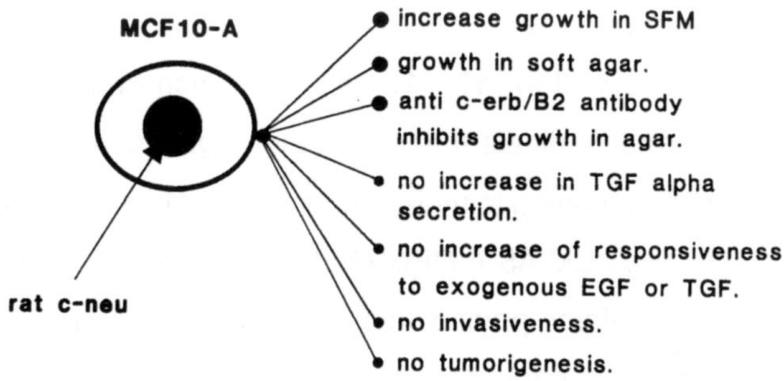

Figure 4: Malignant phenotypes induced by the rat c-neu in MCF-10A cells.

RESPONSE OF MCF-10F CELLS TO CHEMICAL CARCINOGENS

It has been shown that the carcinogens N-methyl-N-nitrosourea (MNU) and 7,12-dimethylbenz(a)anthracene (DMBA) both induce a point mutation of the ras gene that correlates with tumor induction (2). However, there is no evidence that chemical carcinogens are causative agents in the human disease and treatment of human breast epithelial cells with chemical carcinogens in vitro has not succeeded in inducing the full expression of malignant transformation and no point mutation of the ras gene has been reported by this treatment. In our laboratory we have shown that MCF-10F cells treated with different chemical carcinogens such as DMBA, MNU, methylnitroso-nitroguanidine (MNNG) and benz(a)pyrene B(a)P express the following malignant phenotypes: alteration in cell morphology, anchorage independent growth and alteration in duct-like formation in collagen gel (34,35). Interestingly enough we have also found that MCF-10F cells treated with MNU, MNNG, DMBA and B(a)P exhibited a point mutation in codon 12 of the c-Ha-ras gene. The results indicate that chemical carcinogens induce in the immortalized MCF-10F cells malignant phenotypes and point mutation; this latter is also induced by the mutated gene itself when it is transfected to the same cells and the responsible for the induction of the observed malignant phenotypes. Chemical carcinogens and mutated ras gene induce malignant transformation of HBEC. The common element in these experiments is the immortalized cell line MCF-10, what suggests that the critical point in the cell transformation pathway is the immortalization of the cell; when this phenotype is present, transformation, as measured by defined malignant phenotypes is expressed in different degrees. However, when mortal cells obtained from primary cultures were used, malignant phenotypes were not induced. Therefore, the understanding of the mechanism of cell immortalization observed in MCF-10 cells, in which other parameters or phenotypes are still normal, indicate that genes that regulate immortalization are different from those that are related to malignant or transformed phenotype.

THE BUFFERING OF CALCIUM AS A MECHANISM OF IMMORTALIZATION

Culture medium containing physiologic levels of calcium (1.05 mM) induce terminal differentiation and senescence in the mortal cells MCF-10, precursor of MCF-10A and MCF-10F cells, and designated MCF-10M, but it did not retard the growth or induced differentiation in the immortal cell sublines MCF-10A, MCF-10F and oncogene transformed MCF-10AneoT cells (22) (Fig. 5). Intracellular levels of

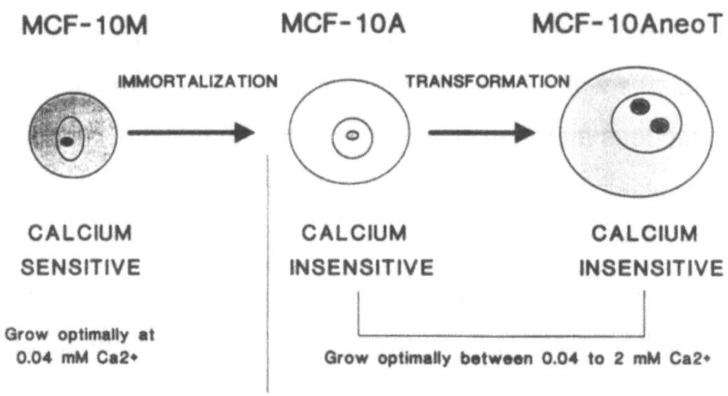

Figure 5: Pathway of calcium dependency in MCF-10 during immortalization and transformation.

calcium were determined in the three cell types grown under two different conditions. The three cell lines were maintained in DMEM/F12 medium containing chelated 5% equine serum and either 0.04 mM (low calcium medium) or 1.05 mM (high calcium) Ca++ (36). There was a significant increase in intracellular calcium (Ca_i) in MCF-10M as Ca++ levels were elevated in the medium from 0.04 to 1.05 mM. The immortal HBEC line, MCF-10A and the transformed MCF-10AneoT cells did not show significant changes in their Ca_i subsequent to the switch. The levels of Ca_i remained increased in MCF-10M cells while they were maintained in high Ca++ medium, but they reversed after the cells switched to low calcium for at least 24 h. MCF-10A and MCF-10neoT cell lines had lower Ca_i while they were maintained in high Ca++ medium, and the concentration of Ca++ did not vary appreciably after switching the cells to low levels. Since increases in Ca_i are normally accompanied by changes in the level of other second messengers such as inositol triphosphate (IP_3), we measured changes in intracellular IP_3 over a three-day period as a function of Ca++ concentration in the medium. At day 0, with all cells in low calcium medium, the IP_3 levels in the three cell lines were at a basal level. By day 1 after switching them to high calcium medium, there was a gradual increase in intracellular IP_3 in MCF-10M, but not in MCF-10A or MCF-10AneoT cells. These data are compatible with the knowledge that increased extracellular calcium acts at the level of cell membrane to activate phospholipase C, resulting in the hydrolysis of phospho inositol 4,5-biphosphate to dyacylglycerol and IP_3. The increased intracellular IP_3 then may be, wholly or in part, responsible for increase in Ca_i (37-39). The increased levels of IP_3 may in turn activate the so-called second messenger operated Ca++ channels (40), resulting in calcium influx from the external milieu. The ability of MCF-10A and MCF-10AneoT cells to strongly buffer changes in Ca_i could be one of the contributing factors if not the only one endowing them into immortality. The inability of the mortal cells to rigorously buffer Ca_i may not only lead to the induction of terminal differentiation but possibly programmed cell death.

CONCLUSIONS AND NEW DIRECTIONS

Our work clearly shows that the mutated c-Ha-ras oncogene is able to induce all the cascade of malignant phenotypes in immortalized HBEC, although transfection of this cell line with other genes, known to be involved in breast cancer, was unable to induce the array of malignant phenotypes induced by the insertion of the mutated c-Ha-ras gene (24). The availability of a cell transformed by a specific agent such as mutated ras, and the fact that different chemical carcinogens also produce a point mutation in the ras gene give as a better tool for understanding in human breast epithelial cells how the carcinogens and oncogenes may interact. In addition it provides a powerful tool for analyzing other physiological functions like the lysosomal trafficking and the production of specific proteolytic enzymes by this gene.

Our findings that immortal and transformed cells are capable of maintaining low intracellular Ca++ levels in the presence of high levels of extracellular Ca++ suggests that the understanding of this mechanism is pivotal in the study of cell immortalization and transformation.

REFERENCES

1. Bishop, J.M. Science 235:305-311, 1987.
2. Barbacid, M. Annu. Rev. Biochem. 56:779-827, 1987.
3. Zarbl, H., Sukumar S, Arthur, A.V., Martin-Zanca, D., and Barbacid, M. Nature 315:382-385, 1985.
4. Balmain, A. and Pragnell, I.B. Nature 303:72-74, 1983.
5. Bos, J.L., Mutat Res. 195:255-271, 1988.
6. Sukumar, S. In: Current Topics in Microbiology and Immunology Vol. 148, Springer-Verlag, Berlin, 1989, pp 93-114.
7. Redmond, S.M.S., Reichmann, E., Muller, R.G., Fris, R.R., Groner, B. and Hynes, N.E., Oncogene 2:259-265, 1988.
8. Hynes, N.E., Jaggi, R., Kozma, S.C., Ball, R., Muellener, D., Whetherall, N.T., Davis, B.W. and Grener, B. Mol. Cell Biol. 5:268-272, 1985.
9. Clark, R., Stampfer, M.R., Milley, R., O'Rouke, E., Walen, K.M., Kriegler, M., Kopplin, J. and McCormick, F. Cancer Res. 48:4689-4694, 1988.
10. Sinn, E., Muller, W., Pattengale, P., Tepler, I., Wallace, R. and Leder, P. Cell 49:465-475, 1987.
11. Sukumar, S., Notario, V., Martin-Zanca, D., and Barbicid, M. Nature (London) 306:658-661, 1983.
12. Dandekar, S., Sukumar, S., Zarbl, H., Young, L.J.T. and Cardiff, R.D. Mol. Cell Biol. 6:4104-4108, 1986.
13. Russo, J., Moussalli, M., Koszalka, M. and Russo, I.H. Proc. Am. Assoc. Cancer Res. 28:471a, 1987.
14. Russo, J., Reina, D., Frederick, J. and Russo, I.H. Cancer Res. 48:2837-2857, 1988.
15. Kumar, R., Sukumar, S., Barbacid, M. Science 248:1101-1104, 1990.
16. Briand, P., Peterson, O.W. and VanDeurs, B.A. In Vitro Cell Dev. Bio. 23:181-188, 1987.
17. Chang, S.E., Keen, J., Lane, E.B. and Taylor-Papadimitriou, J. Cancer Res. 42:2040-2053, 1982.
18. Gaffney, E.V., Cell Tissue Res 227:563-568, 1982.
19. Stampfer, M.R. and Bartley, J.C. Proc. Natl. Acad. Sci. USA 82:2394-2398, 1984.
20. Band, V. and Sager, R. Proc. Natl. Acad. Sci. USA 86:1249-1253, 1989.
21. McGrath, C.M. and Soule, H.D. In Vitro Cell Dev. Biol. 20:652-662, 1984.
22. Soule, H.D., Maloney, T.M., Wolman, S.R., Peterson, W.P., Brenz, R., McGrath, C.M., Russo, J., Jones, R.F., Brooks, S.C. Cancer Res. 50:6075-6086, 1990.
23. Tait, L., Soule, H.D. and Russo, J. Cancer Res. 40:6087-6094, 1990.
24. Basolo, F., Elliott, J., Tait, L., Chen, X.Q., Maloney, T., Russo, I.H., Pauley, R., Momiki, S., Caamano, J., Klein-Szanto, A.J.P., Koszalka, M. and Russo, J. Mol. Carcinogenesis 4:25-35, 1991.
25. Spandidos, D.A., Wilkie, N.M. Nature 310:469-475, 1984.
26. Zhang, P.L., Elliott, J.W., Basolo, F. and Russo, J. Proc. Am. Assoc. Cancer Res. 32:687a, 1991.
27. Ochieng, J. Basolo, F., Albini, A., Melchiori, A., Watanabe, J., Elliott, J.W., Raz, A., Parodi, S. and Russo, J. Invasion and Metastasis 261:1-10, 1990.
28. Goustin, A.S., Leaf, E.G., Shipley, G.D. and Moses, H.L. Cancer Res. 46:1015-1029, 1986.

29. Derynck, R., Cell 54:593-595, 1988.
30. Bringman, T.S., Lindquist, P.B. and Derynck, R. Cell 48:429-440, 1987.
31. Ciardello, F., McGeady, M.L., Kim, N., Basolo, F., Hynes, N., Langton, B.C., Yokozaki, H., Saeki, T., Elliott, J.W., Maruii, H., Mendelsohn, J., Soule, H., Russo, J. and Salomon, D.S. Cell Growth and Differentiation 1:407-420, 1990.
32. Rozhin, J., Moin, K., Russo, J. and Sloane, B.F., Proc. Am. Assoc. Cancer Res. 32:392a, 1991.
33. Slamon, D.J., Godolphi, W., Jones, L.A., Holt, J.A., Wang, S.G., Keith, D.E., Levin, W. Stuart, S.G., Udove, J., Ulrich, A. and Press, M.F. Science 244:707-712, 1989.
34. Calaf, G. and Russo, J. Proc. Am. Assoc. Cancer Res. 32:690a, 1991.
35. Calaf, G., Tait, L. and Russo, J. Proc. Am Assoc. Cancer Res. 32:676a, 1991.
36. Ochieng, J., Tahin, Q.S., Booth, C.C and Russo, J. J. Cell. Biochem. 46:1-5, 1991.
37. Berridge, M.J. and Irvine, R.F. Nature 312:315-321, 1984.
38. Janken, S. and Yupsa, S.H. Carcinogenesis 9:1033-1038, 1988.
39. Hennings, H., Kreizewski, F.H. and Yuspa, S.H. Carcinogenesis 10:777-780,1989.
40. Meldolesi, J, Pozzan, T. Exp. Cell Res 171:271-283, 1987.

ACKNOWLEDGEMENTS

We thank Vivian Powell and Jeanne Nace for typing this manuscript and Rocio M. Rivera for her photographic assistance.

This investigation was supported by Public Health Service Grant CA-38921, awarded by the National Cancer Institute.

INTERACTIONS BETWEEN MALIGNANT AND NON-MALIGNANT COMPONENTS OF THE BREAST

W.R. MILLER
Imperial Cancer Research Fund, Medical Oncology Unit, Western General Hospital, Edinburgh EH4 2XU, U.K.

INTRODUCTION

Breast cancers primarily develop within the terminal lobular-alveolar units of the breast(1). As a result there has been considerable interest in the relationship between normal and malignant epithelium and the processes which may destabilize normal epithelium and lead to carcinogenesis. However, it is important to realise that the breast is a complex organ in which, apart from during pregnancy and lactation, parenchymal elements constitute only a minor compartment(2). Thus glandular tissue constitutes only about 20-30% of the mature breast and after the menopause it rapidly diminishes to represent merely 5% of the organ in senility (Figure 1). In contrast, other components such as stroma and adipose tissue form the bulk of the breast although their proportions vary markedly at different stages of development. These elements are not inert and the potential exists for inter-communication between the various compartments of the breast.

The aim of this paper is to present evidence for paracrine interaction between malignant and non-malignant components of the breast and illustrate how this might influence the natural history and progression of breast cancer.

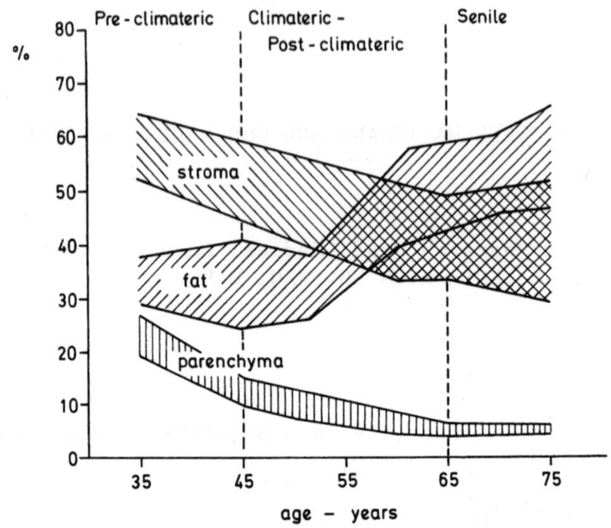

Fig. 1. Variation with age in the proportion of the major elements in the female breast.

STROMA AND BREAST CANCER

Conventionally the major function of breast stroma is attributed to the passive mechanical support of the mammary glandular system but there is reason to believe that connective tissue elements may also play a more active role(3). Thus, in rodents, stroma may mediate steroidal effects on epithelial (de)differentiation(4) and in vitro studies show that fibroblasts may enhance oestrogen responses in mammary epithelium(5).

Fibroblast behaviour may be abnormal in patients either at risk to or with familial breast cancer(6). This is based on the observation that foetal and adult human skin fibroblasts display distinctive migratory phenotypes when cultured on 3-dimensional collagen gels. Fibroblasts from about one half of breast cancer patients without a family history of the disease display foetal type behaviour but this incidence rises to almost 100% in those with familial breast cancers; age-matched controls invariably show the adult-phenotype. These studies have recently been extended and indicate that (i) foetal fibroblast behaviour is also found in unaffected first-degree relatives of breast cancer patients(7),

(ii) a soluble factor (MSF) secreted by foetal-type fibroblasts can transform the migratory behaviour of normal adult fibroblasts(8) and (iii) fibroblasts from interlobular stroma can differ from their intralobular counterparts(9).

It is also clear that fibroblasts can increase the take-rate and growth of breast cancers innoculated into the mammary fat pad of immunosuppressed mice(10). These effects appear to be mediated by growth factors secreted by fibroblasts; media conditioned by growth with fibroblasts can markedly stimulate the growth of breast cancer cells(11).

Recently a novel metallo-proteinase gene (Stromelysin 3) has been identified in the stromal cells immediately surrounding the neoplastic cells of the invasive, but not the *in situ*, component of breast carcinomas or fibroblasts more distant from invading cells(12). The pattern of expression suggests that the enzyme may play a part in the lytic processes involved in breast cancer progression. The data also would be consistent with an interaction between invasive epithelial cells and surrounding stromal cells supporting the hypothesis that fibroblasts in the neighbourhood of cancer cells are activated by an inductive stimulus eminating from the cancer cell - interestingly Stromelysin 3 could be induced by a series of growth factors(12), many of which may be produced by breast cancer cells(13).

ADIPOSE TISSUE AND BREAST CANCER

Compared with other glands in the body, the adult human breast is unusual in being invested in an abundance of fat. This is most marked in older women, the ratio of breast adipose tissue to glandular elements increasing with age(2). The role of mammary adipose tissue is not well understood but there is evidence of a link with the development of mammary cancer in both animals and humans. Thus, mammary cancer exists only in animal species with well-developed fat pads(14). and, in rodents, animals with little mammary adipose tissue or experimentally-cleared fat pads appear resistant to mammary neoplasms(15). The mammary fat pad thus appears to be essential for the development of hyperplastic lesions and cancers. "Take" and growth rates of human breast cancer cells are also increased when implanted into the mammary fat pad of immunosuppressed animals as compared with other body sites(16).

Epidemiological evidence implicates mammary fat with risk of human breast cancer. Obesity, which increases the amount of adipose tissue in the breast(17) is associated with an increased risk of breast cancer in postmenopausal women(18). Similarly, the relative proportion of adipose tissue increases with age in parallel with the incidence of breast cancer. A comparison of Japanese immigrants to Hawaii with native Japanese women also showed a similar positive correlation between the proportion of mammary adipose tissue and the incidence of hyperplastic breast lesions and breast cancer(19).

There are several potential mechanisms by which breast fat may influence the natural history of breast cancer. Firstly by nature of its lipid content it could act as a sponge for organic carcinogens. Secondly, adipose tissue is not metabolically inert and it may synthesize factors capable of stimulating both normal and malignant epithelium. Finally, high concentrations of steroid hormones may be extracted from breast fat(20). At this stage it is not clear whether these represent stores absorbed and concentrated from the circulation or if they result from local biosynthesis. However, as will be discussed in the next section, breast adipose tissue has the potential to synthesize and metabolise steroid hormones and this capacity may be influenced by the presence and stage of breast cancer.

STEROID METABOLISM IN MAMMARY FAT IN RELATION TO BREAST CANCER

Oestrogens have a central role in the development of the breast and are implicated in the promotion of breast cancers(21).

Two of the major pathways by which oestradiol may be synthesized within the breast are illustrated in Figure 2. These involve the activity of 17β hydroxysteroid dehydrogenase(s) which transforms 17-oxosteroids into 17β-hydroxy-steroids (including the conversion of oestrone to oestradiol) and the aromatase complex which catalyses the transformation of androgens to oestrogens. Both activities are present in breast fat but their level varies markedly between different specimens(22). Studies have therefore been performed to elucidate the factors influencing steroid metabolism in mammary adipose tissue and to determine whether there are relationships with breast cancer.

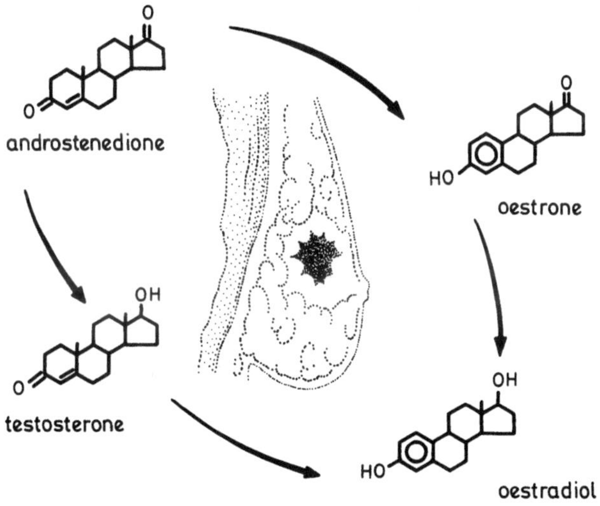

Fig. 2. Oestrogen biosynthesis within the breast involving the aromatization of androgens (androstenedione and testosterone being converted to oestrone and oestradiol respectively) and 17β-hydroxysteroid dehydrogenase activity (the interconversion of (a) androstenedione and testosterone and (b) oestrone and oestradiol).

STEROID METABOLISM AND THE PRESENCE OF BREAST CANCER:

Comparisons have been made between adipose tissue derived from breast cancer patients and that from women with benign conditions. The results are shown in Figure 3. Despite a large overlap in values between the groups, aromatase activity was significantly higher in patients with breast cancer, the median value in the cancer group being over two-fold higher than that of the benign group. No significant difference was detected in 17β hydroxysteroid dehydrogenase activity in mammary fat between women with benign breast disease or breast cancer (Figure 3).

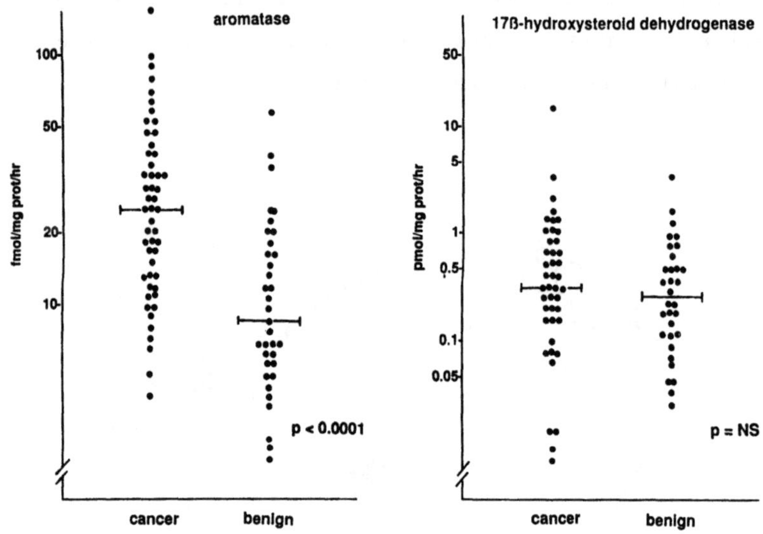

Fig. 3. Aromatase (left panel) and 17β hydroxysteroid dehydrogenase activity (right panel) in adipose tissue from the breasts of women with either breast cancer or benign breast disease. Bars represent median values p value by Wilcoxon Rank test. N.S. = non-significant.

These studies have been taken further by comparing steroid metabolism in fat taken from the periphery of each quadrant of 12 consecutive mastectomy specimens from patients being treated for breast cancer (Figure 4).

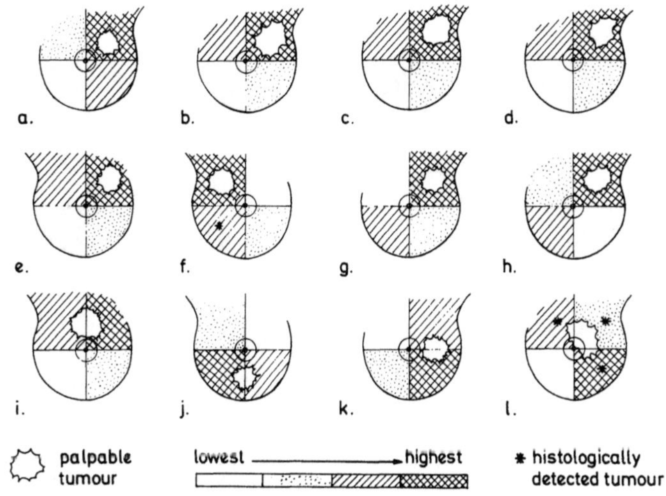

Fig. 4. The relationship between aromatase activity in mammary adipose tissue and tumour locations in the breasts of women with breast cancer. Relative levels of activity are diagrammatically represented by shading.

In all 12 mastectomy specimens examined, the quadrant displaying the highest level of aromatase activity always contained palpable tumour and conversely the quadrant with the lowest activity never contained tumour. Furthermore, in those breasts in which tumour was present in more than one quadrant, tumour-bearing areas always had higher aromatase activity than those without tumour. This variation in aromatase activity was not a simple reflection of increased steroid metabolism, 17β-hydroxysteroid dehydrogenase activity showing no relation with tumour site in the same mastectomy specimens (Figure 5).

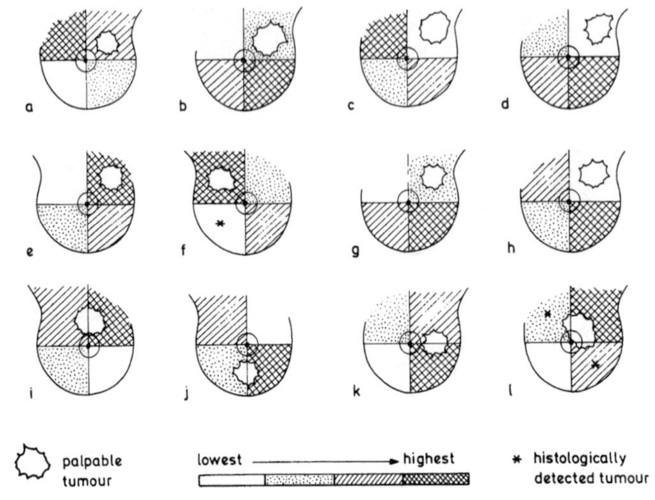

Fig. 5. The relationship between 17β-hydroxysteroid dehydrogenase activity in mammary adipose tissue and tumour location in the breasts of women with breast cancer. Relative levels of activity are diagrammatically represented by shading.

There are several potential explanations for the foregoing observations. First, as breast cancers invariably display higher aromatase activity than adipose tissue(23), samples taken in tumour-bearing quadrants might be more likely to contain microscopic deposits of tumour. This possibility cannot be totally excluded, but samples of fat adjacent to those taken for aromatase assay showed no evidence of gross abnormalities.

It is also possible that regionally increased aromatase activity preceded the appearance of the tumour. Indeed, it could be postulated that enhanced aromatase could lead to a locally high concentration of oestrogen which in turn would encourage malignant growth at that particular site. This conjecture can neither be confirmed nor refuted at this stage.

However, if induction of aromatase preceded the appearance of overt cancer it might be expected to be elevated in mammary fat from breasts at high risk of cancer. We have examined a series of risk factors for breast cancers including family history, obesity, age at menarche, parity and age at first pregnancy and been unable to show increased levels of aromatase in fat from the high risk sub-groups(24).

However, in the context of the present discourse, the possibility with the most relevance is that breast tumours secrete factors into their local environment which either induce or stimulate aromatase activity. In support of this it has been shown that breast cancer cells may secrete growth factors such as epidermal growth factor (EGF), transforming growth factors α and β (TGF-α and TGF-β)(13) and that these factors have the potential to influence aromatase activity in adipose tissue(25).

We also have preliminary data which would be consistent with paracrine secretion of tumour factors influencing steroidogenesis in adipose tissue cells. These results are summarized in Figure 6 and relate to a fibroblast (pre-adipocyte) cell line derived from breast fat.

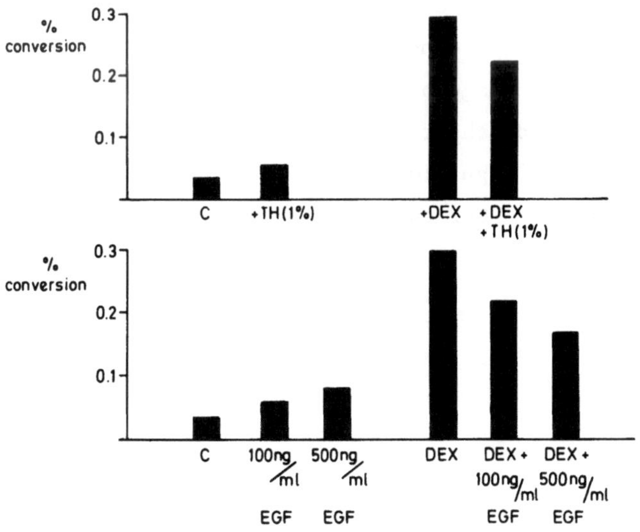

Fig. 6. Aromatase activity in human breast fat fibroblasts cultured in the absence of additives (C) with a homogenate (1%) of breast cancer (TH) with dexamethasone (DEX) with both dexamethasone and breast cancer homogenate (DEX + TH) with varying concentrations of epidermal growth factor (EGF) and with both dexamethasone and epidermal growth factor (DEX + EGF).

This cell line displayed aromatase activity which could be markedly induced by culturing in the presence of dexamethasone for 48 hours. The inclusion of EGF in the medium produced different effects dependent upon whether dexamethasone was present or not. In the absence of dexamethasone, EGF was stimulatory; in its presence, aromatase was inhibited by EGF. Of particular interest was the effect of including a homogenate of breast cancer for the 48 hour culture period in the same fibroblast cell line. Effects again were dependent upon whether dexamethasone was present. In its absence, the tumour homogenate caused an increase in fibroblast aromatase activity whereas in the presence of dexamethasone the homogenate was inhibitory. The effects of the addition of material derived from this breast cancer were therefore similar to those of EGF. The inference is that the active principle within the tumour has properties compatible with the action of a growth factor.

Steroid metabolism and stage of cancer:

While there is no evidence that aromatase activity in breast fat changes as breast cancers become more advanced, circumstantial data suggest that stage of disease is related to levels of 17β-hydroxysteroid dehydrogenase. Thus the activity in breast fat is positively and significantly related to the size of the cancer in the breast(26). Our own results are shown in Figure 7.

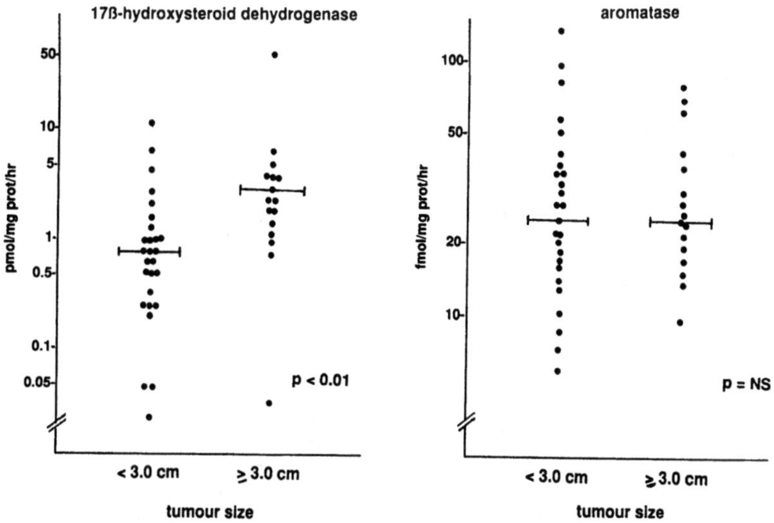

Fig. 7. 17β-hydroxysteroid dehydrogenase (left panel) and aromatase (right panel) activities in breast adipose tissue from patients with small (<3cm) and large (≥3cm) breast cancers. The horizontal bars denote the median activity for the group. The p value is for the difference between the groups as derived from the Wilcoxon rank test. NS = non significant.

These show that adipose tissue associated with large tumours (≥ 3cm) has significantly increased levels of 17β hydroxysteroid dehydrogenase activity (but not aromatase) compared with those in fat surrounding smaller tumours (< 3cm).

Similarly as is shown in figure 8, levels of 17β hydroxysteroid dehydrogenase activity were found to be significantly higher in breast fat from women whose cancers had spread to axillary lymph nodes as compared with activity in breast fat from those who were pathologically node-negative. Aromatase activity showed no such relationship.

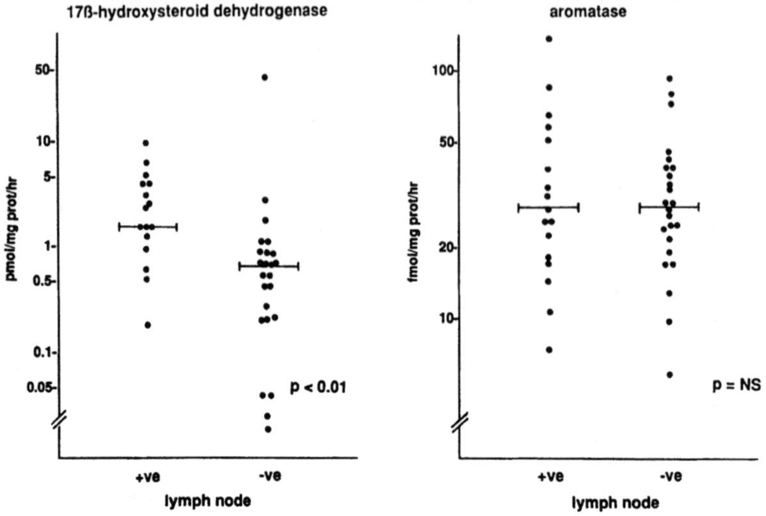

Fig. 8. 17β-hydroxysteroid dehydrogenase (left panel) and aromatase (right panel) activities in breast adipose tissue from breast cancer patients with lymph nodes shown pathologically either to be invaded with tumour (+ve) or disease free (-ve). The horizontal bars denote the median activity for the group. The p value is for the difference between the groups as derived from the Wilcoxon rank test. NS = non significant.

These data are consistent in that 17β-hydroxysteroid dehydrogenase activity is elevated in breast fat associated with tumours of a more advanced stage (in terms of size and lymph node involvement). Whether this relationship is casual or causal is unknown, but again the observations are compatible with the concept that more aggressive tumours secrete increased levels of different factors into their surrounding compartments compared with cancers of an earlier stage or of a less aggressive nature. It is therefore pertinent that homogenates of breast cancer and growth factors known to be secreted by tumours are able to affect 17β-hydroxysteroid dehydrogenase activity when added to cultures of breast fat(27). (Conversely conditioned media from breast fibroblasts are able to induce 17β-hydroxysteroid dehydrogenase activity in MCF-7 cancer cells)(28).

However since aromatase but not 17β-hydroxysteroid dehydrogenase is associated with the presence of tumour whereas dehydrogenase but not aromatase is associated with advancement of disease, it must be assumed that different factors (or spectrum of factors) are involved in early and late stages of tumour progression.

GROWTH MODULATING AGENTS IN BREAST FLUIDS

From the previous sections it is clear that experimental observation suggests that the growth and development of breast cancers may be influenced by other compartments of the breast and such effects may be mediated by locally produced factors. It is equally clear that the addition of known hormones and growth factors to experimental systems may affect events within cancer cells. The link can therefore be made that such agents are the modulators of these paracrine effects. To do this it is appropriate to demonstrate that the local concentrations of growth factors and steroids within the breast are sufficient to elicit promotional events. In this respect we have undertaken a systematic study of the composition of breast cyst fluids and nipple aspirates.

Whilst palpable cysts are not a normal feature of the breast, microcysts are sufficiently frequent within normal breast to be regarded as at the extreme end of the range of normality(29). Furthermore, the composition of fluids aspirated from palpable cysts can resemble that found in breast lobular units and secretion aspirated under negative pressure from the nipple(30). We have therefore measured constituents within cyst fluids in the hope that they may give some reflection of the ambient environment within the breast. These analyses have been extremely revealing in that both hormones and growth factors have been detected in large concentrations. For example, as is shown in figure 9, median

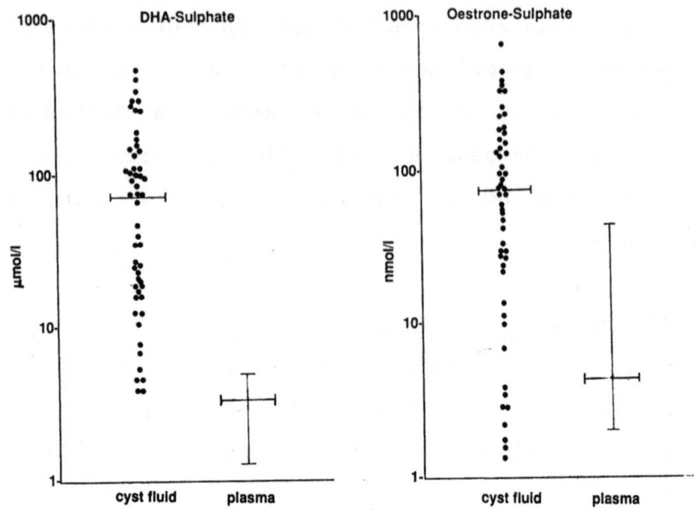

Figure 9. Concentrations of DHA sulphate (left panel) and oestrone-sulphate (right panel) in breast cyst fluids. Horizontal lines represent median values. Vertical line is the reference range in plasma.

levels of steroid conjugates such as DHA sulphate and oestrone sulphate in cyst fluid are at least 30-fold higher than those in plasma. There is also an enormous range of values in cyst fluids, the significance and cause of which is unknown, although in the case of DHA sulphate, values appear to be associated with the histology of the cyst lining epithelium(31). Whilst these steroid conjugates are substantially less biologically active than unconjugated steroids it may be relevant that breast cancer cells possess sulphatases which could catalyse the local synthesis of more potent hormones(32). In this way the steroid conjugates and the sulphatase systems could act to regulate the local environment of active steroids.

Similarly levels of growth factors such as EGF are markedly higher in cyst fluids than in circulating plasma. Again an intriguing feature is the enormous range of values between different cyst fluids. In part these are related to different cyst types and there is a positive association between EGF levels and those of DHA-sulphate(33). The source of EGF-like material within cyst fluid is as yet unknown but levels would be sufficient to cause proliferation of epithelial cells if the material was biologically active(34).

To determine whether cyst fluids contain material capable of stimulating cellular proliferation, studies have been performed in which cyst fluids have been added to cell lines of breast cancer cells growing in culture. Examples of these results are shown in figure 10.

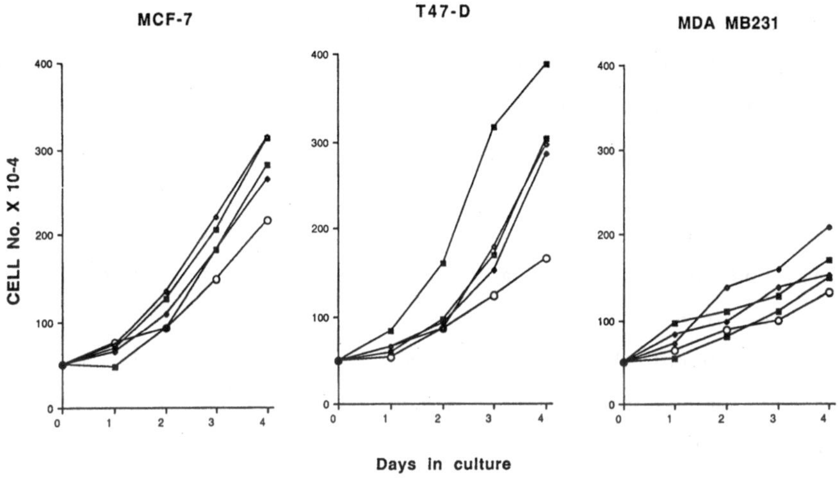

Fig. 10. Effects of adding 4 different breast cyst fluids diluted x 1,000 (filled symbols) to cultures of MCF-7 (left panel), T47-D (middle panel) and MDA MB231 (right panel) breast cancer cells. Control cultures in the absence of cyst fluid (open circles).

Thus all the cyst fluids so far examined have been able to stimulate the growth of established breast cancer cell lines including the MCF-7, T47-D and MDA-MB-231. It is important to note that these cell lines show differing hormone sensitivity, the MCF-7 line being oestrogen receptor-positive and sensitive to both oestrogens and progestogens, the T47-D being oestrogen receptor-poor but progestogen receptor-rich and sensitive to progestogens but not to oestrogen and the MDA-MB-231 being devoid of steroid receptors and displaying little responsiveness to hormones. The cell lines did show some quantitative difference in sensitivity to cyst fluids, the T47-D in general being more responsive. Interestingly the quantitative order of potency of cyst fluids varied between cell lines suggesting that there might be a cocktail of growth promotors within cyst fluids whose mix may differentially affect different cell lines.

SUMMARY

Evidence has been reviewed that non-epithelial components of the breast such as stroma and adipose tissue are not merely inert support structures but have the capacity to elaborate and secrete biologically active agents such as growth factors and steroid hormones. Since these factors may have the potential to influence the differentiation of epithelial cells and the progression of malignant cells it is relevant that behaviour and response of both stroma and adipose tissue may vary according to the risk, presence and stage of breast cancer.

The concept that the development and evolution of breast cancer is dependent upon "cross-talk" with the "soil" in which the malignancy is developing is supported by the additional observations that (i) growth factors and steroid hormones may be present in breast fluids, extracts and media conditioned from breast cell lines in amounts capable of producing profound biological responses and (ii) in experimental systems, tumour-derived factors can influence the metabolism of non-malignant elements of the tumour and conversely factors derived from mammary stroma and adipose tissue can modify the growth of malignant cells. This reciprocity also extends to the trophic factors involved in such paracrine communication. Thus it is clear that steroid hormones are capable of influencing the production and pattern of growth factors elaborated by the breast and conversely growth factors also have the potential to modify local mammary steroid biosynthesis. As a result one can visualise a series of complex and extended paracrine loops within the breast involving cancer cells, non-malignant parenchyma, stroma and adipose tissue and mediated by hormones, growth factors and extracellular matrix. Since these loops might have both positive and negative effects on tumour evolution, the future challenge must be to harness such communication processes to the therapeutic advantage of patients with breast cancer.

REFERENCES

1. Wellings, S.R., Jensen, H.M. and Marcum, R.G. J. Natl. Cancer Inst. 55: 231-273, 1975.
2. Preschtel, K. Fortschr Med. 89: 1312-1315, 1971.
3. Tanzer, M.L. and Spring-Mills, B. J. Natl. Cancer Inst. 73: 999-1001, 1984.
4. Durnberger, H., Henberger, B., Schwartz, P., Wasner, G. and Kratochwil, K. Cancer Res. 38: 4066-4070, 1978.
5. Haslam, S.Z. Cancer Res. 46: 310-316, 1986.
6. Schor, S.L., Haggie, J.A., Durning, P., Howell, A., Smith, L., Sellwood, R.A.S. and Crowther, D. Int. J. Cancer 37: 831-836, 1986.
7. Haggie, J., Howell, A., Sellwood. R.A., Birch, J.M. and Schor, S.L. The Lancet i: 1455-1457, 1987.
8. Schor, S.L., Schor, A.M., Grey, A.M. and Rushton, G.M. J. Cell Science 90: 391-399, 1988.
9. Schor, A.M., Rushton, G., Schor, S.L., Picardo, M., Ferguson, J.E. and Redford, J. Proc. 4th Int. Symp. Benign Breast Disease. Parthanon Press. In press, 1991.
10. Horgan, K., Jones, D.L. and Mansel, R.E. Br. J. Surg. 74: 227-229, 1987a.
11. Ryan, M.C., Jones, D.L. and Horgan, K. Br. J. Cancer 63: suppl XIII 70, 1991.
12. Basset, P., Bellocq, J.P., Wolf, C., Stoll, I., Hutin, P., Limarcher, J.M., Podhajcer, O.L., Chenard, M.P., Rio, M.C. and Chambon, P. Nature 348: 699-704, 1990.
13. Lippman M.E. and Dickson R.B. Proc Ro Socy (Edin) 95B: 89-106, 1989.
14. Beer, A.E. and Billingham, R.E. Lancet 2: 296, 1978.
15. Deome, K.B., Franklin, L.J. and Bern, H.A. Cancer Res. 19: 515-520, 1959.
16. Price, J.E., Polyzos, A., Zhang, R.D. and Daniels, L.M. Cancer Res 50: 717-721, 1990.
17. Strombeck, J.O. Acta Chirugia Scand. (Suppl) 34: 33-36, 1964.
18. DeWaard, F. and Trichopoulos, D. Int. J. Cancer 41: 666-669, 1988.
19. Sasano, N., Tateno, H. and Stemmerman, G.N. Preventative Medicine 7: 196-204, 1978.
20. Deslypere, J.P., Verdonck, L. and Vermeulen, A. J. Clin. Endocrinol. Metab. 61: 564-570, 1985.
21. Miller, W.R. Brit. Med. Bulletin 47: 470-483, 1990.
22. Miller, W.R. and O'Neill, J.S. Proc. R. Soc. Edinburgh 95B: 203-217, 1989.

23. Perel, E., Wilkin, D. and Killinger, D.W. J. Steroid Biochem. 13: 89-94, 1980.
24. Miller, W.R. and O'Neill, J.S. J. Steroid Biochem. Molec. Biol. 37: 317-325, 1990.
25. Simpson, E.R. and Mendelson, C.R. Proc. Roy. Soc. Edinburgh 95B: 153-159, 1989.
26. Berenek, P.A., Folkerd, E.J., Newton, C.J., Reed, M.J., Ghilchik, M.W. and James, V.H.T. Int. J. Cancer 36: 685-687, 1985.
27. McNeill, J.M., Reed, M.J., Berenek, P.A., Newton, C.J., Ghilchik, M.W. and James, V.H.T. Cancer Letters 31: 213-219, 1986.
28. Adams, E.F., Newton, C.J., Braunsberg, H., Shaikh, N., Ghilchik, M. and James, V.H.T. Breast Cancer Res. Treat. 11: 165-172, 1988.
29. Hughes, L.E. Brit. Med. Bulletin 47: 251-257, 1990.
30. Dixon, J.M. Brit. Med. Bulletin 47: 258-271. 1990.
31. Miller, W.R., Dixon, J.M. and Forrest, A.P.M. Ann. N.Y. Acad. Sci. 464: 275-287, 1986.
32. Miller, W.R. In: Breast Cancer: Treatment and Prognosis (Ed. B.A. Stoll), Blackwell Scientific Publications, Oxford, 1986, pp. 156-172.
33. Smith, K., Miller, W.R., Fennelly, J.A., Matthews, J.N.S., Scott, W.N. and Harris, A.L. Int. J. Cancer 44: 229-232, 1989.
34. Osborne, C.K., Hamilton, B., Titus, G., Livingstone, R.B. Cancer Res. 40: 2361-1366, 1980.

INVOLVEMENT OF HEPARANASE AND EXTRACELLULAR MATRIX-BOUND FIBROBLAST GROWTH FACTOR IN TUMOR PROGRESSION

I.Vlodavsky, R. Ishai-Michaeli, M. Mohsen, G. Korner and R. Catane
Department of Oncology, Hadassah University Hospital, Jerusalem 91120, Israel

The pluripotent angiogenic factor, basic fibroblast growth factor (bFGF) was extracted from the extracellular matrix (ECM) produced by cultured endothelial cells (EC) and was identified in epithelial and endothelial basement membranes of the rat fetus, bovine cornea and human blood vessels. Despite the ubiquitous presence of bFGF in normal tissues, EC proliferation in these tissues is usually very low with turnover time measured in years. This raises the question of how these heparin-binding growth factors are prevented from acting on the vascular endothelium and in response to what signals they become available for stimulation of EC proliferation. Our studies demonstrate that bFGF binds specifically to heparan sulfate (HS) and heparin-like molecules in the ECM and cell surfaces, as indicated by its displacement by heparin, HS, or HS-degrading enzymes, but not by unrelated GAGs or GAG degrading enzymes. Heparanase activity expressed by intact cells (i.e. platelets, mast cells, neutrophils, lymphoma cells) was found to degrade the ECM-HS and to release active bFGF from ECM and basement membranes of bovine cornea. Elevated levels of heparanase were detected in highly metastatic tumor cells and in tumor biopsies of cancer patients. Moreover, treatment of experimental animals with heparanase inhibitors (i.e. non-anticoagulant species of heparin) markedly reduced the incidence of lung metastasis induced by B16 melanoma, Lewis lung carcinoma and mammary adenocarcinoma. Our results indicate that heparanase mediated degradation of HSPG is involved in cell invasion and release of ECM-resident angiogenic factors, both critical events in tumor progression. Heparanase inhibiting molecules are therefore expected to have a significant anticancerous effect. We propose that restriction of bFGF bioavailability due to its lack of a signal peptide and sequestration by HS, as well as local regulation of its release in the vicinity of EC, provides a novel mechanism for regulation of capillary blood vessel growth in processes such as wound repair, inflammation and tumor development.

INTRODUCTION

Basement membranes and extracellular matrices are the natural substrates upon which cells migrate, proliferate and differentiate *in vivo*. Historically, the extracellular matrix (ECM) was regarded as a relatively inert scaffolding which stabilizes the physical structure of tissues. Subsequent studies aimed to elucidate the mode of cellular responses to ECM indicated that the ability of cells to respond to various growth and differentiation factors is determined to a large extent by their shape and orientation and that these are modulated by components of the ECM through interaction with specific transmembrane cell surface receptors (1,2). In the case of epithelial tissues with a high rate of cell turnover, such as the epidermis or the corneal epithelium, active cell proliferation is restricted to their basal layer, composed of tall and columnar cells. These cells respond to epidermal growth factor (EGF) and are in close contact with a basement membrane. In contrast, cells in the upper layers, which are no longer associated with a basement membrane loose their ability to proliferate and gradually adopt a flattened configuration. Corneal epithelial cells, for example, adopt a flattened configuration when maintained on plastic and are sensitive to fibroblast growth factor (FGF), but not to EGF. When maintained on collagen, on the other hand, they adopt their characterisitic tall and columnar configuration and respond primarily to EGF (1).

Based on these observations it is now recognized that basement membrane plays an active and complex role in regulating the morphogenesis of cells that contact it, influencing their development, migration, proliferation and metabolic functions. These effects are exerted by the combined action of basement membrane macromolecules (i.e. collagen IV, laminin, nidogen/entactin, proteoglycans) and active molecules (i.e. growth factors, enzymes) that are immobilized and stored in the ECM by means of binding to its macromolecular constituents, primarily to heparan sulfate proteoglycans (HSPG) (3,4).

In vivo, all epithelial cells capable of proliferation or long term survival are found in contact with a basement membrane which separates organ parenchymal cells from the underlying interstitial stroma. Likewise, cultured cells, in order to proliferate and express their normal phenotype, require, in addition to nutrients and growth factors, an appropriate substratum upon which they can attach and spread (5-7). Based on these and other observations, the extracellular matrix (ECM) is regarded as an insoluble complex of factors that regulate cellular growth, morphogenesis and differentiation. Basement membranes are also of particular importance in the development of epithelial malignancies since they are the first barrier encountered in the invasive process of carcinomas. In fact, basement membranes are usually defective or absent in carcinomas, suggesting that partial or total loss of basement membranes is characteristic for invasive tumors, but not for their preinvasive or benign counterparts (8). The lack of an adequate substrate similar to that with which the cells are closely associated *in vivo* and of a proper cell orientation is therefore thought to be responsible for the fact that most of the established cell lines originating from normal tissues, exhibit, despite their different origins, similar morphologies and growth characteristics. This applied not only to normal human cells but also to those derived from malignant tissues, because in order for a tumor to develop, the cells must find a favorable environment in terms of neighboring tissues and extracellular matrices (8).

Tumor cells can synthesize matrix components which are generally of the same type produced by the normal cell counterpart. The amount and type of matrix accumulated depend on the type of tumor and its state of differentiation. Whereas actively growing and poorly differentiated tumors frequently produce less matrix than the normal counterpart, highly differentiated tumors synthesize and accumulate matrix in large amounts. In fact, the ECM produced by such tumors has been used as a convenient source for the isolation and characterization of various matrix constituents such as laminin, nidogen, collagen type IV and heparan sulfate proteoglycans (HSPG) (9). Tumor cells can also induce an increased production of matrix components by host cells in response to the local presence of the tumor. Such excessive accumulation of connective tissue (desmoplasia) is thought to be mediated by diffusable chemotactic or mitogenic host factors elaborated in response to the tumor cells (8). A central issue in tumor biology is therefore the interaction between tumor cells and their local environment occurring at multiple stages during tumor progression. A better understanding of tumor cell interaction with extracellular matrices may clarify the need for stromal and fibroblastic support for tumor cell growth; the mechanism through which various artificial substrates introduced into the animal results in the production of malignant mesothelioma and fibrosarcoma, and the ability of tumor cells to reorganize their local environment in order to grow and invade.

Our studies on the control cell proliferation and tumor progression by its local environment, focused on the interaction of cells with the ECM produced by cultured corneal and vascular endothelial cells (EC). This ECM closely resembles the subendothelium *in vivo* in its morphological appearance and molecular composition. It contains collagens (mostly type III and IV, with smaller amounts of types I and V), proteoglycans (mostly heparan sulfate- and dermatan sulfate- proteoglycans, with smaller amounts of chondroitin sulfate proteoglycans), laminin, fibronectin and elastin (6,7). Moreover, because the ECM is secreted in a polar fashion, exclusively underneath the endothelial cell monolayer, and because it is firmly attached to the entire area of the tissue culture dish, the cell layer can be removed while leaving the underlying ECM intact and free of nuclei, cytoskeletal elements and other cellular debris. We have demonstrated that cells plated in contact with ECM, attached, proliferated and expressed differentiated functions to a much greater extent as compared to cells plated on regular tissue culture plastic (10). A general feature was that cells plated on ECM required less serum or no serum at all and often were no longer dependent on exogenous factors in order to proliferate and express their differentiated functions (11). In an attempt to use the ECM substrate for the growth of human mammary epithelial cells, whether normal or carcinomatous, we have developed a routine procedure for tissue dissociation and cell culture under conditions which suppress the growth of stromal fibroblasts. This procedure combines the high plating efficiency obtained on ECM and the use of a serum free medium supplemented with high density lipoprotein (HDL) (12).

The present article focuses on the identification and properties of ECM-bound growth factors and enzymes which may function in tumor angiogenesis and metastasis. We propose that in addition to macromolecular constituents, the ECM provides a storage depot for active molecules such as growth factors and enzymes which are thereby stabilized and protected. Clearly, ECM-bound molecules may exert more localized and persistent effects as compared to the same molecules in a fluid phase. Our studies demonstrate that degradation of ECM components by invasive tumor cells, liberates active endothelial cell (EC) growth factors which may participate in tumor angiogenesis. We suggest that alterations in basement membrane structure and turnover that are associated with tumor progression may also be responsible for the onset of angiogenic activity upon the transition of an *in situ* carcinoma from the prevascular to the vascularized state (13).

Involvement of Heparanase in Cell Invasion and Metastasis

Extravasation of blood-borne cells, whether normal or malignant, is initiated by specific adhesive interactions between circulating cells and the vascular endothelium. These interactions are mediated by an array of a diverse family of cell surface adhesion molecules expressed by endothelial cells (EC), cells of the immune system and tumor cells. Among these are molecules of the integrin subfamily which recognize both ECM and cell surface glycoproteins, and lectin cell adhesion molecules (LEC-CAM) which utilize protein-carbohydrate interactions. Metastatic tumor cells often attach at or near the intercellular junctions between adjacent EC followed by rupture of the junctions, retraction of the EC borders and migration through the breach in the endothelium toward the exposed underlying basal lamina (14). Signals to trigger EC retraction are believed to be cell surface proteins and physiologic constituents of the blood-borne cells. Since cells adhere more tightly to the basal lamina than to the vascular endothelium, it is conceivable that a gradient of increasing cellular adhesion results in the net migration of cells from the circulation into the surrounding tissue. Once enveloped between EC and the basal lamina, the invading cells must degrade the subendothelial glycoproteins and proteoglycans in order to escape into the extravascular tissue(s) where they establish metastasis (14).

Several cellular enzymes (i.e., collagenase IV, plasminogen activator, cathepsin B, elastase) are thought to be involved in degradation of basement membranes (8,15). Among these enzymes is an endo-β-D-glucuronidase (heparanase) that cleaves HS at specific intrachain sites (16,17). HSPG have been isolated from a variety of basement membranes and cell surfaces of normal and malignant cells (18,19). In large vessels they are concentrated mostly in the intima and inner media whereas in capillaries they are found mainly in the subendothelial basement membrane where they support proliferating and migrating endothelial cells and stabilize the structure of the capillary wall. Cleavage of heparan sulfate (HS) may therefore result in disassembly of the subendothelial ECM and hence may play a decisive role in extravasation of blood borne cells. The ability of cells to degrade HS in the ECM was studied by allowing cells to interact with a metabolically sulfate labeled ECM, followed by gel filtration (Sepharose 6B) analysis of degradation products released into the culture medium (16,17). While intact HSPG are eluted next to the void volume of the column, ($Kav<0.2$, $Mr \sim 0.5x10^6$), labeled degradation fragments of HS side chains are eluted more toward the V_t of the column ($0.5<kav<0.8$, $Mr = 5\text{-}7x10^3$) (17). Expression of a HS degrading endoglucuronidase (heparanase) was found to correlate with the metastatic potential of various tumor cells (16,17) and with the ability of activated cells of the immune system to leave the circulation and elicit both inflammatory and autoimmune responses (20).

Heparanase activity was found to correlate with metastatic potentials of mouse lymphoma (17), fibrosarcoma and melanoma (16). Moreover, elevated levels of heparanase were detected in sera from metastatic tumor bearing animals and melanoma patients (16) and in tumor biopsies of cancer patients (21). Immunohistochemical staining of frozen tissue sections revealed that heparanase is localized preferentially in metastatic murine and human melanomas (22).

Heparanase mediated degradation of HS is inhibited by heparin, both when exerted by intact cells or soluble heparanase (16,23). We investigated the heparanase inhibitory effect of various non-anticoagulant species of heparin that might be of potential use in preventing extravasation of blood-borne cells. Inhibition of heparanase depended on the size and degree of sulfation of the heparin molecule, the position of sulfate groups and the occupancy of the N-position of the hexoseamines. Inhibition of heparanase was best achieved by heparin species containing 16 sugar units or more and having sulfate groups at both the N and O positions. Low sulfate oligosaccharides were less effective heparanase inhibitors than medium and high sulfate fractions of the same size oligosaccharides. While O-desulfation abolished the heparanase inhibiting effect of heparin, O-sulfated, N-acetylated heparin retained a high inhibitory activity, provided that the N-substituted molecules had a molecular size of about 4000 daltons or more. A synthetic pentasaccharide, representing the binding site to antithrombin III, was devoid of inhibitory activity (23). A further indication that the heparanase inhibitory and anticoagulant activities of heparin are unrelated was obtained by using heparin fractions with high and low affinity for anti-thrombin III. These heparins differed about 200 folds in their anticoagulant activity, but had a similar high heparanase inhibitory activity.

Treatment of tumor cells and animals with heparanase inhibitors markedly reduced the incidence of lung metastases induced by B16 melanoma, Lewis lung carcinoma and mammary adenocrcinoma cells (13,16,24). A single injection (I.V. or S.C.) of native or modified heparins, decreased the number of melanoma lung metastases to about 5% of control, but there was no effect to totally desulfated heparin. Heparin fractions with high and low affinity to anti-thrombin III exhibited a comparable high anti-metastatic activity, indicating that the heparanase inhibiting activity of heparin rather than its anticoagulant activity plays a role in the anti-metastatic properties of the polysaccharide. Most efficient inhibition of tumor cell metastasis was obtained when the melanoma cells and heparin were injected at the same time. Around 75% inhibition of metastasis was achieved when heparin was given 6 h before or 2 h after the tumor cells, suggesting that the polysaccharide interferes with the passage of tumor cells across the capillary wall (13). Similar results were reported by Nakajima et al (16) and Parish et al (24).

Heparanase Activity Expressed by Normal and Malignant Cells Releases Active bFGF from ECM

Fibroblast growth factors are a family of structurally related polypeptides characterized by high affinity to heparin (25). They are highly mitogenic for vascular EC and are among the most potent inducers of neovascularization and mesenchyme formation (25,26). Basic fibroblast growth factor (bFGF) has been extracted from the subendothelial ECM produced *in vitro* (27) and from basement membranes of the cornea (28), suggesting that ECM may serve as a reservoir for bFGF. Immunohistochemical staining revealed the localization of bFGF in basement membranes of diverse tissues (29) and blood vessels (30). Despite the ubiquitous presence of bFGF in normal tissues, EC proliferation in these tissues is usually very low, suggesting that bFGF is somehow sequestered from its site of action. Studies on the interaction of bFGF with ECM revealed that bFGF binds to HSPG in the ECM and can be released by heparin-like molecules, HS degrading enzymes (31,32), or plasmin (33). These results suggest that the ECM HSPG provide a natural storage depot for bFGF and possibly other growth promoting factors (3,13). Displacement of bFGF from its storage within basement membranes and ECM may therefore provide a novel mechanism for induction of neovascularization in normal and pathological situations. To investigate whether heparanase, expressed by various normal and malignant cells, is involved in release of bFGF from ECM, we first identified molecules which inhibit the enzyme but do not release the ECM-bound bFGF. Using these inhibitors (i.e. carrageenan lambda, N-acetylated heparin), we have demonstrated that heparanase activity expressed by platelets, neutrophils, and lymphoma cells is involved in release of active bFGF from ECM and basement membranes of bovine corneas (32). Regardless of the source of heparanase and of whether release of bFGF was brought about by a pure enzyme, intact cells, or cell lysates, inhibition of bFGF-release correlated with inhibition of heparanase activity, measured by release from ECM of sulfate labeled HS degradation products (32) . We suggest that heparanase activity expressed by tumor cells may not only function in cell migration and invasion, but at the same time may also elicit an indirect neovascular response by means of releasing the ECM-resident FGF. Likewise, platelets, mast cells and activated cells of the immune system (i.e. macrophages, neutrophils, T lymphocytes) that are often attracted by tumor cells may indirectly stimulate tumor angiogenesis by means of their heparanase activity. These cells may also elicit an angiogenic response in the process of inflammation and wound healing.

Several studies indicate that μg quantities of heparin and HS inhibit the mitogenic activity of bFGF, but at the same time stabilize and protect the molecule from inactivation (34,35). It is therefore proposed that bFGF is stored in ECM in a highly stable but relatively inactive form, as also indicated by the highly stable ECM-resident growth-promoting activity, as compared to that of bFGF in a fluid phase. Release from ECM of bFGF as a complex with HS fragment is likely to yield a form of bFGF that is more stable than free bFGF and yet capable of binding to high affinity plasma membrane receptors (Fig. 1). A recent study indicate that cell surface and/or soluble heparin and HS are required for binding of bFGF to high affinity cell surface receptors. While bFGF failed to bind to HS-deficient CHO mutant cells, binding to high affinity receptor sites was restored by the addition of ng quantities of heparin and HS (36). It is therefore conceivable that binding of heparin or HS imposes on the bFGF molecule the conformation necessary for optimal interaction with its high affinity cell surface receptor (36). We propose that restriction of EC growth factors in ECM prevents their systemic action on the vascular endothelium, thus maintaining a very low rate of EC turnover and vessel growth. On the other hand, release of bFGF from storage in ECM may elicit a localized EC proliferation and neovascularization in processes such as wound healing, inflammation and tumor development (3, 13) (Fig. 1).

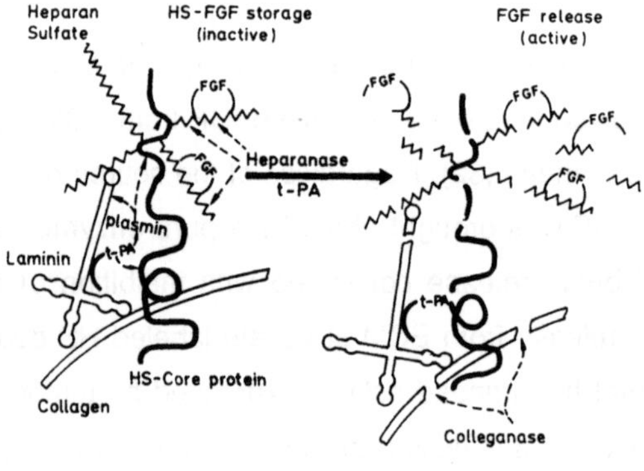

Figure 1. Scheme describing the presence of heparan sulfate-bound FGF in ECM and release of FGFby heparanase. The ECM also contains plasminogen activator which participates in sequential degradation of heparan sulfate in ECM.

Structural Requirements for Release of ECM-bound bFGF by Heparin

Heparin exhibits a high degree of heterogeneity due to variations in the size of the polysaccharide chains and in the degree and distribution of sulfate groups. We investigated structural requirements for release of ECM- and cell surface- bound bFGF by heparin and heparin-like molecules. For this purpose ECM was incubated with ^{125}I-bFGF, washed free of unbound bFGF and exposed to various size homogeneous oligosaccharides prepared from heparin by nitrous acid depolymerization. Maximal release of ^{125}I-bFGF was achieved already by the octasaccharide. Exposure of ECM to higher oligosaccharides containing up to 16 sugar units and to intact heparin yielded results which were, on a weight basis, similar to those obtained with the octasaccharide (31,37).

In order to analyze the involvement of O-sulfate and N-sulfate residues of heparin in release of ECM-bound bFGF, both intact heparin and low Mr heparin were either totally desulfated or N-desulfated. N-sulfate groups of these heparins were also partially or fully substituted with acetyl groups. It was found that both totally desulfated and N-desulfated heparin failed to release the ECM-bound bFGF. In contrast, N-resulfation of totally desulfated heparin restored its bFGF releasing activity to a large extent. Total N-acetylation of heparin and low Mr heparin resulted in an almost complete inhibition of their bFGF releasing activity. Over sulfation of these N-acetylated molecules resulted in partial restoration of their ability to release bFGF from ECM. These results indicate that N-sulfate groups of heparin are critical for efficient release of ECM-bound bFGF (37).

The ability of a given compound to release bFGF from ECM was dependent primarily on the position of the sulfate group rather than on the total level of sulfation (i.e. % sulfur). Thus, N-resulfated, O-desulfated heparin (% sulfur= 5.3) exhibited a higher bFGF releasing activity than N-desulfated- or N-acetylated- heparin containing 9.7% and 8.7% sulfur, respectively. In order to correlate the anticoagulant activity of heparin to its bFGF releasing activity, heparin was separated on an antithrombin-Sepharose column into a nonbinding fraction of virtually no anti-FXa activity and a binding fraction of high anti-FXa activity. Heparin fractions with high and low affinity to antithrombin III exhibited a similar high bFGF releasing activity, despite a nearly 200 fold difference in their anti-FXa activity (37).

Different Structural requirements for release of ECM-bound bFGF and inhibition of heparanase by heparin. Different structural properties of heparin were required for release of ECM-bound bFGF and for inhibition of heparanase activity. For example, while substitution of the N-sulfates of heparin with acetyl groups had little or no effect on its ability to inhibit heparanase, it greatly reduced its ability to release ECM-bound bFGF. On the other hand, heparin derived oligosaccharides containing 6-8 sugar units exhibited a high bFGF releasing activity, but failed to inhibit the heparanase enzyme. Likewise, release of bFGF from ECM, but little or no inhibition of heparanase activity were brought about by O-desulfated, N-resulfated heparin (37). These results indicate that different effects of heparin are mediated by unique sugar sequences and that specific heparin-like molecules can be designed to elicit or inhibit a specific effect. For example, N-substituted species of heparin, rather than native heparin, could be applied to inhibit tumor metastasis, since their efficient inhibition of heparanase activity was not associated with a significant release of active bFGF from cells and ECM. These compounds are therefore expected to inhibit metastases formation by certain tumor cells, correlated with their inhibition of heparanase activity (16,24), with little or no potential induction of tumor angiogenesis in response to bFGF release. On the other hand, heparin derived oligosaccharides containing 6-8 sugar units may be applied to stimulate bFGF release and neovascularization in the process of tissue repair.

Our studies on the sequestration and release of bFGF suggest that bFGF may acquire an immobilized storage form that is stable but relatively inactive, and a soluble form that is labile but highly active. Release of HS-bound bFGF by heparin derived oligosaccharides containing 6-10 sugar units, as well as by heparin- and HS- degrading enzymes may yield an intermediate type of molecule that is relatively stable (34,35) and may readily diffuse through the stroma (38), as compared to free bFGF. This released form is also capable of binding to high affinity plasma membrane receptors (33), resulting in proliferative and differentiation responses in endothelial cells and other mesoderm derived cells. Sequestration and release of FGF-like factors may thus provide a novel mechanism for regulation of capillary blood vessel growth. Under normal conditions it may prevent them from acting on the vascular endothelium, while perturbation of the ECM and/or exposure to heparin-like molecules may elicit localized EC proliferation and neovascularization.

ECM-bound Plasminogen Activators

The serine proteases tissue plasminogen activator (t-PA) and urinary plasminogen activator (u-PA) convert the zymogen plasminogen into the serine protease plasmin (39). Whereas plasminogen activators (PAs) possess a greatly restricted substrate specificity, plasmin cleaves a wide range of proteins and thereby has been implied in various physiological and pathological processes including fibrinolysis, cellular migration, neuronal outgrowth, ovulation, activation of latent collagenase, and tumor metastasis (39). Our studies on degradation of HS in ECM by normal and malignant cells have demonstrated a synergistic involvement of both protease and heparanase activities. This degradation was markedly enhanced by plasminogen and inhibited by aprotinin, suggesting a role for plasminogen activator (PA) in sequential degradation of the ECM-HS (40). Subsequent studies revealed that PA activity is associated with the ECM itself (Fig. 1). Incubation of plasminogen on ECM, but not on regular tissue culture plastic, resulted in plasmin generation, as evidenced by its ability to degrade fibrin upon subsequent incubation with ^{125}I-fibrin coated wells. Heating the ECM inactivated its ability to generate plasmin from plasminogen, but this activity was not inhibited when the matrix was preincubated with DFP or aprotinin (13,40). We have demonstrated that most of the ECM-resident PA was deposited as a function of time by intact endothelial cells together with other constituents of the ECM. To characterize the ECM associated PA, ECM extracts were subjected to SDS-PAGE zymography. Two main bands of proteolytic activity were observed when the gel was co-polymerized in the presence, but not in the absence of plasminogen. The high molecular weight protein cross-reacted with anti-human t-PA antiserum while the lower band of PA activity cross reacted with anti-human u-PA antibodies (13). The presence of t-PA and u-PA in the subendothelial ECM was also demonstrated by inhibition of the ECM mediated plasminogen activation in the presence of both anti t-PA and anti u-PA antibodies. PA was also found to be associated with the ECM produced by EHS tumor, kidney epithelial cells and neurons (41). Our preliminary results indicate that PA, like many of the other ECM-bound molecules, is sequestered primarily by the ECM-HS. Exposure of ECM to highly purified preparations of bacterial heparitinase or mammalian heparanases (i.e. human hepatoma, human placenta) resulted in release of PA activity inhibitable by anti u-PA and anti t-PA antibodies. Moreover, heparanase mediated release of the ECM resident PA was blocked in the presence of heparanase inhibiting molecules. In addition to its role in fibrinolysis, the ECM PA may be involved in turnover of some ECM components and in local dissolution of ECM and basement membranes in tumor metastasis, inflammation and other processes involving cell migration and tissue remodeling. Modification of specific matrix constituents by PA and plasmin may alter cellular responses to ECM and thus play an important role in the control of cell-matrix interactions.

We have demonstrated that ECM-bound bFGF is released upon degradation of the ECM HS by heparanase (32). Stimulation of this degradation by the ECM-PA may accelerate the release of ECM-bound FGF. The released FGF may then stimulate the ECM producing EC to secrete PA and type IV collagenase (42), resulting in a more efficient matrix degradation by invasive cells. The released FGF will at the same time stimulate EC migration and proliferation. Angiogenesis may be further controlled locally through modulation of the ECM adhesivity and structural integrity which affect capillary growth, differentiation, and involution (2). Altogether, these results further indicate that the ECM provides a solid-phase regulatory system for complex processes such as cell invasion and angiogenesis. It may ensure that the involved enzymes and growth factors will function at a given location and time while being stabilized and protected from inactivation by circulating factors.

Other Effects on Tumor Progression

ECM storage of growth promoting factors may effect tumor development not only through induction of neovascularization, but also through a direct effect on the tumor cells themselves. It has long been postulated that secondary tumor growth in certain organs is the result of a favorable environment afforded by certain tissues ('seed and soil' theory) . It has been demonstrated that host tissues themselves may exert an effect on metastasizing cancer cells that helps to determine the eventual outcome of tumor growth patterns (43). Thus, although a similar number of metastatic tumor cells may reach several sites, certain tumors are often developed in certain organs, but not in others. Organ preference of metastasis can be attributed, among other factors, to storage and release of growth promoting and growth inhibiting factors in certain tissues. A lung derived growth factor has recently been purified and found to stimulate the growth of tumor cells metastatic to the lung (44). The microenvironment may also suppress tumor growth as reported for murine melanocytes transformed by bFGF cDNA. When placed into the cutaneous environment of host animals, the transformants reverted to having a normal melanotic phenotype and restricted growth. It was suggested that *in vivo* the bFGF produced by the transformed cells is released into the ECM and thus stimulates the cell surface receptors which then trigger the expression of differentiated functions (45). Recently, a gene, stromelysine, has been identified that is expressed specifically in stromal cells immediately surrounding the neoplastic cells of the invasive, but not the *in situ* , component of breast carcinomas. This new member of the metalloproteinase enzymes is thought to be one of the stroma- derived factors that have long been postulated to play an important part in progression of epithelial malignancies (46).

We have previously reported that activated T-lymphocytes capable of inducing experimental autoimmune encephalomyelitis (EAE), respond to ECM-bound myelin basic protein with a 4-5 fold stimulation of heparanase activity (47). This may result in the preferential extravasation of these cells in brain as compared to other organs. It is therefore conceivable that ECM-bound antigens, growth promoting and growth inhibiting factors may, among other factors, determine the site of extravasation and render some organs more conducive to neoplastic growth then other tissues.

Acknowledgements. This work was supported by Public Health Service Grants CA-30289 awarded to I.V.by the National Cancer Institute, DHHS, and by grants from the USA-Israel Binational Science Foundation and the German-Israel Foundation for Scientific Research and Development.

REFERENCES

1. Gospodarowicz, D., Greenberg, G., and Birdwell, C.R. Cancer Res. 38:4155-4171, 1978.
2. Ingber, D.E. Proc. Natl. Acad. Sci. USA 87:3579-3583, 1990.
3. Vlodavsky, I., Ishai-Michaeli, R., Bashkin, P., Korner, G. and Bar-Shavit, R. TIBS 16:268-271, 1991.
4. Ruoslahti, E., and Yamaguchi, Y. Cell 64:867-869, 1991.
5. Enat, R., Jefferson, D.M., Ruiz-Opazo, N., Gatmaitan, Z., Leinwand, L., Reid, L.M. Proc. Natl. Acad. Sci. USA 81:1411-1415, 1984.
6. Gospodarowicz, D., Delgado, D. and Vlodavsky, I. Proc. Natl. Acad. Sci USA 77:4094-4098, 1980.
7. Vlodavsky, I., Liu, G.M. and Gospodarowicz, D. Cell 19:607-616, 1980.
8. Barsky, S.H., Siegal, G., Janotta, F. and Liotta, L.A. Lab. Invest. 49:140-148, 1983.
9. Kleinman, H.K., McGarrey, M.L., Hassel, J.R., Star, V.L., Cannon, F.B., Laurie, G.W. and Martin, G.R. Biochemistry 25:312-318, 1986.
10. Vlodavsky, I., Levi, A., Lax, I., Schlessinger, J. and Fuks, Z. Develop. Biol. 93:285-300, 1982.
11. Gospodarowicz, D. and Ill, C.R. Proc. Natl. Acad. Sci. USA 77:2726-2730, 1980.
12. Biran, S., Horowitz, A.T., Fuks, Z., and Vlodavsky, I. Int. J. Cancer 31:552-566, 1983.
13. Vlodavsky, I., Korner, G., Ishai-Michaeli, R., Bashkin, P., Bar-Shavit, R. and Fuks, Z. Cancer Met. Rev. 9:203-226, 1990.
14. Nicolson, G.L. Cancer Met. Rev. 7:143-188, 1988.
15. Jones, P.A. and DeClerk, Y.A. Cancer Met. Rev. 1:289-317, 1982.
16. Nakajima, M., Irimura, T. and Nicolson, G.L. J. Cell Biochem. 36:157-167, 1988
17. Vlodavsky, I., Fuks, Z., Bar-Ner, M., Ariav, Y. and Schirrmacher, V. Cancer Res. 43:2704-2711, 1983.

18. Hassell, J.R., Kimura, J.H. and Hascall, V.C. Ann. Rev. Biochem., 55: 539-567, 1986.
19. Hook, M., Kjellen, L., Johansson, S. and Robinson, J. Ann. Rev. Biochem. 53:847-869, 1984.
20. Lider, O., Baharav, E., Mekori, Y., Miller, T., Naparstek, Y., Vlodavsky, I. and Cohen, I.R. J. Clin. Invest. 83:752-756, 1989.
21. Vlodavsky, I., Ishai-Michaeli, R., Bar-Ner, M., Fridman, R., Horowitz, A.T., Fuks, Z. and Biran, S. Is. J. Med. 24:464-470, 1988.
22. Jin, L., Nakajima, M. and Nicolson, G.L. Int. J. Cancer 45:1088-1095, 1990.
23. Bar-Ner, M., Eldor, A., Wasserman, L., Matzner, Y. and Vlodavsky, I. Blood 70:551-557, 1987.
24. Parish, C.R., Coombe, D.R., Jakobsen, K.B. and Underwood, P.A. Int. J. Cancer 40:511-517, 1987.
25. Burgess, W.H. and Maciag, T. Annu. Rev. Biochem. 58:575-606, 1989.
26. Folkman, J. and Klagsbrun, M. Science 235:442-447, 1987.
27. Vlodavsky, I., Folkman, J., Sullivan, R., Fridman, R., Ishai-Michaeli, R., Sasse, J. and Klagsbrun, M. Proc. Nat. Acad. Sci. USA, 84:2292-2296, 1987.
28. Folkman, J., Klagsbrun, M., Sasse, J., Wadzinski, M., Ingber, D. and Vlodavsky, I. Am. J. Pathol. 130:393-400, 1988.
29. Gonzalez, A-M., Buscaglia, M., Ong. M. and Baird, A. J. Cell Biol. 110:753-765, 1990.
30. Cardon-Cardo, C., Vlodavsky, I., Haimovitz-Friedman, A., Hicklin, D. and Fuks, Z. Lab. Invest. 63:832-840, 1990.
31. Bashkin, P., Klagsbrun, M., Doctrow, S., Svahn, C-M., Folkman, J. and Vlodavsky, I. Biochemistry 28:1737-1743, 1989.
32. Ishai-Michaeli, R., Eldor, A. and Vlodavsky, I. Cell Reg. 1:833-842, 1990.
33. Saksela, O. and Rifkin, D.B. J. Cell Biol. 110:767-775, 1990.
34. Gospodarowicz, D. and Cheng, J. J. Cell. Physiol. 128:475-484, 1986.
35. Saksela, O., Moscatelli, D., Sommer, A. and Rifkin, D.B. J. Cell Biol. 107:743-751, 1988.
36. Yayon, A., Klagsbrun, M., Esko, J.D., Leder, P. and Ornitz, D. Cell 64: 841-848, 1991.
37. Ishai-Michaeli, R., Svahn, C-M., Chajek-Shaul, T., Korner, G., Ekre, H.-P.T. and Vlodavsky, I. I Biochemistry. Submitted 1991.
38. Flaumenhaft, R., Moscatelli, D. and Rifkin, D.B. J. Cell Biol. 111:1651-1659, 1990.
39. Laiho, M. and Keski-Oja, J. Cancer Res. 49:2533-2553, 1989.
40. Bar-Ner, M., Mayer, M., Schirrmacher, V. and Vlodavsky, I. J. Cell Physiol. 128:299-307, 1986.
41. McGuire, P.G. and Seeds, N.W. J. Cell Biochem. 40:215-227, 1989.
42. Rifkin, D.B. and Moscatelli, D. J Cell Biol.. 109:1-6, 1989.
43. Morikawa, K., Walker, S. M., Nakajima, M., Pathak, S., Jessup J. M. and Fidler, I.J. Cancer Res. 48: 6863-6871, 1988.
44. Gavanaugh, P. G. and Nicolson, G. L. Cancer Res. 49: 3928-3933, 1989.
45. Basset, P., Bellocq, J. P., Wolf, C., Stoll, I., Hutin, P., Limacher, J. M., Podhajcer, O. L., Cjhenard, M.P., Rio, M. C. and Chambon, P. Nature 348: 699-704.
46. Naparstek, Y., Cohen, I.R., Fuks, Z. and Vlodavsky, I. Nature 310:241-243, 1984.

SECTION IV

HORMONE RESPONSIVENESS
AND
ORAL CONTRACEPTIVES

ESTROGEN AND PROGESTERONE RECEPTOR ACTIVITY IN BREAST CANCER CELLS

SAVERIO BETTUZZI*, ALAN ROBINSON#, ROBIN FUCHS-YOUNG#, AND GEOFFREY L. GREENE#

***Universita di Modena, Istituto Chimica Biologica, 41100 Modena, Italy**
#University of Chicago, Ben May Institute, Chicago, Illinois 60637

INTRODUCTION

The elucidation of the molecular mechanisms responsible for the hormonal control of cell proliferation in breast cancer has been the object of intense research. Because most breast cancers are initially dependent upon estrogens for continued growth, much of this research has focused on the role of estrogen receptor (ER) in the control of gene expression and mitosis (1), and on its use as a marker for hormone responsiveness and prognosis (2). In addition, progesterone receptor (PR), as both a mediator of hormonal responses and as a product of estrogen action on breast cancer cells, has been studied extensively as a tumor marker (3) and in terms of its regulation by estrogen agonists and antagonists (4). Although its function in breast cancer is unknown, the presence as well as the induction of PR has been coupled to estrogen-induced proliferative responses in breast cancer cells. An improved understanding of the function and regulation of expression of these transcription factors is emerging from studies of the structure, composition and dynamics of the receptor proteins and the genes that encode them. The cloning and molecular analysis of all of the known steroid receptors has led to the definition of common functional domains and a proposed mechanism by which they interact with responsive genes, via *cis*-acting DNA enhancer elements, in normal and neoplastic tissues (5, 6) (7). For ER and PR, these studies have been aided by the availability of a number of monoclonal antibody probes directed against specific regions of each receptor (8, 9). In addition, the same antibodies have been used to develop validated quantitative and histochemical immunoassays for ER and PR in a variety of hormone-responsive tissues and related cancers. Such assays have proved particularly useful in the evaluation of ER and PR in breast tumor extracts (10), in frozen and paraffin-embedded tissues and tumor sections (11, 12, 13) (14) (15) and in needle biopsies (16) (17). This paper summarizes the results of recent studies on ER and PR structure, composition and activity in breast cancer cells as a function of agonist and antagonist binding.

STEROID RECEPTORS - General Considerations

The estrogen and progesterone receptors, like all of the steroid receptors, are members of a large family of trans-activating transcription factors that are activated by a ligand and bind with high affinity and specificity to short DNA enhancer elements called hormone response elements (HREs). Interaction of steroid-receptor complexes with responsive genes in vivo can result in either up or down regulation of transcription, depending upon the target gene and the tissue (5, 6). The molecular mechanisms by which either pathway occurs are still unclear, although it is generally believed that for transcriptional activation, receptor-DNA complexes recruit, or allow the recruitment of, other transcription factors that comprise a functional transcription complex. This process might involve protein-protein interactions between receptor and other factors, resulting in the formation of DNA loops (18) to accommodate long stretches of DNA between promoters and HREs, or possibly by altering the local chromatin organization (19) to permit access of other transcription factors; obviously, both processes could occur. Transcriptional inhibition by steroid receptors may also involve more than one mechanism. Recent data suggest that in some systems (eg. prolactin gene) (20), suppression may involve interaction of receptor regions outside of the DNA-binding domain with promoter elements and tissue-specific factors, whereas in other systems (eg. osteocalcin gene) (21), receptor may bind to specific HREs and sterically hinder the binding of a trans-activator. Similar results were observed for an ovalbumin-globin reporter gene (OV-GLOB), which was used to assess the effect of the B and A forms of chicken PR (cPR) on the transcriptional regulation of OV-GLOB in the presence of human ER (hER) (22). The B form of cPR partially suppressed the hER-mediated induction of OV-GLOB in transfected chicken embryo fibroblasts, whereas the smaller A form of cPR actually enhanced the hER effect. However, for an MMTV-CAT reporter gene, cPR B and A were both stimulatory, although B was five times more efficient than A; hER had no effect. A third possibility is that receptor may interact directly, or indirectly, with other transcription factors (eg. Jun) or steroid receptors to form heteromers that can have both positive and negative transcriptional activity (23). In addition, one or more members of a heteromeric complex may interact with mixed DNA elements or half sites in a responsive gene. It seems likely that control of transcriptional activity is a complex process that reflects the cooperative interaction of receptors, other specific and nonspecific transcription factors, various combinations of *cis*-DNA elements, and chromatin structure.

HUMAN ESTROGEN RECEPTOR

Structure and Properties

The isolation, sequencing, and expression of ER cDNA from MCF-7 human breast cancer cells has provided a wealth of information about the composition and organization of various functional domains in the estrogen receptor (24). A comparison of amino acid sequences among all members of the steroid receptor family, coupled with functional analyses of *in vitro* generated mutants, has identified regions essential for at least four functions of steroid receptors, namely ligand binding, nuclear localization/translocation, DNA binding, and transcriptional activation. The most highly conserved region is now known to be the 66 amino acid DNA-binding domain (Fig. 1) and it is this region that has been used to define the members of a superfamily of regulatory proteins that includes the steroid receptors. This region can be further divided into two subregions of cysteine clusters tetrahedrally coordinated to zinc, analogous to the zinc 'fingers' found in the *Xenopus* transcription factor IIIA. The hydrophobic region in the carboxy terminal portion of the ER molecule contains not only the ligand binding domain, but also a ligand-dependent transcription activating

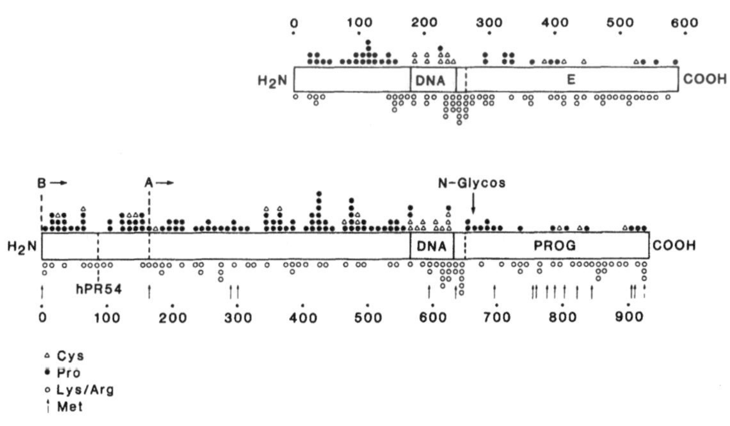

Fig. 1. Schematic amino acid comparison between MCF-7 human estrogen receptor (upper) and T47D human progesterone receptor (lower). The two representations are aligned to make the 66-amino acid DNA-binding domains coincide. The putative initiation ATGs for the B and truncated A forms of hPR are shown.

region that is responsible for the dimerization of ER (27).

region, as well as a constitutive (hormone-independent) translocation signal (25). In addition, it is probably this general region, by analogy to GR (26), that interacts with the hsp90 heat shock protein *in vitro,* although this has not been demonstrated for ER. It is also this region that is responsible for the dimerization of ER (27). The amino terminal portion of ER appears to be required for maximal ER transcriptional activity and may contain more than one transcription activating region, one of which may be cell type specific (28). Multiple transactivation domains may be a general feature of steroid receptors.

In regard to defining the structure and function of the hormone binding domain of ER, we have succeeded in locating one possible contact point (cys 530) by covalently labeling human ER either with ^{3}H-tamoxifen aziridine (an antagonist) or ^{3}H-ketononestrol aziridine (an agonist) (29) Following fragmentation of labeled ER with CNBr, trypsin, or V8, sequence analysis of purified peptides revealed that the site of attachment for both ligands had to be a cysteine at position 530, which is very close to the carboxyterminal end of the defined hormone binding domain (position 538) (30). We have therefore demonstrated that an estrogen agonist and antagonist can bind to the same site on the ER molecule, suggesting that these molecules regulate ER activity by differential alteration of the conformation of ER.

Interaction of hER with DNA

As described above, the DNA binding domain of each steroid receptor appears to contain all of the information needed for target-specific interaction with an appropriate HRE, although the nature of this interaction remains to be better defined. It has been suggested that the first finger motif is responsible for sequence specificity and that the second finger may stabilize protein-DNA interaction through nonspecific DNA binding (31). Several recent studies (32) have more precisely localized specificity and DNA contact to the region between and immediately following the second pair of cysteines in the first finger. For estrogen receptor, the known response elements (EREs), such as those found in the chicken and *Xenopus* vitellogenin A2 genes, are palindromic sequences with 5 bp stems separated by a 3 bp spacer (33). Single copies of these elements are able to confer significant estrogen inducibility to reporter genes containing heterologous promoters, such as the chloramphenicol acetyltransferase (CAT) gene fused to the thymidine kinase promoter, when transfected into ER-containing cells. A half-site ERE (34) that may involve the Fos/Jun complex (35) has been found in the chicken ovalbumin gene and more recently in the human PR gene (36)(37). By gel shift analysis, the specific, high affinity interaction of purified MCF-7 ER (>90% pure) with the perfect palindromic vitellogenin A2 ERE contained in a 27-mer synthetic oligonucleotide was demonstrated (38). Both halves of the ERE palindrome appear to be in contact with the receptor complex, which suggests the formation of a complex containing a head to head dimer of ER bound to the ERE, with each monomer recognizing one half of the palindrome. These results are consistent with extensive *in vitro* data that indicates the formation of a 5 S homodimer of ER when receptor is activated. Purified ER has also been characterized by us as an activated dimer. Interestingly, it was recently reported that binding of ER to ERE may require a 45-kDa single-stranded DNA-binding protein (39). However, we have not observed a similar phenomenon with the purified human ER.

Expression of Human ER in Heterologous Cells

A major goal has been to express hER cDNA in various eukaryotic cells in order to study the properties and dynamics of human ER in homologous as well as heterologous systems, and to produce large quantities for structural studies. High level expression (3-6 x 10^6 molecules per cell) of functional full-length human ER was achieved by cadium selection of chinese hamster ovary (CHO-k1) cells stably cotransfected with plasmids encoding MCF-7 hER and metallothionein (24) (40). The human ER isolated from these cells forms a classical 8-9S complex under hypotonic

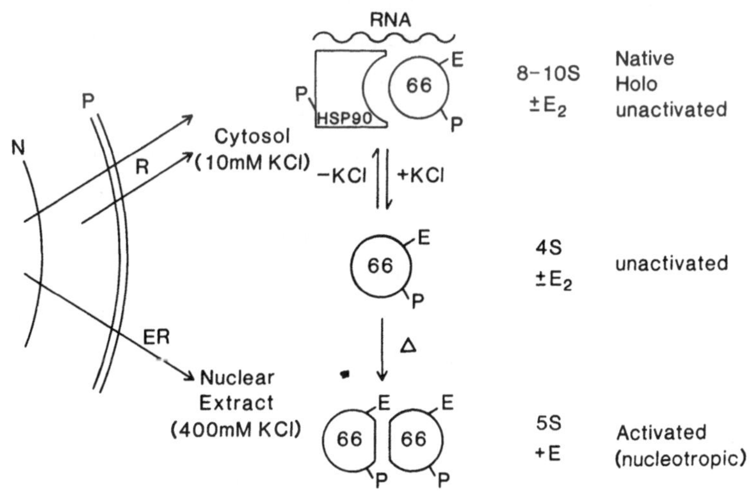

Fig. 2. Model of various *in vitro* forms of estrogen receptor isolated from a hormone responsive cell. E = estrogen; E_2 = estradiol; P = phosphorylation site(s); Δ = heat. See text for details.

conditions, which suggests that associated nonsteroid-binding components (eg. heat shock protein hsp90) are present in nontarget cells in sufficient quantity to complex ER that is 50-100 times more abundant than in MCF-7 cells. The human ER appears to be fully functional in CHO cells, even though it contains an artifactual mutation (gly → val) at residue 400 that results in a 10-fold lower affinity for estradiol at 25 C (41). An unexpected, but intriguing, observation was the sensitivity of CHO-ER cells to estrogens. In cells expressing the highest levels of hER, estrogens were cytotoxic. The partial antagonist hydroxytamoxifen was equally toxic, whereas the complete antagonist ICI-164 was not. It is still not clear whether some form of ER-mediated squelching is occurring, or whether induction or suppression of a gene(s) involved in replication might be occurring. Studies designed to address this question are in progress.

Regardless of whether the unoccupied receptor is present in the cytoplasm or nucleus of a target cell, it is proposed to exist as a complex consisting of one steroid-binding protein, a dimer of hsp90, and possibly one or more small RNA molecules, as has been reported for unactivated rat glucocorticoid receptor (42). A schematic representation of the possible composition of the different forms of ER observed *in vitro* is shown in Fig. 2. Phosphorylation sites exist on both the hsp90 and receptor proteins. In CHO-ER cells, estrogens induce rapid increased levels of phosphorylation of ER (unpublished data). Also, preliminary data suggests that serine residues are involved; no evidence of tyrosine phosphorylation has been observed, although it has been reported that tyrosine phosphorylation of ER is required for steroid binding (43). Recent experiments have shown a synergistic action of estradiol and cAMP on the induction of various ERE-tk-CAT reporter plasmids in Hela, CHO, and MCF-7 cells that express either recombinant or natural hER. This response has both hormone dependent and independent components. However, the presence of hER is absolutely required. What is not yet clear is whether hER is being directly phosphorylated in response to cAMP, or whether hER is interacting with another protein whose activity is stimulated by cAMP. We are attempting to elucidate the mechanism of this phenomenon.

In regard to the subcellular location of ER in the absence of hormone, a wealth of data now supports the idea that this receptor, and probably all other characterized members of this family except the glucocorticoid and mineralocorticoid receptors, are nuclear proteins (8). Overexpressing CHO cells transfected with human ER cDNA show a nuclear localization of ER when stained with the H222 antibody by an indirect immunoperoxidase technique in cells that were grown in phenol red-free medium containing charcoal-stripped serum (44). Little or no specific ER staining is observed in the cytoplasm of any of these cells, unless the cell is undergoing mitosis. Thus, the translocation signal(s) encoded within the ER molecule does not appear to require hormone to be active, unlike the glucocorticoid receptor (45). Recently, Picard et al. (25) demonstrated that the human ER contains only one constitutive nuclear localization signal, located in the hinge region (aa 256-303), whereas the glucocorticoid receptor contains a second signal in the hormone binding domain which is dominant and requires hormone. Apparently, the progesterone receptor also contains two nuclear localization signals (46), of which the one located in the hinge region is dominant and constitutive. However, unlike GR, the second signal in PR involves both the DNA and hormone binding domains.

Regulation of ER Expression

The regulation of ER mRNA and protein levels in breast cancer cells is complex and apparently dependent upon the hormonal history of the cells. In studies carried out in collaboration with Benita Katzenellenbogen (47), both up (T47D) and down (MCF-7) regulation of ER by estrogens were observed, although only MCF-7 cells that were maintained in normal calf serum displayed down regulation of ER. MCF-7 cells grown in charcoal-stripped serum were basically unaffected by short term estrogen treatment. Differential regulation of ER by estrogen antagonists, progestins, and progestin antagonists was also observed, whereas several growth factors had only minimal effects on ER levels. Thus, it appears that the steroid hormones themselves are the dominant factors in ER regulation, at least in the breast cancer cell lines tested. Other laboratories have reported estrogen-mediated down regulation of ER in MCF-7 cells (48) and one of these groups (49) observed no regulation of ER in the particular T47D cell line used in their study. Progestin-mediated down regulation of ER mRNA in MCF-7 and T47D cells has also been reported (50). A close correlation between protein and mRNA levels has been observed in all of these studies, consistent with transcriptional regulation, although post-transcriptional effects have been proposed (48).

HUMAN PROGESTERONE RECEPTOR

Purification and Immunochemical Analysis

The purification of human PR by steroid affinity chromatography and/or immunoadsorption, and the characterization of 14 rat and mouse monoclonal antibodies has been described (9). PR from T47D human breast cancer cells consists of two steroid-binding forms (A: 88-93 kDa; B: 109-119 kDa); the origin of these forms remains controversial, as discussed below. Highly purified PR migrates as 93 kDa and 119 kDa progestin-binding proteins in SDS gels. In all, 13 monoclonal antibodies have been obtained that recognize epitopes shared by both forms of PR. One mouse immunoglobulin (KC146) is completely specific for the larger B form. The epitope for this antibody is present on all PRs tested, including the B form from chicken oviduct, whereas nine other antibodies recognize only human or nonhuman primate PR and the remaining four cross react with rabbit PR. Interestingly, two antibodies (KD67 and KD68) do not recognize PR in monkey oviduct and thus appear to be specific for human PR. This discrimination between a human and nonhuman primate steroid receptor has not been observed previously for any of the characterized receptor antibodies.

Cloning of Human Progesterone Receptor cDNAs and Chromosomal DNAs

As part of our effort to understand the structural and molecular aspects of hPR gene regulation by several receptor-ligand complexes, genomic DNA and T47D cDNA clones encompassing the entire translated portion of hPR mRNA and approximately 7 kb of 5' untranslated sequence have been isolated, sequenced, and used to create CAT reporter plasmids as well as expression vectors for hPR isoforms. A comparison of corresponding human PR and rabbit PR sequences shows considerable homology in

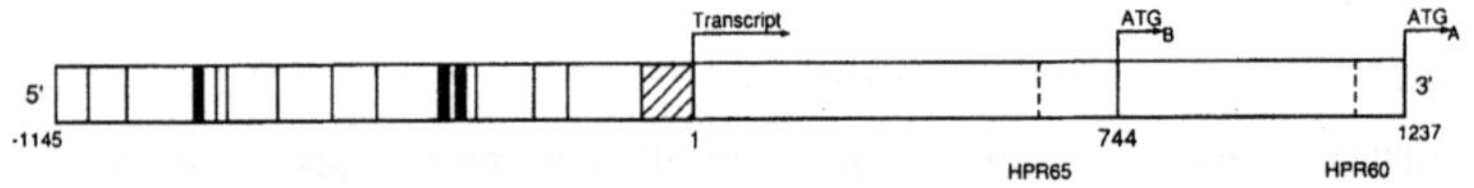

Fig. 3. Schematic drawing showing the organization of genomic hPR DNA. Positions of the putative initiation site for transcription (n 1146) and the first two ATGs in the open reading frame are shown. ATG_A begins at position +493 relative to ATG_B. Start sites for the HPR65 and HPR60 cDNAs are also indicated.

the 5' untranslated portion of the two PR genes. In contrast, the corresponding region of the chicken PR mRNA (366 bp) is not homologous to either mammalian PR mRNA. The transcription start site for the full length B form of T47D hPR has been reported (36). A long 5' untranslated sequence (743 bp) containing several small open reading frames and an in-frame stop codon precede the AUG_B initiation codon for hPR (Fig. 3). Like the rPR genomic sequence, the hPR genomic sequence upstream from the putative transcription start site contains several possible regulatory elements, including a CAACT sequence at position -98 which may correspond to a CAAT box. Both genes have a high GC content in this region and both have putative binding sites (TGGGCGGGCC) for the transcription factor Sp1. When aligned with human ER *via* the DNA-binding domains, all of the additional PR sequence appears as an extension of the amino terminal portion of the molecule (Fig. 1). Like ER, the PR protein contains a high proportion of prolines in the amino terminal half of the receptor, as well as a cluster of 10 cysteines in theDNA-binding domain, 9 of which are conserved with respect to ER, and a cluster of basic residues in and around the DNA-binding domain. The amino acid sequence homology between human ER and PR is about 56% in the 66-amino acid DNA binding domain and about 28% in the hormone-binding region. There is little homology between ER and PR 5' to the DNA binding domain.

Because progesterone receptor expression can be induced by estrogens and variably suppressed by progestins in reproductive tissues and several breast cancer cell lines, it is of interest to determine the role of the corresponding receptor proteins in this regulation. Several studies suggest that both ER and PR may directly modulate the level of transcription of the human PR gene in MCF-7 and/or T47D cells. We therefore analyzed the 5' untranslated hPR sequence for the presence of potential ER response elements (EREs) and PR response elements (PREs). Although reporter plasmids containing portions of this region have been shown to respond to ER in co-transfection experiments (37), well defined ERE/PRE sites have not yet been identified. Interestingly, a 600 bp region (-2.3 to -1.7 kb) that occurs only in the human hPR gene contains several striking palindromic sequences, including a possible PRE, . Recently, this putative PRE was shown to bind hPR selectively in vitro, suggesting that it may play a role in autoregulation of hPR gene expression. Several other potential estrogen receptor (ER) and hPR binding sites, some of which coincide with similar sites in the rPR gene, were also found in the 3 kb region preceeding the hPR promotor.

Regulation of PR expression

In collaboration with Benita Katzenellenbogen (4), we have studied the effects of estrogens, progestins and their antagonists on PR protein and mRNA levels in several breast cancer cell lines. By Northern blot analysis with human PR cDNA probes,

PR mRNA appears as five species of 11.4, 5.8, 5.3, 3.5, and 2.8 kb; these species are absent in the PR-negative MB-231 and LY2 cell lines. In T47D cells, both the receptor and its mRNA levels are reduced by 90% within 48 hr of treatment with the synthetic progestins R5020 or ORG2058. In contrast, treatment with RU38,486, a progestin antagonist, reduces receptor and mRNA only transiently. In MCF-7 cells, PR mRNA and protein are virtually absent in the absence of estrogens. Treatment with estradiol induces both, in parallel, about 10 to 40-fold within three days. Antiestrogens (eg. LY117018) block this effect completely. Interestingly, progestins and progestin antagonists both reduce receptor and mRNA levels in MCF-7 cells, although only by 40-60%. Clearly, the regulation of PR expression is different in the two cell lines. However, there is a close correlation between protein and mRNA levels and the changes appear to be directly mediated by the ligands, presumably via their cognate receptors.

Expression of B and A forms of hPR

An issue that still remains unresolved is the relationship, derivation, and functional differences of the two reported hormone-binding forms of mammalian and avian PR. Among the members of the steroid receptor transcription factor family, only PR and possibly androgen receptor are reported to exist in two ligand-binding forms. Estimates of PR molecular weights vary from 78-95 kDa for the smaller A form and from 108-120 kDa for the larger B form. Gene cloning data for chicken, rabbit, and human PR indicate the existence of only one gene for these PRs, although multiple forms of PR mRNA have been observed. The most likely explanations for the appearance of A in cell-free extracts are: 1) that A is a proteolytic fragment of B, as suggested for rabbit and human PR (51), 2) that A is derived by translation of PR mRNA from an internal methionine initiation codon, as suggested for chicken PR (52, 53), or 3) that there are two classes of mRNA, one containing AUG_B and one containing AUG_A, as suggested recently for both chicken (54) and human (36) PR. The putative translation start sites for the B and A forms of T47D PR are identified in Figs. 1 and 3. Although rabbit and human PR have been reported to occur exclusively as 110-kDa species in extracts or translation mixtures containing protease inhibitors, most studies show that mammalian and avian PRs exist in both forms under a variety of tested conditions. In fact, we have never observed the conversion of the T47D B form to A in any cell-free system. An alternative explanation is that the cleavage of B to A occurs *in vivo* via a specific proteolysis mechanism, although there is no data to support this hypothesis.

To determine whether the B and A forms of human PR are derived from the same mRNA via two independent translation initiation sites, full length (hPR65) and N-terminal truncated (hPR60) expression vectors were created and tested in an *in vitro* translation system and in transiently transfected Cos-1 cells. When the hPR65 transcript was translated *in vitro* and the ^{35}S-labeled products were analyzed by SDS-PAGE in 10% gels, the dominant ^{35}S-labeled protein produced was the full length B form (120 kDa) of hPR; less than 5% of the smaller A form was observed. When the hPR60 transcript was similarly translated, a major 90-kDa ^{35}S-labeled protein was observed, along with a very weak band migrating just behind the 90-kDa protein. We have been unable to convert the full length B protein produced *in vitro* to the 95-kDa A protein, even after prolonged incubation at 37 C in cytosol or nuclear extracts from T47D cells. In fact, both translated proteins were stable under all tested *in vitro* conditions. This data is consistent with the hypothesis that A cannot be generated from the mature B protein, at least not *in vitro*.

When hPR65 and hPR60 were expressed in Cos-1 cells, the 120-kDa and 90-kDa B and A forms of hPR were obtained in both cytosol and nuclear extracts of cells transiently transfected with the pSVL vectors. Western blot analysis with antibodies (JZB39 and KD68) that recognize both hPR forms revealed a dominant 120-kDa protein for hPR65 and a minor, but significant (ca. 5-20%), amount of immunoreactive 90-kDa protein, especially in the hypotonic cytosol extract. Therefore, the full length transcript appears to be capable of producing the smaller A form of hPR, presumably via initiation from AUG_A, even though B is dominant. For hPR60, the dominant immunoreactive species was a 90-kDa protein in both extracts. COS cells transfected with empty pSVL plasmid do not contain any hPR-immunoreactive protein in either extract. Although transfected cells were grown in charcoal-stripped serum to remove any endogenous progestins, a significant percentage of both immunoreactive hPR forms was found in the high salt (400 mM KCl) "nuclear" extract. When cells were treated with 10 nM ^3H-ORG2058 for 30 min at 37 C, a portion of both forms of expressed hPR became more tightly associated with nuclear components, as judged by the disappearance of immunoreactive hPR from the low salt extract. Interestingly, an upward shift in the migration rate of some of the hPR was observed for both forms after hormone treatment. These small changes in apparent molecular weight may represent increased levels of phosphorylation of the two proteins, as has been observed for progesterone receptor derived from various mammalian and avian tissues and breast cancer cell lines treated with progestins.

Transcriptional Activity of the B and A forms of hPR

To assess the relative ability of the B and A forms of hPR to regulate the transcriptional activity of a progestin-responsive gene, Cos-1 cells were cotransfected with an MMTV-CAT reporter plasmid (pMSG-CAT) and PR65 and/or hPR60. The MMTV long terminal repeat contains a hormone response element that is sensitive to both glucocorticoid receptor and progesterone receptor stimulation of transcriptional initiation. When comparable amounts of either form of hPR are expressed transiently in Cos-1 cells cotransfected with MMTV-CAT, the B form of PR is four- to six-fold more effective than the A form of PR in stimulating hormone-dependent CAT expression. The progestin antagonist RU486 significantly inhibited the hormone-induced stimulation of CAT expression and had little or no effect on CAT activity when used alone. Thus, both expressed forms of hPR are capable of stimulating the transcription rate of a progestin-sensitive reporter gene, at least in heterologous Cos-1 cells. However, the full length B isoform is significantly more efficient than the A form in regulating the PRE present in the MMTV long terminal repeat fused to CAT cDNA. These results are consistent with the observed preferential regulation of a similar MMTV-CAT reporter construct by the chicken PR B protein in cotransfected HeLa cells and in primary chicken embryo fibroblast (CHEF) cells (22). Similar results were reported recently for human PR (36). Thus, at least in transfected heterologous cells, the N-terminal domain of chicken and human PRs can specify target gene activation. What is not resolved by these studies is whether the B or A forms of PR preferentially regulate the expression of different target genes in the same cell under physiologic conditions. More information about the activities of other promoter elements and/or additional tissue-specific factors will be required to better define the role of the N-terminal domain in the differential activation of target genes.

Obviously, there are still a number of key dynamic and molecular aspects of receptor activity that are not resolved at this time. With the antibody, cDNA and genomic DNA probes that are now available for ER and PR, it is now feasible to define both biochemical and genetic aspects of receptor activity in the coordinate regulation of gene expression in hormone responsive tissues and cancers.

ER AND PR IMMUNOASSAYS

The development of immunoassays for hER and hPR in hormone responsive tissues and neoplasms has provided a wealth of information about receptor dynamics, such as nuclear localization in the absence of hormone, and about the existence and location of target cells for estrogens and progestins. We have continued to use our monoclonal antibodies to measure, characterize and localize ER and PR in normal and neoplastic target tissues and their extracts from human, nonhuman primate, and rodent sources. Many of these studies are collaborative. Both quantitative and histochemical immunoassays continue to be evaluated extensively on breast cancer specimens throughout the world. Several studies (14)(12)(17)(15) have shown that both ER-and PgR-ICA are predictors of endocrine response in patients with advanced mammary carcinoma, and survival in women with Stage I or Stage II disease. Although studies such as these indicate that ICA analyses for ER and PR may be more informative than conventional ligand binding assays, the numbers are still relatively small and additional data is required to establish their clinical value. These methods have also proved useful for the evaluation of breast tumor needle biopsies (16), endometrial cancers (55), and ovarian cancers. A particularly promising application of ER and PR immunocytochemistry has been the mapping of ER- and PR-expressing cells in the brain and pituitary of guinea pigs (56), rats, and some species of monkey. Correlations of ER expression with neurological and endocrine signalling in these tissues will allow detailed assignment of control mechanisms in the central nervous system. Clearly, immunocytochemical analysis of PR in target tissues and cell lines is proving to be a powerful analytical tool for studying hormone responses.

ACKNOWLEDGEMENTS

These studies were supported by Abbott Laboratories, the American Cancer Society (BC-86) and the NCI (CA-02897).

REFERENCES

1. R. Dickson, M. McManaway, M. Lippman, *Science* **232**, 1540-1543 (1986).
2. E. DeSombre, et al., *N. Engl. J. Med.* **301**, 1011-1012 (1979).
3. G. Clark, W. McGuire, C. Hubay, O. Pearson, J. Marshall, *N. Engl. J. Med.* **309**, 1343-1347 (1983).
4. L. Read, C. Snider, J. Miller, G. Greene, K. Katzenellenbogen, *Mol. Endo.* **2**, 263-271 (1988).
5. R. Evans, *Science* **240**, 889-8895 (1988).
6. M. Beato, *Cell* **56**, 335-344 (1989).
7. M. Carson-Jurica, W. Schrader, B. O'Malley, *Endo. Rev.* **11**, 201-220 (1990).
8. G. Greene, N. Sobel, W. King, E. Jensen, *J. Steroid Biochem.* **20**, 51-56 (1984).
9. G. Greene, et al., *Mol. Endocrinol.* **2**, 714-726 (1988).
10. G. Greene, M. Press, in *Immunological Approaches to the Diagnosis and Therapy of Breast Cancer* R. Ceriani, Eds. (Plenum Publishers, New York, NY, 1987) pp. 119-137.
11. M. Press, G. Greene, *Endocrinology* **122**, 1165-1175 (1988).
12. L. Kinsel, E. Szabo, G. Greene, J. Konrath, K. McCarty, *Cancer Res.* **49**, 1052-1056 (1989).
13. C. DeRosa, L. Ozzello, D. Habif, J. Konrath, G. Greene, *Ann. Surg.* **210**, 224-228 (1989).
14. L. P. Pertschuk, et al., *Cancer* **66**, 1663-1670 (1990).
15. L. Ozzello, C. DeRosa, D. Habif, G. Greene, *Cancer* **67**, 455-462 (1991).

16. M. Lozowski, et al., *Acta Cytol.* **34**, 27-30 (1990).
17. U. Berger, et al., *Cancer Res.* **51**, 239-244 (1991).
18. B. Théveny, et al., *Nature* **329**, 79-84 (1987).
19. H. Richard-Foy, G. Hager, *EMBO J.* **6**, 2321-2328 (1987).
20. S. Adler, M. Waterman, X. He, M. Rosenfeld, *Cell* **52**, 685-695 (1988).
21. N. Morrison, et al., *Science* **246**, 1158-1161 (1989).
22. L. Tora, H. Gronemeyer, B. Turcotte, M.-P. Gaub, P. Chambon, *Nature* **333**, 185-188 (1988).
23. S. Tsai, M.-J. Tsai, B. O'Malley, *Cell* **57**, 443-448 (1989).
24. G. Greene, et al., *Science* **231**, 1150-1154 (1986).
25. D. Picard, V. Kumar, P. Chambon, K. Yamamoto, *Cell Regul.* **1**, 291-299 (1990).
26. W. Pratt, et al., *J. Biol. Chem.* **263**, 267-273 (1988).
27. S. Fawell, J. Lees, R. White, M. Parker, *Cell* **60**, 953-962 (1990).
28. L. Tora, et al., *Cell* **59**, 477-487 (1989).
29. K. Harlow, D. Smith, J. Katzenellenbogen, G. Greene, B. Katzenellenbogen, *J. Biol. Chem.* **264**, 17476-17485 (1989).
30. S. Fawell, J. Lees, M. Parker, *Mol. Endo.* **3**, 1002-1005 (1989).
31. S. Green, V. Kumar, I. Theulaz, W. Wahli, P. Chambon, *EMBO J.* **7**, 3037-3044 (1988).
32. J. Berg, *Cell* **57**, 1065-1068 (1989).
33. L. Klein-Hitpass, G. Ryffel, E. Heitlinger, A. Cato, *Nucl. Acids Res.* **16**, 647-663 (1988).
34. M.-E. Meyer, et al., *Cell* **57**, 433-442 (1989).
35. M.-P. Gaub, M. Bellard, I. Scheure, P. Chambon, P. Sassone-Corsi, **63**, 1267-1276 (1990).
36. P. Kastner, et al., *EMBO J.* **9**, 1603-1614 (1990).
37. P. Kastner, et al., *J. Biol. Chem.* **265**, 12163-12167 (1990).
38. L. Klein-Hitpass, et al., *Mol. and Cell. Biol.* **9**, 43-49 (1989).
39. R. Mukherjee, P. Chambon, *Nucl. Acids. Res.* **18**, 5713-5716 (1990).
40. P. Kushner, E. Hort, J. Shine, J. Baxter, G. Greene, *Mol Endocrinol* **4**, 1465-1473 (1990).
41. L. Tora, et al., *EMBO J.* **8**, 1981-1986 (1989).
42. A. Unger, R. Uppaluri, S. Ahern, J. Colby, J. Tymoczko, *Mol. Endo.* **2**, 952-958 (1988).
43. A. Migliaccio, et al., *Mol. Endo.* **3**, 1061-1069 (1989).
44. G. Greene, P. Gilna, P. Kushner, in *Immunological approaches to the diagnosis and therapy of breast cancer II* R. L. Ceriani, Eds. (Plenum, New York, NY, 1989) pp. 119-129.
45. D. Picard, K. Yamamoto, *EMBO J.* **6**, 3333-3340 (1987).
46. A. Guiochon-Mantel, et al., *Cell* **57**, 1147-1154 (1989).
47. L. Read, G. Greene, B. Katzenellenbogen, *Mol. Endo.* **3**, 295-304 (1989).
48. M. Saceda, et al., *Mol. Endo.* **2**, 1157-1162 (1988).
49. A. Berkenstam, H. Glaumann, M. Martin, J.-A. Gustafsson, G. Norstedt, *Mol. Endo.* **3**, 22-28 (1989).
50. I. Alexander, J. Shine, R. Sutherland, *Mol. Endocrinol.* **4**, 821-828

(1990).
51. M. Misrahi, et al., *Nucl. Acids Res.* **16**, 5459-5472 (1988).
52. M. Carson, et al., *Mol. Endo.* **1**, 791-801 (1987).
53. H. Gronemeyer, et al., *EMBO J.* **6**, 3985-3994 (1987).
54. J.-M. Jeltsch, *J. Biol. Chem.* **265**, 3967-3974 (1990).
55. J. Soper, et al., *Gyne. Oncol.* **36**, 363-368 (1990).
56. L. DonCarlos, G. Greene, J. Morrell, *Neuroendocrinology* **50**, 613-623 (1989).

ORAL CONTRACEPTIVES AND BREAST CANCER: THE SCOPE FOR A HYPOTHESIS-ORIENTED APPROACH

CARLO LA VECCHIA

Istituto di Ricerche Farmacologiche "Mario Negri", Via Eritrea 62, 20157 Milano, Italy, and Institute of Social and Preventive Medicine, University of Lausanne, 1005 Lausanne, Switzerland.

Over the last two decades, a substantial amount of epidemiological data has been published on the oral contraceptive/breast cancer issue, but the topic is still open, and seems still to be attracting interest: about half of the over two dozen studies published to date have appeared during the last two years alone (1-3).

This increasing attention is certainly justified by the major public health relevance of the issue, and probably by a few points open to debate in published data, too. Though the global evidence for oral contraceptive use in all age groups, is in fact, largely reassuring, with an overall relative risk based on over 12,000 cases of 1.07 (95% confidence interval 0.81 to 1.26 (4)), there are consistent indications that long-term pill use increases the risk of breast cancer in women before age 35 or 40 - in the absence of any evidence of an association in middle aged women.

This pattern of risk could be interpreted in terms of a

cohort effect (since only the most recent generations of women have had the opportunity to accumulate long-term pill use from younger age), hence projecting a spread of the association in the future to middle-aged and older women, with a consequent major public health impact (5).

Alternatively, it would seem equally reasonable to predict a flattening off or even a reversal of the association in the medium-long term, with a pattern of risk similar to that observed for parity, which increases breast cancer risk for a few year period, but subsequently results in long-term protection (6).

In the absence of data on long-term pill use from younger age in women now in their middle age, various hypotheses seem thus equally reasonable, including the persistence of an increased risk, their flattening off towards unity, or even a reversal in the medium-long term, as recently suggested by a case-control study conducted in Northern Italy (7), as well as by a larger WHO Collaborative Study of Neoplasms and Steroids Contraceptives from ten different countries (8).

This presentation provides an update of the Italian data, and discusses some of the open questions for current and future research.

THE ITALIAN BREAST CANCER CASE-CONTROL

Design and methods of this ongoing case-control investigation of breast cancer have already been described. Briefly, from January 1983 to April 1990, 1941 cases of incident, histologically confirmed breast cancer in women below age 60 were recruited and interviewed in a network including major teaching and general hospitals in the Greater Milan area, northern Italy. The comparison group consisted of 1623 women admitted for acute, non-neoplastic, non-hormone-related diseases (33% traumas, 30% other orthopaedics, 15% surgical, 22% other miscellaneous) to the network of hospitals where cases had been identified. The catchment area of cases and controls was comparable, since over 85% of subjects interviewed cases and controls came from the same region, Lombardy. Participation was almost complete, since less than 3% of subjects refused to be interviewed.

Within a structured questionnaire, including information on socio-demographic factors and general risk factors for breast cancer, information was collected on oral contraceptive use, including time and duration of each episode of use and the brand name, whenever available.

Statistical analysis was based on standard methods for case-control studies, including age- and sex-adjusted relative risks (RR) and the corresponding 95% confidence intervals (9).

The age distribution of women with breast cancer and the comparison group is given in Table 1. Median age was 47 years for both cases and controls.

Table 1. Distribution of 1941 cases of breast cancer and 1623 controls according to age. Milan, Italy, 1983-1990.

	Breast cancer		Controls	
	Number	%	Number	%
Age (years)				
< 35	112	5.8	176	10.8
35-44	564	29.1	431	26.6
45-54	861	44.4	674	41.5
55-59	404	20.8	343	21.1

Table 2 gives the relative risk of breast cancer in relation to various measures of oral contraceptive use. Ever use was reported by 15% of the cases and 13% of the controls; the corresponding RR estimate was 1.2, of borderline statistical significance (95% CI 1.0 to 1.4). The risk, however, was not related to duration, since the highest RR was observed for the shortest period (< 2 years, RR=1.6). The RR was 1.2 for 2 to 5 years, and 0.8 for 5 years or more. No clear pattern of risk was observed in relation to time since first or last use, and the risk was not elevated for women who had used oral contraceptives before their first birth (RR=0.9, 95% CI 0.6 to 1.5).

The relation between oral contraceptives and breast cancer is further considered in Table 3 in two separate age groups (<45 and ≥ 45 years; the prevalence of O.C. in this population was too low for meaningful analysis under age 35). Although the risk estimates were somewhat higher above age 45, no formal statistical heterogeneity was observed across age strata.

Table 2. Relative risk of breast cancer in relation to various measures of oral contraceptives use. Milan, Italy, 1983-1990.

	Breast cancer	Controls	Relative Risk estimates (95% CI)+
Ever use			
No	1650	1409	1 *
Yes	291	214	1.2
			(1.0-1.4)
Duration of use (months)			
< 24	153	90	1.6
			(1.2-2.1)
24-59	79	58	1.2
			(0.8-1.3)
≥ 60	58	63	0.8
			(0.6-1.2)
Unknown	1	3	-
X^2_1 (trend)			0.73
			(n.s.)
Time since first use (years)			
< 10	120	95	1.3
			(0.9-1.8)
10-14	68	51	1.2
			(0.8-1.7)
≥ 15	103	66	1.1
Unknown	-	2	(0.8-1.6)
Time since last use (years)			
< 5	69	55	1.3
			(0.9-1.9)
5-9	87	65	1.2
			(0.9-1.7)
≥ 10	132	85	1.3
			(1.0-1.8)
Unknown	3	6	
O.C. use before first birth			
Ever	43	39	0.9
			(0.6-1.5)

+) Mantel-Haenszel estimates adjusted for age *) Reference category

Table 3. Relative risks+ of breast cancer in relation to oral contraceptive use in separate strata of age. Milan, Italy, 1983-1990.

	Age group	
	< 45	≥ 45
Ever use	1.1 (0.8-1.4)	1.6 (1.1-2.3)
Duration of use (months)		
< 24	1.3 (0.9-1.8)	2.0 (1.1-3.7)
24-59	1.3 (0.8-1.8)	1.3 (0.7-2.6)
≥ 60	0.7 (0.5-1.2)	1.0 (0.5-2.0)

+) Mantel-Haenszel estimates adjusting for age. Reference category : never oral contraceptives users.

DISCUSSION

The update results of this study are in agreement with most published evidence since they show no consistent association between oral contraceptives and breast cancer risk, although, on account of the limited prevalence of use in this population, they are of limited value for investigating the most widely reported issue, i.e. the potential association in younger women (10).

Still, they offer further reassurance, particularly since there was no evidence of direct relation with duration and time since first or last use, and hence they do not support the hypothesis that any potential association may become evident with a considerable lag-time after exposure to oral contraceptives.

The role of various time factors in the relationship between oral contraceptives and breast cancer should nonetheless be further investigated. These include calendar period of diagnosis, age at diagnosis, age at starting and stopping use, duration of use, time since first and last use, and calendar period of use.

These time factors are clearly interrelated, and it is consequently difficult to disentangle the separate effect of each factor. For instance, when age at diagnosis and duration are defined, age at starting tends to be defined as well, and this is strongly correlated with calendar period of use, and hence type of preparation as well.

For some of these temporal relationships, information in the studies conducted to date is inevitably scant or lacking. For instance, while an association between long-term oral contraceptive use at younger age and breast cancer risk has been observed in women below age 35 or 40, no data are available on the possible impact of this use on middle-aged or older women simply because oral contraceptives were not available when those generations of women were younger. Thus, reliable information on the impact of oral contraceptives on women aged 40 to 60 is now of outstanding importance.

In the absence of a precise understanding of the underlying biological mechanism(s), epidemiology can nonetheless try to develop integrated hyppotheses for hormonal and reproductive factors in breast carcinogenesis, which could be tested using the large amount of data already collected. Further, the apparent discrepancies in published data should not only be considered in terms of chance or bias (11), but also viewed within the framework of the complex, and sometimes contradictory, age and time effects of various (hormone-related) risk factors in breast carcinogenesis (3).

The elucidation of the timing of the oral contraceptive-breast cancer relationship is, of course, still essential for defining the long-term implications of oral contraceptives in breast cancer risk as well as on ovarian and endometrial cancer, and ultimately for quantifying any risk-benefit analysis of oral contraceptives and disease (12). Only continued monitoring, moreover, will make it possible to study the long-term impact of early, long lasting oral contraceptives use, and hence to provide a reliable assessment of this major public health issue.

Acknowledgements: This work was conducted within the framework of the CNR (Italian National Research Council) Applied Project "Oncology" (Contract No.87.01544.44) and "Prevention and Control of Disease Factors", and other specific support from the "Europe Against Cancer Program of Commission of the European Communities and of the Italian Ministry of Health". The contribution of the Italian League Against Tumours and the Italian Association for Cancer Research, Milan, Italy are gratefully acknowledged. We wish to thank Ms. J.Baggott, Ms. M.P.Bonifacino, and G.A. Pfeiffer Memorial Library staff for editorial assistance.

REFERENCES

1. Prentice R.L., Thomas D.B. On the epidemiology of oral contraceptives and disease. Adv. Cancer Res. 1987; 49: 285.
2. Olsson H. Oral contraceptives and breast cancer. A review. Acta Oncol. 1989; 28: 849.
3. La Vecchia C., Bruzzi P., Boyle P. Some further consideration on the role of oral contraceptives in breast carcinogenesis. Tumori 1990; 76: 220.
4. Thomas D.B. The breast. In: Symposium on Improving Safety Requirements for Contraceptive Steroids. World Health Organization: Geneva, 1988.
5. McPherson K., Coope P.A., Vessey M.P. Early oral contraceptive use and breast cancer: Theoretical effects of latency. J. Epidemiol. Community Health 1986; 40: 289.
6. Bruzzi P., Negri E., La Vecchia C., Decarli A., Palli D., Parazzini F., Rosselli Del Turco M. Short-term increase in breast cancer risk of full-term pregnancy. Br. Med. J. 1988; 297: 1096.
7. La Vecchia C., Parazzini F., Negri E., Boyle P., Gentile A., Decarli A., Franceschi S. Breast cancer and combined oral contraceptives: An italian case-control study. Eur. J. Cancer Clin. Oncol. 1989; 25: 1613.
8. The WHO Collaborative Study of Neoplasia and Steroid Contraceptives. Breast cancer and combined oral contraceptives: Results from a multinational study. Br. J. Cancer 1990; 61: 110.
9. Breslow N.E., Day N.E. Statistical Methods in Cancer Research. I. The Analysis of Case-Control Study. IARC Sci. Publ. 1980; 32.
10. La Vecchia C., Decarli A., Parazzini F., Gentile A., Negri E., Franceschi S. Determinants of oral contraceptive use in Northern Italy. Contraception 1986; 34: 145.
11. Skegg D.C.G. Potential for bias in case-control studies of oral contraceptives and breast cancer. Am. J. Epidemiol. 1988; 127: 205.
12. La Vecchia C., Franceschi S., Bruzzi P., Parazzini F., Boyle P. Incidence, aetiology and prevention of adverse effects of oral contraceptives. Drugs Safety, in press.

SECTION V

RISK FACTORS; MONITORING OF BREAST CANCER PROGRESSION AND REGRESSION

BENIGN BREAST DISEASE: LINKS TO RISK OF CANCER

David L. Page, M.D. and William D. Dupont, Ph.D.
Vanderbilt University Medical Center
Nashville, Tennessee 37232

Benign Breast Disease (BBD) is a term with unspecific reference. It has utility in that it denies the presence of cancer, and probably any but remote threat to life. However, the term "disease" should include some element of discomfort or indicate an association with threat to life (malignancy). Thus, the term <u>benign breast disease</u> should not be applied to trivial changes present in the majority of the population, which do not have a negative impact on the quality of life. It will be impossible to define this broad-sweeping phrase (BBD) more tightly, and it probably should remain as a term with broad and ill-defined reference. For that reason, it should specifically not be used to implicate an elevated risk of carcinoma developing in the patient without specification of magnitude and nature of risk assessment.

The specific associations of BBD particularly with implications of cancer risk are defined primarily by method of detection, whether by the patient, physician, or a specific diagnostic or screening test such as mammography. The precise or even fairly well-understood relationships between the different categories are not currently available, but are under study. For example, it is possible that the palpably firm breast, with irregular and relatively stable lumps which has a nodular pattern of densities by mammography, actually indicates an increased risk of carcinoma (1). If so, in which women would it be of most predictive importance? Although histologic determinants of breast cancer risk have recently been accepted, it is still not clear if these anatomic markers are more than slightly increased in clinically lumpy breasts (2) and mammographically dense breasts (3,4). Several studies have implicated the cancer association of these anatomic markers which are hyperplastic lesions (5). The interaction between these implicated and methodologically defined risk indicators and some more specifically defined ones which have met the test of reproducibility in several epidemiologic studies is awaited with interest. Recent studies (6) would indicate that there is some association between mammographic density, particularly with irregular nodular densities, and risk. The association of histopathologically defined risk factors and mammographic densities was strongest for older women(1).

Basically, most studies which have been done indicating an association between any risk factor and breast cancer have been concurrent studies. From this study design, one may view a positive association between any marker and breast cancer as only a suggestion for the more rigorous test of prospective studies (7). The most complete of these concurrent studies were those of Jensen and Wellings (5,8). Their studies gave us many histologic guidelines used in later studies with prospective design (see below).

Basically, if any predictive element is to be used to derive clinically relevant information with regard to patient management in women currently without cancer, the studies to be referred to must be prospective and thus provide predictive parameters for the subsequent development of clinically important breast cancer. The study design for follow-up studies based on histologic information from benign breast biopsies is prospective with regard to histologic data because the histologic changes are present as they were initially. This study design is also known as a cohort study done in retrospect. Such studies are weaker with regard to associations other than with histology because the information such as family history, etc. is obtained in a retrospective fashion.

Concurrent Studies:

In this study design, changes present at the same time a carcinoma is initially diagnosed are evaluated for their association with cancer and compared to cases without cancer. This study design is valuable because it allows for the entire breast to be evaluated because mastectomy specimens from surgery or autopsy are usually utilized. However, for statements of risk to be clinically valuable it is necessary for the study design to be related to breast biopsies without the concurrent presence of carcinoma as noted below.

The many studies of concurrent design were well-reviewed in the works of Jensen and Wellings (5,8) as a backdrop to the most complete studies of this type. The histologic classifications utilized by Dupont and Page (9,10) are an outgrowth of the classifications used by Jensen and Wellings. The approaches have been compared, at least for the "ductal" pattern lesions (11) with the approach utilizing the combined cytologic and pattern definitions of"atypical hyperplasia" being selective of a higher risk of cancer than the approach of Wellings et al. (5).

Predictive Studies:

The study of Kodlin et al. (12) is the largest study reviewing benign breast biopsies and then using a cohort design with subsequent patient follow-up prior to the Nashville-based studies. That study used the criteria of Black and Chabon (13) for premalignant lesions and in the analysis had to group some lesions together. Although very small, their group of most severe change just less than carcinoma in situ did attain a very high risk (Table 1).

Of great interest is a study of Carter et al. (14) in which data from a form filled out by hospital-based pathologists was used to test predictiveness of subsequent carcinoma development in women who had been screened in the Breast Cancer Detection Demonstration Projects of the United States National Cancer Institute and the American Cancer Society. When these diagnoses, which were not derived from any stated criteria but were recorded as pathologists would suspect included diagnoses of atypical hyperplasia and when grouped together in a three tiered system to most closely approximate the criteria of the Nashville-based studies noted below, risk figures were found as detailed in the accompanying chart. Note that the spread of risk is not as great, but the further corroboration more complex examples of hyperplasia were associated with increased risk is apparent. A recent similar study from Italy(15) is also supportive of these observations.

The Nashville-based studies used quite strict histologic criteria of cytology and histologic pattern combined with extent of lesion to produce lesions termed atypical ductal and atypical lobular hyperplasis. These terms were derived from the parentage of the analogous carcinoma in situ lesions. Some may regard many, but not all of the atypical hyperplastic lesions as smaller examples of DCIS or LCIS. This precise approach or a closely analogous approach have now been used in several other studies (16). Most recently, the nurses health study under the guidance of the Harvard School of Public Health has reviewed benign breast biopsies of women in their cohort and indicated that the risk of subsequent carcinoma development using the same criteria noted above are very similar in this group of patients (17). Connolly et al. used the precise histologic criteria of the Dupont and Page studies. This extends the relevance of AH because the initial studies (9,10) involved a cohort biopsied in the 1950's and 1960's. Also, Tavassoli and Norris have documented the experience of a reference center with atypical hyperplasia(18).Using criteria similar to those of Page et al (9,10), but including a criterion of size up to 2-3 mm. in greatest dimension, they found similar risks for later carcinoma development. Also, Eusebi et al (19), analyzed histologic alterations similar to AH, termed clinging carcinoma, and found a similar magnitude of cancer risk elevation.

Epidemiologic Associations and Risk Assessment:

Many risk factors for breast cancer have been identified, predominantly related to specifics of menstrual and pregnancy history as well as family history of breast cancer. Most of these risk factors indicate a magnitude of cancer risk less than two times that of comparable women from the general population (20-23), and are correctly not considered determinant premalignant conditions. The diagnostic phrase <u>proliferative breast disease</u> (PBD) indicates that there are proliferative alterations noted by histology, and that they indicate a disease by their demonstrated link to an increased risk of subsequent carcinoma development (21). This is a term which may be used to knit together the histologic and risk statements found in Table 2 for slight and greater risk lesions.

There is an elevated risk of subsequent invasive carcinoma after biopsies demonstrating specific AH. The magnitude of this risk has been characterized as moderate (24-26) because it is intermediate between that recognized by proliferative disease without atypia (10) (slightly increased risk of 1.5-2 x general population) and that recognized by LCIS (27,28) and small examples of DCIS (29,30) 9-11 x that of the general population.

Atypical hyperplastic lesions (AH) have been found in approximately 4% of otherwise benign biopsies and were found to indicate a relative risk of subsequent breast carcinoma development of 4-5 times that of the general population (9). Note that this relative risk of later invasive carcinoma. applies to the studied group of women and analogous women of similar age followed for a similar period of time, and that in mammographically indicated breast biopsies that incidence of AH is higher (31) than in these studies predating extensive use of mammography. This means that this relative risk cannot be applied to the risk of breast carcinoma over a lifetime. The absolute risk (certainly for women in the most frequently biopsied age group, perimenopausal) would be 8 to 10% in ten to fifteen years. This is a magnitude of risk very similar to that for the contralateral breast after invasive carcinoma development and treatment in one breast. The two types of atypical hyperplasia (ductal and lobular patterns) demonstrated little difference from each other except in age incidence, with ALH decreasing in incidence after menopause. Each recognized an equal incidence of later carcinoma in each breast. Most of our knowledge about AH relates to women in perimenopausal age, and that we really know little about the young and older women.

The relationship between relative risk (RR) and absolute risk (AR) is poorly understood. RR always compares one group with another and is thus of less direct relevance than determining the experience of comparable women and relaying the information in a more direct way as in AR, e.g., "10% likelihood of developing invasive carcinoma in 10-15 years" is a direct statement of risk in absolute terms. A specific period of time is necessary in the statement. In general terms we do not feel that prediction of breast cancer risk should be extended beyond 10 to 15 years (32) because the stability of risk with time is unproven. It is our experience, particularly with older women, that these elevated risks will fall (at least in relative terms) 10 to 15 years after detection (32).

There is such a strong interaction with family history and AH that it is relevant to consider women with atypical hyperplasia separately from those who do not. The definition of a positive FH in these studies was at least a first degree relative (mother, daughter, sister) with proven breast cancer. The absolute risk of breast cancer development in women with atypical hyperplasia without a family history was 8% in 10 years, whereas, those with a positive family history experienced a risk of 20-25% at 15 years. This strong interaction with family history has been supported in a recent study (23). This magnitude of risk for women with AH and FH is closely analogous to that accorded lobular carcinoma in-situ (33-36).

Molecular Markers:

New markers of the cell surface, growth factors or hormone receptors, proliferation, etc. have not yet found clear relevance in the premalignant sphere and breast cancer risk predictiveness. We have suggested that if there is any sharp divide within the non-invasive proliferative lesions, that it would be between comedo DCIS and lesser examples of in-situ disease (37), and this is supported by the demonstration of over-expression of the oncogene c-erbB-2 in comedo DCIS as well as by the few studies of DNA content (ploidy)(38).

Many studies of c-erB-2 protein in non-invasive proliferative diseases have shown remarkable uniformity of over-expression in comedo DCIS, and lack of expression in LCIS and non-comedo examples of DCIS(39-42). Apparently the mechanism for this is most often gene amplification(43).

There have been few studies of the presence of estrogen or progesterone receptors in the in situ proliferative diseases(44). Although there is no known clinical or therapeutic correlate of the demonstration that estrogen receptor protein is present in most AH and CIS lesions, the demonstration certainly would support the current interest in preventive trials using antiestrogens.

Conclusion:

Benign breast disease is a broad arena in which many elements interact in poorly understood ways. Specific definitions of these elements within each diagnostic domain should be sought. Mammography and histology are the best current measures of links to cancer risk prediction.

TABLE 1
SUMMARY OF THE RESULTS FROM COHORT STUDIES OF HISTOLOGICALLY DEFINED BENIGN BREAST DISEASE

Histological Diagnosis	No. Patients	RR*
Dupont and Page(10)		
Entire group	3,303	1.5
Atypical hyperplasia (AH)	232	4.4
Proliferative disease without atypia	1,693	1.6
Lacking proliferative change	1,378	0.89
Kodin et al (12)		
Entire group	2,931	2.7
Black-Chabon atypia-4	49	6.0
Black-Chabon atypia-3	262	2.4
Black-Chabon atypia-1-2	2,092	2.3
Papilloma, intraductal	80	5.0
Carter et al (14)		
Entire group	16,692	2.7
Non-proliferative	3,914	1.5
Proliferative	8,772	1.9
Atypical hyperplasia	1,305	3.0
Tavassoli and Norris (18)		
AH (ductal pattern)	82	4-5 (range)
Eusebi et al (19)		
Entire group	4,397	
"Clinging carcinoma"	21	4.3

*Relative risk calculated with respect to the general population. Different external reference populations used in each study.

TABLE 2

RELATIVE RISK FOR INVASIVE BREAST CARCINOMA BASED ON PATHOLOGIC EXAMINATION OF BENIGN BREAST TISSUE

NO INCREASED RISK

Women with any lesion specified below in a biopsy specimen are at no greater risk for invasive breast carcinoma than comparable women who have had no breast biopsy:

- Adenosis
- Apocrine metaplasia
- Cysts, macro and/or micro
- Hyperplasia (mild, more than 2 but not more than 4 epithelial cells in depth)
- Duct ectasia
- Fibroadenoma
- Fibrosis
- Mastitis (inflammation)
- Periductal mastitis
- Squamous metaplasia

SLIGHTLY INCREASED RISK (1.5 to 2 Times)

Women with any lesion specified below in a biopsy specimen are at slightly increased risk for invasive breast carcinoma relative to comparable women who have had no breast biopsy:

- Hyperplasia, moderate or florid, solid or papillary
- Papilloma with fibrovascular core
- Sclerosing adenosis, well-developed

MODERATELY INCREASED RISK (4-5 times)

Women with a lesion specified below in a biopsy specimen are at moderately increased risk for invasive breast carcinoma relative to comparable women who have had no breast biopsy:

- Atypical hyperplasia (borderline lesion)
- Specific patterns of atypical ductal hyperplasia
- Specific patterns of atypical lobular hyperplasia

Notes for Table 2:

1. All forms of adenosis were accepted in 1985 as having no indication of increased cancer risk. Since that time, well-developed examples of sclerosing adenosis, apart from other associations, indicate a slightly increased risk (16,45).

2. Cysts were placed in this category in 1985 and probably should remain there, although there is some interest in analyzing special subsets of cysts identified biochemically or by apocrine cytology. These studies are in progress. There is a suggestion that women with a family history and cysts (presumably large and palpable) have a slightly greater risk than identified by their family history alone, but the effect does not as much as double the familial indicator, and has not been controlled for the simultaneous presence of hyperplastic lesions.

3. There is a suggestion from large epidemiologic studies that women with fibroadenomas (FA) have a slightly increased risk of later carcinoma, about 1.7 times. This is "slight", less than double that of comparable women. Note that the absolute risk of cancer for these young women is not greatly changed, i.e., women under 40 y.o. in North America have less than a 0.1% incidence of breast cancer per year.

REFERENCES

1. Bartow,S.A., Pathak,D.R. and Mettler,F.A. Cancer 66: 1721-1725, 1990.
2. Bartow,S.A., Pathak,D.R., Black,W.C., Key,C.R. and Teaf,S.R. Cancer 60: 2751-2760, 1987.
3. Page,D.L. and Winfield,A.C. Am J Roentgen 147: 487-490, 1986.
4. Goodwin,Pamela J. and Boyd,Norman F. Am J Epidemiology 127: 1097-1108, 1988.
5. Wellings,S.R., Jensen,H.M. and Marcum,R.G. J. Natl. Cancer Inst. 55: 231-273, 1975.
6. Saftlas,A.F., Hoover,R.N., Brinton,L.A., Szklo,M., Olson,D.R., Salane,M. and Wolfe,J.N. Cancer 67: 2833-2838, 1991.
7. Dupont,W.D., Rogers,L.W., Vander Zwaag,R. and Page,D.L. Pathol. Res. Pract. 166: 471-480, 1980.
8. Jensen,H.M., Rice,J.R. and Wellings,S.R. Science 191: 295-297, 1976.
9. Page,D.L., Dupont,W.D., Rogers,L.W. and Rados,M.S. Cancer 55: 2698-2708, 1985.
10. Dupont,W.D. and Page,D.L. N. Engl. J. Med. 312: 146-151, 1985.
11. Page,D.L., Dupont,W.D. and Rogers,L.W. Cancer Detect. Prev. 9: 441-448, 1986.
12. Kodlin,D., Winger,E.E. and Morgenstern,R.G. Cancer 39: 2603-2607, 1977.
13. Black,E.M. and Chabon,A.B. Pathol Annu 4: 185-210, 1969.
14. Carter,C.L., Corle,D.K., Micozzi,M.S., Schatzkin,A. and Taylor,P.R. Am. J. Epidemiol. 128: 467-477, 1988.
15. Palli,D., Rosselli del Turco,M., Simoncini,R. and Bianchi,S. Int. J. Cancer 47: 703-706, 1991.
16. McDivitt,R.W., Rubin,G.L., S tevens,J.A. and Wingo,P.A. Lab Invest 58: 62A, 1988.
17. Connolly,J.L.,Schnitt,S.J.,London,S.J.and Colditz,G. Lab Invest 64: 10a, 1991.(Abstract)
18. Tavassoli,F.A. and Norris,H.J. Cancer 65: 518-529, 1990.
19. Eusebi,V., Foschini,M.A., Cook,M.G., Berrino,F. and Azzopardi,J.G. Sem. Diag. Path. 6: 165-173, 1989.
20. Faccini,J.M. Exp. Pathol. 37: 177-180, 1989.
21. Page,D.L. and Dupont,W.D. Cancer 66: 1326-1335, 1990.
22. Page,D.L. and Dupont,W.D. Surg. Clin. N. A. 70: 831-851, 1990.
23. Carter,C.L., Corle,D.K. and Micozzi,M.S. Am J Epidemiology 128: 467-477, 1988.
24. Hutter,R.V.P. Arch Pathol Lab Med 110: 171-173, 1986.
25. Winchester,D.P. Bull Am Coll Surg 71: 29-31, 1986.
26. McFadyen,I.J., Raab,G.M., Macintyre,C.C.A. and Forrest,A.P.M. Br. Med. J. 298: 931-931, 1989.

27. Rosen,P.P.,Lieberman,P.H.,Braun,D.W.,Jr., Kosloff,C. and Adair,F. Am. J. Surg. Pathol. 2: 225-251, 1978.
28. Haagensen,C.D., Lane,N., Lattes,R. and Bodian,C. Cancer 42: 737-769, 1978.
29. Page,D.L., Dupont,W.D., Rogers,L.W. and Landenberger,M. Cancer 49: 751-758, 1982.
30. Betsill,W.L.,Jr., Rosen,P.P., Lieberman,P.H. and Robbins,G.F. J. A. M. A. 239: 1863-1867, 1978.
31. Rubin,E., Alexander,R.W., Visscher,D.W., Urist,M.M. and Maddox,W.A. Cancer 61: 2077-2082, 1988.
32. Dupont,W.D. and Page,D.L. Hum Pathol 20: 723-725, 1989.
33. Frykberg,E.R., Santiago,F., Betsill,W.L. and O'Brien,P.H. Surg Gynecol Obstet 164: 285-301, 1987.
34. Wapnir,I.L., Rabinowitz,B. and Greco,R.S. Surg. Gynecol. Obstet. 171: 171-184, 1990.
35. Gump,F.E. Surg. Clin. N. A. 70: 873-883, 1990.
36. Hutter,R.V.P. Cancer 53: 798-802, 1984.
37. Page,D.L. and Dupont,W.D. Cancer 66: 1326-1335, 1990.
38. Norris,H.J., Bahr,G.F. and Mikel,U.V. Analytical and Quantitative Cytol Histol 10: 1-9, 1987.
39. Lodato,R.F., Maguire,H.C., Greene,M.I., Weiner,D.B. and LiVolsi,V.A. Modern Pathol 3: 449-454, 1990.
40. Bartkova,J.,Barnes,D.M.,Millis,R.R. and Gullick,W.J. Hum Pathol 21: 1164-1167, 1990.
41. Miller,A.B., Howe,G.R., Sherman,G.J., Lindsay,J.P., Yaffe,M.J., Dinner,P.J., Risch,H.A. and Preston,D.L. N. Engl. J. Med. 321: 1285-1289, 1989.
42. Borg,A., Linell,F., Idvall,I., Johansson,S., Sigurdsson,H., Ferno,M. and Killander,D. Lancet 1: 1268-1269, 1989.
43. Iglehart,J.D., Kraus,M.H., Langton,B.C., Huper,G., Kerns,B.J. and Marks,J.R. Cancer Res. 50: 6701-6707, 1990.
44. Barnes,R. and Masood,S. Am. J. Clin. Pathol. 94: 533-537, 1990.
45. Jensen,R.A., Page,D.L., Dupont,W.D. and Rogers,L.W. Cancer 64: 1977-1983, 1989.

PROLIFERATION RATE IN DIFFERENT CELL TYPES IN BENIGN BREAST DISEASE.

Sapino A., Macrì L., Gugliotta P., Manini C. and Bussolati G.

Dept. of Biomedical Sciences and Human Oncology University of Turin, Italy.

ABSTRACT

The histological patterns of Benign Breast Disease (BBD) are related to structural interaction of different cell types i.e. epithelial, myoepithelial, apocrine and "null" undifferentiated cells.

To identify the type of the proliferating cell, we devised a dual immunostaining procedure: the proliferating nuclei were labelled by 5-bromo-2'-deoxyuridine (BrdU) and/or PCNA (cyclin) and stained in brown with an immunoperoxidase reaction, while we employed alkaline phosphatase anti-alkaline phosphatase (APAAP) (red staining) or, alternatively, ß-galactosidase (blu staining) procedures to visualize specific cytoplasmic markers. Luminal epithelial cells were identified by a monoclonal antibody against keratin (AE1); myoepithelial cells were specifically recognized by α–sm-actin antibody and apocrine cells were stained by serum directed against GCDFP-15, a glycoprotein of cystic disease fluid. Cells unstained by these antibodies were defined "null" or undifferentiated. Fifteen cases of BBD were studied and different lobular lesions (epitheliosis, blunt duct adenosis, sclerosing adenosis and apocrine cysts) were identified in H&E stained sections. On serial sections stained with the double immunocytochemical procedure the different cell types constituting the lesions were counted. Within each cytotype, the absolute and relative number of proliferating cells was evaluated.

The results indicate that apocrine cells in cystic lesions do not proliferate representing therefore terminally differentiated cells. In typical ductal "hyperplasia" (epitheliosis) and in sclerosing adenosis, proliferation was negligible in all type of cells.

We conclude that terms such as ductal or lobular "hyperplasia" are misnomers; we could not confirm the hypothesis that these processes represent precursors to highly proliferative carcinomatous lesions.

INTRODUCTION

Benign breast disease (BBD) is comprehensive of a complex of histological lesions related to hormonal imbalance and resulting of structural interactions of cell types.

Preliminary to a study of BBD lesions is the question of the relationship, in mammary gland, between differentiation and proliferation. According to various authors (1, 2) the different cell types of the mammary gland originate from a common, basally located undifferentiated stem cell, the target of proliferation regulating factors. These cells would then differentiate towards the epithelial (luminal) myoepithelial (basal) and secretory (lactating) cytotypes.

Proliferative activity in the human mammary gland of menstruating women and in cases of benign cystic disease had previously been investigated by the thymidine labelling procedure (1, 3-5). Recently, Christov and co-workers (6) demonstrated the proliferative activity of normal breast epithelial cells after "in vivo" labeling of BrdU in pre- and post-menopausal women undergoing partial mastectomy for breast carcinoma. These studies indicate variations of proliferative activity during the menstrual period; maximal activity was found in the secretory phase. Evidence of post-menopausal proliferation was obtained either by in vitro thymidine labeling (5) or in vivo BrdU uptake (6).

However, all these studies failed to identify the proliferating cytotype, since only the "proliferation" parameter, and not the "cell type" was considered.

We have recently afforded the problem of the relationship between differentiation and proliferation in the mouse mammary gland, by using a double immunocytochemical staining procedure: proliferating cells were identified by the uptake of BrdU which was then revealed by a specific monoclonal antibody in a immunoperoxidase reaction (brown color), while differentiated cell types were marked by cytoplasmic staining with antibodies against keratin (AE1 monoclonal, recognizing epithelial cells), actin ($\alpha-$sm1 monoclonal identifying myoepithelial cells) and α-lactalbumin (the milk protein proper of secretory cells) (7).

These cytoplasmic markers were revealed by a color alternative of the brown nuclear staining, i.e. either red, as a result of an immunoalkaline phosphatase procedure or blue, the indigo product of ß-galactosidase activity. Cells negative with the differentiation markers were designated as "null" cells. The various proliferating and/or differentiated cell types present in the different segment of the gland were counted and a proliferation index of the different cells could be established. The results of this study indicate that hormonal stimulations in the mouse mammary gland induce cell differentiation and proliferation.

In the present study we analyzed 15 cases of BBD using an immunocytochemical staining procedure similar to that used to study the mouse mammary gland (7). The nuclei of proliferating cells were marked by BrdU uptake (8-10) and/or PCNA staining (11).

To identify the cell type, we employed selective markers for the different cytotypes and the reaction was developed by labelling with enzymes (either alkaline phosphatase or ß-galactosidase) producing a color precipitate (either red or blue) alternative to the brown diaminobenzidine precipitate revealing nuclear positivity.

MATERIAL AND METHODS

Material for investigation was obtained from 15 cases of

pre-menopausal women (age 22-50, mean 40.8) operated for cosmetic reasons (2 cases) or from histologically-proven benign cystic disease (13 patients) not associated with malignancy.

Lobular lesions were identified on H and E stained sections; serial sections were stained with a dual immunocytochemical procedure to reveal proliferating cells and, the different cell types building up the lesion.

To demonstrate cell proliferation serial sections of BBD were dewaxed through xylene and passed through a graded series of ethanols to distilled water, then incubated for 1 h at room temperature with monoclonal anti-BrdU antibody (previous BrdU uptake (Amersham, kit dilution) or PC-10 (Dako, dilution 1:200) to mark PCNA. After washing in PBS, sections were treated with peroxidase anti-mouse IgG (Amersham) for 30 min., washed in PBS and developed for 5 min. with 25 mg of 3.3' diaminobenzidine, 0.3% H_2O_2 and 0.3% nickel chloride/cobalt chloride in 50 ml of phosphate buffer at pH 7.4.

The specific markers employed to stain epithelial, myoepithelial and apocrine cells selectively are listed in table 1. We have been employing AE1 monoclonal a marker of epithelial cells, in analogy with our previous study in the mouse mammary gland (7). Myoepithelial cells are instead specifically identified by monoclonal α–sm1 recognizing the alpha isoform of smooth muscle actin (12, 13). Apocrine cells can be identified by rabbit antiserum against a 15000 M.W. glycoprotein of cystic disease (GCDFP-15) (14). Cells that were not stained by any of these markers were indicated as "null" undifferentiated cells. Sensitive procedures employing either alkaline phosphatase and mouse anti-alkaline phosphatase (APAAP) of alternatively ß-galactosidase-labeled anti-mouse secondary serum and an immunogalactosidase procedure were used as a second step.

Briefly, in the APAAP sistem the sections were incubated with nonimmune serum, then with primary antibody at the appropriate dilution (see table 1) overnight at room temperature. After washing in PBS, sections were treated with anti-mouse IgG (Dakopatts, Glostrup, Denmark, 1/50 in PBS) or biotinylated anti-rabbit IgG (Vector Laboratories, Burlingame, USA; 1/200 in PBS) respectively. Specimens were then incubated with mouse APAAP complex (Dakopatts,1/50 in PBS) or with monoclonal anti-biotin antibody diluted 1/20 (Dakopatts). A second step was performed with anti-mouse IgG and finally with mouse APAAP complex.

The reaction was developed with a substrate solution containing 50 mg of FAST Red TR salt (Sigma) dissolved in 1 ml of dimethylformamide (DFM), 36 mg of Naphthol AS-BI phosphoric acid sodium salt (Sigma) dissolved in 1 ml of DMF and 18 mg of levamisole (Sigma) in 50 ml of 1.3-propanediol buffer at pH 9.5 (Merck, Daemstadt, FRG). The solution was then filtered and used immediately. Incubation of the sections was continued on a shaker at room temperature for 5-10 min.

Nuclei were lightly counterstained with methyl green or with haemalum. The slides were mounted in water-soluble mountant and kept in the dark.

Alternatively, ß-galactosidase labelled anti-mouse secondary anti-serum (Carlo Erba, Milan, Italy) was used in the immunogalactosidase procedure at kit dilution. Sections were then washed in PBS and the enzyme activity was revealed using 5-bromo-4-chloro-5-indolyl-ß-D-galactoside (IbGA) (Serva, Heidelberg, West Germany) 0.044% in PBS containing 1.1 mM $MgCl_2$ and potassium ferri- and ferrocyanide 3 mM each. Specimens were incubated with this working solution for 1 h at 37°C. Nuclei were counterstained with neutral red; sections were then dehydrated and mounted in Canada balsam.

Selected areas were counted on serial sections under the light microscope by two persons independently. The relative percentage of the different cytotypes in the different BBD lesions was evaluated and the proliferative activity of various cell types in different structures of the gland tree were considered.

Table 1. Specific cytoplasmic markers.

Marker	Reagent	Source	Dilution	Cell specificity
α–smooth muscle actin	1A4 (MAb)	Sigma (St. Louis, MO)	1:1000	myopithelial
Keratin	AE1 (MAb)	Cambridge Research (Cambridge, MA)	1:200	epithelial
GCDFP-15	antiserum	Dr. D.E. Haagensen (Boston, MA)	1:5000	apocrine

RESULTS

The results indicate that, in histologically "normal" lobules, the proliferating cells mostly corresponded to AE1-positive epithelial cells, while proliferation in myoepithelial cells was recorded as a rare event (Fig. 1). In agreement with other authors (4, 6) we found a variability in the distribution of labeled cells within different lobular structures.

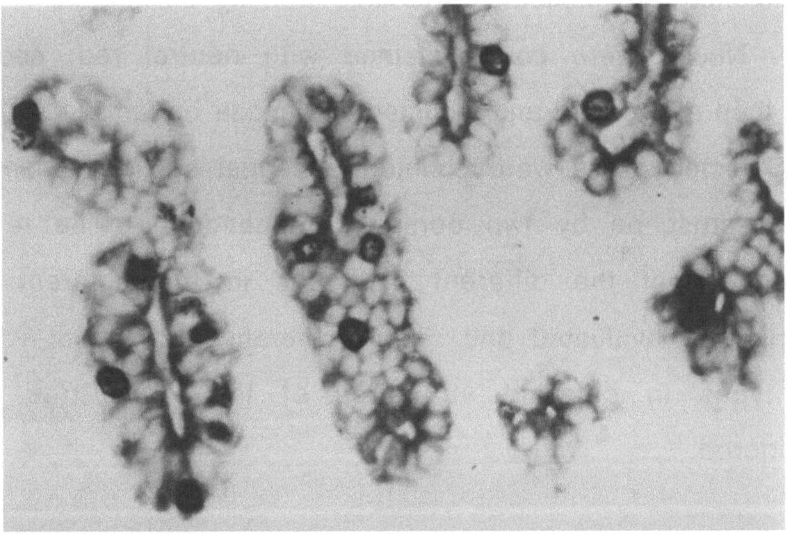

Fig. 1. Ductules in a histologically normal lobule in case of BBD. Double immunochemical staining with AE1 MoAb anti-keratin (blue cytoplasm, in the original slide) and anti-BrdU MoAb (dark brown). Stained proliferating nuclei mainly correspond to keratin-expressing epithelial cells (400 x).

In apocrine cyst 0.55% of total cells were proliferating and all of them were undifferentiated ("null"). Apocrine cells in cystic lesions were never seen to proliferate.

No proliferation activity was detected in areas of sclerosing adenosis; we noted that cell identification in this type of lesion was rather uncertain: some overlapping of the counted number of epithelial and myoepithelial cells was observed. This phenomenon is probably related to the co-expression of luminal-type of keratin and of α-actin by the elongated cells featuring this lesion. In ductal adenosis 1.53% of total cells were proliferating: of these 68% were epithelial, 29% "null" and only 2.5% myoepithelial in nature. In typical ductal hyperplasia s.c. "epitheliosis", only 0.12% of total cells were proliferating and 91% were "null" and 9% myoepithelial (Table 2).

Table 2. Proliferation rate and identification of proliferating cell type(s) in different lesions of BBD.

Lesion	% Proliferation	Proliferating cytotype
apocrine cysts	0.55	"null" (100%)
duct adenosis	1.53	epithelial (68.5%) "null" (29%) myoepithelial (2.5%)
sclerosing adenosis	0	0
duct hyperplasia	0.12	"null" (91%) myoepithelial (9%)

CONCLUSIONS

Cytological analysis of the different histological lesions of benign breast disease helps to understand the complex structural organization and bears diagnostic interest. The interaction between epithelial, myoepithelial and apocrine cell types and the regional prevalence of single cell types characterizes different lesions. However, these data do not allow to draw conclusions on the pathogenesis and evolution of the lesions. Cell proliferation might add a novel functional parameter which might help to answer the question on the preneoplastic nature of BBD.

Meyer and Connor (4) measured cell proliferation in fibrocystic disease by thymidine labelling (TLI). This study was conducted in histologically defined lesions from 49 patients; the results, expressed as mean values of the "percentage of labelled cells" obtained in various lesions, were compared to those observed in "normal women" and in patients with infiltrating or in situ carcinoma. The results obtained indicated a low and remarkably similar TLI in all benign histological entities in contrast with the high values observed in in situ carcinomatous lesions.

Our results, obtained with more complex procedure, allowing not only the evaluation on the proliferative activity, but the interpretation as well on the proliferating cell types, are only partly in agreement with the conclusions of Meyer and Connor (4). These authors observed a relatively low, but appreciable proliferative activity in cells lining cystic lesions. However, they failed to recognize the apocrine nature of the cells and might therefore have been referring to other non-apocrine cysts. Our data do not indicate a proliferation activity in apocrine cells, which seem therefore to represent a terminally differentiated cell. The questions related to the preneoplastic potential BBD and on which cell type might possibly represent the precursor of in situ cancerous lesions, remains unanswered. However, our data do not indicate an excessive proliferation in s.c. ductal or lobular hyperplasia.

The hypothesis that these "hyperplastic" processes represent precursors to highly proliferative carcinomatous lesions is not confirmed by the present study. The histologic feature of filling up of ducts and ductules rather than the result of enhanced cell proliferation (which we were unable to confirm) might rather be related to decreased cell turnover.

REFERENCES (in ordine di citazione)

1. Ferguson, D.J.P. Virchows Arch. (Pathol. Anat.) 407:379-385, 1985.
2. Joshi, K., Smith, J.A., Perusinghe, N. and Monoghan, P. Am. J. Pathol. 124:199-206, 1986.
3. Meyer, J.S. Human Pathol. 8:67-81, 1977.
4. Meyer, J.S. and Connor, R.E. Cancer 50:746-751, 1982.
5. Russo, J., Calaaf, G., Roj, L. and Russo, I.H. J. Natl. Cancer Inst. 78:413-417, 1987.
6. Christov, K., Chew, K.L., Ljung, B.M., Walda, F.M., Duarte, L.A., Goodson III, W.H., Smith, H.S. and Mayall B.H. Am. J. Pathol. 138:1371-1377, 1991.
7. Sapino, A., Macrì, L., Gugliotta, P. and Bussolati, G. J. Histochem. Cytochem. 38:1541-1547, 1990.
8. De Fazio, A., Leary, J.A., Hedley, D.W. and Tattersall, N.H. J. Histochem. Cytochem. 35:571-577, 1987.
9. Hayashi, Y., Koile, M., Matsutani, M. and Hoshino, T. J. Histochem. Cytochem. 36:511-514, 1988.
10. Meyer, J.S., Nauert, J., Koehm, S. and Huges, J. J. Histochem. Cytochem. 37:1449-1454, 1989.

11. Galand, P. and Degraef, C. Cell Tissue Kinet. 22:383-392, 1989.
12. Skalli, O., Ropraz, P., Trzeciak, A., Benzonana, G., Gillessen, D. and Gabbiani G. J. Cell. Biol. 103:2787-2796, 1986.
13. Gugliotta, P., Sapino, A., Macrì, L., Skalli, O., Gabbiani, G. and Bussolati, G. J. Histochem. Cytochem. 36:659-663, 1988.
14. Mazoujian, G., Pinkus, G.S., Davis, S. and Haagensen, D.E. Am. J. Pathol. 110:105-112, 1983.

ASPECTS OF CELL MEDIATED IMMUNITY IN MONITORING BREAST CANCER

URSULA KOLDOVSKY

Department of Gynaecology, Immunological Laboratory, University Düsseldorf, Germany

The host immune response to transformed cells is an important factor in protection against the growing tumor. This defense mechanism should not be understood as a strict, well defined tumor specific response but rather as a regulatory instrument in the fight against transformed somatic cells. It goes beyond the limit of a discussion of cell mediated immunity in breast cancer to speak about the whole problematic of altered cell membrans and the quantitative and qualitative changes of surface antigens after malignant transformation. Since tumor cells have the property to be not always very different in the expression of their surface antigens from their normal counter cells the evaluation of the tumor immunological regulation mechanisms may turn out to be cumbersome. Straightforward answers are not easy to give to questions how the immune system works against the growing tumor. The situation is even more complicated, as some immune reactions can apparently faciliate the tumor growth. Nevertheless the simplified statement can be made that these surface changes on the tumorcells can induce an anticancer reaction of the patient.

Dividing cell mediated and serological immune response is artificial; in the organism these compartements of the immune response exist together and influence each other. Cellulare immunity seems to be the most important primary host response to the growing tumor but must not necessarily be dominant in all clinical stages of the disease.

The clinical tumorimmunology has two major objectives: 1) to monitore the immune reaction and relate it to the clinical status and to the conventional treatment. 2) to use the results for non specific and specific cancer immuno therapy. Both aspects can not be separated, because they intervene by logistic experimental designes and methods and benefit from each other.

The immunological monitoring related to clinical tumor-immunology covers four categories: 1) assessment of the antigenic make up of the tumor cells (gain and loss of antigen, quantitative changes that are capable to induce an immune reaction), 2) measurement of tumor associated substances in body fluids, produced either directly by the tumor or indirectly by the patient in response to the tumor growth, 3) evaluation of the cellulare and humoral response to the tumor associated antigens (point 1 and 2), 4) evaluation of the overall competence of the different arms of the immune system.

For the evaluation of the immune reaction of tumor patients in vivo and in vitro tests can be performed.
The in vivo tests recognize the general immunocompetence of the patient. So called recall antigens (bacterial or candida antigens) and synthesized antigens (DNCB) are

used. The specific antitumor reaction can be seen by injection of small doses of tumor extract or TAA into the skin as a type of delayed hypersensitivity test or by the skin window assay of M. Black (1). In vitro tests include testing of percentage and absolute number of lymphocytes and their subpopulations and the response of the lymphocytes to different stimuli. Sources for the lymphocytes are the peripheral blood, lymphnodes and the tumor itself. The results are seen as a proliferative response, a cytotoxic reaction or a production of mediators (cytokines, lymphokines).

The topic of this section asks for discussion of the cellulare immunity in breast cancer. Therefore attempts will be made to give short comments about monitoring cellmediated immunity in breast cancer and the likely influence of conventional therapy on it. The possibility of its use as a prognostic factor and the consequences for an immunotherapy will be discussed shortly.

Determination of lymphocytes and their subpopulations

Since a long time pathologists have talked about tumor infiltrating lymphocytes (TIL). A classical picture is that of a medullary breast carcinoma. In 1946 Foote and Stewart (2) suggested that lymphocyte infiltration of the stroma may represent a host reaction to this tumor. 1949 Moore and Foote (3) proposed this as a good prognostic sign. 1968 Iris Hamlin (4) gave an overall picture of host defence reaction in 272 fully documented radical mastectomy specimens. She related survival after 15 years to the histological features present in tumor and lymphnode and to the density of lymphocytes and plasma cells in tumor and lymphnode. Scores for the host defense reaction indicated the density of the immune cells in and around the tumor as well as the intensity of reaction in the lymphnode. From 55 patients with a high grad malignancy but also a high graded host defence reaction 29 were still alive after more than 15 years in comparison to 88 patients with high grad malignancy and low grad host defense reaction, where only 3 were still alive.

Black (1955-5) and Berg (1959-6) suggested that infiltration of immune cells into breast cancer other than medullary carcinoma represents host resistance. Examinations of the 1980 s revealed T cells as the main component of the infiltrates. With monoclonal antibodies the phenotypic characteristic was determined (Table 1).

Author	year	Predominance CD4+	CD8+	
Bhan et al.	1983		+	J. Natl. Cancer Inst. 71, 507
Görno et al.	1983		+	Arch. Pathol. Lab. Med. 107, 415
Rowe et al.	1984		+	Br. J. Cancer 49, 149
Whitwell et al.	1984	+		Br. J. Cancer 49, 16
Götlinger et al.	1985	+		Int. J. Cancer 35, 199
Hurliman et al.	1985		+	Int. J. Cancer 35, 753
Horny et al.	1986	+		Virchows Archiv 409, 275
Ben Ezra et al.	1987	+		Cancer 59, 2037
von Kleist et al.	1987	+		Int. J. Cancer 40, 18
Bilik et al.	1989		+	Cancer Immunol. Immunother. 28, 143
Salch et al.	1990	+		Arch. Surg. 125, 200
Whitford et al.	1990		+	Br. J. Cancer 62, 971
Küppers et al.	1991		+	Biennial Meeting of the International Association for Breast Cancer Research

Table 1: Phenotypic characterization of TIL in breast cancer.

Note: Lymphocytes carry cluster of differentiation (CD).
The numbers correspond to various subsets.
CD3 = all T-cells; CD4 = helper cells, CD8 = T-cytotoxic/suppressor cells;
CD2, CD57 = T-cells, NK-cells; CD16 = KN-cells

Predominance of CD4+ cells is found as often in the biopsies as predominance of CD8+ cells. This may depend upon the different methods. Whitford (7) for example used flow cytometry on eluated cells, while others used the different kinds of immunohistochemistry (8, 9). Variations in the amount of cells and lymphocytes from section to section within a block of tissue and heterogenity may be part of the discrepancy.

Not only tumor infiltrating lymphocytes can be examined but also tests can be done on the evaluation of the amount of peripheral blood lymphocytes and their subpopulations. A 10 year follow up study reveals for example that a low pretreatment lymphocyte count with a steady rise after surgery carries a good prognostic sign, while a high presurgery count with a fall thereafter is indicative of a recurrence (10). In our laboratory 9 years ago a prospective study was started to find out if the amount of lymphocyte subpopulations may be used for prognosis (11). After five years four groups of breast cancer patients were compared to age matched controls (presurgery for primary breast cancer, in therapy, in post therapy, in progressiv). The lowest depression of CD3+, CD4+ and CD8+ cells is seen mainly during therapy and in progression. The lowest levels are found for CD8+ cells in patients in progression. A certain number of patients but not all have depressed T-cells even at the time of primary diagnosis.

<u>Detection of T Cell mediated immunity</u>

The search for evidence of specific lymphocyte activation by the growing breast cancer is mainly done with assays of T cell proliferation. T cell proliferation is measured by incorporation of the DNA precursor 3H thymidin into lymphocytes after stimulation with autologous tumor extract or mitogenetic lectins (mitogens). Helper, suppressor or cytotoxic T cell subsets can proliferate. Helper T cells can be recognized by their ability to be restimulated by the autologous tumor extract and by the production of the lymphokine Il 2. Suppressor cells and especially their supernatant can inhibit the primary lymphocyte proliferation through mitogens. The cytotoxic function is assayed by the so called Cr 51 release, whereby Cr 51 is set free from prelabeled tumor cells after they had been in contact with the cytotoxic cell. The cytokine production is measured by several inhibition, migration or adherence assays.

Lymphoproliferative responses to autologous breast cancer material have mainly been described between 1970 and 1980 and impairment has been shown in some breast cancer patients. 1977 for example Dean et al (12) showed that 12 of 34 breast carcinoma patients of all clinical stages reacted with proliferation of their lymphocytes to autologous tumor extract. After 10 and more years 9 of 16 patients, whose lymphocytes had not responded postsurgery had died compared to 1 of 20 who had responded.

The overall T cell activity, seen in the proliferative response to stimulation with mitogens, was tested by the same group as above (13). It was demonstrated that one third of 107 breast cancer patients had a depressed proliferative answer to at least one mitogen. More recent lymphoproliferative studies (14) employ lymphocytes from tumor draining lymphnodes. Lymphocytes from the more proximal node proliferate less after stimulation with mitogen or lymphokine (Il 2) than the more distant ones. Also differences could be seen in the response on mitogen stimulation of axillary lymphnode lymphocytes (LNL) versus peripheral lymphocytes (PBL) from nonmetastatic and metastatic mammary carcinoma patients. The ability of the LNL to proliferate was always stronger than of the PBLs.

The cytotoxic T-lymphocyte (CTL) attack on the tumor cell can occur on the basis of recognition of foreign (tumor associated) antigens on the tumorcell and their presentation to T cells in connection with MHC antigens. CTLs are generated in these steps of antigen presentation and by enlargement of the relevant receptor carrying clones to blast cells. The expression of MHC class I antigens on tumor cells is therefore necessary for the task of CTLs to kill the relevant tumor cell. This expression of MHC class I antigens varies on tumor cells and especially on breast cancer cells. The necessity of the cytotoxic T cell to recognize tumorassociated antigens and MHC class I on the target cell in order to lyse this cell shows the difficulty of the search for specific cytotoxic T cells in the laboratory. However very recently in two Japanese laboratories the identification of such cytotoxic T lymphocyte clones against autologous breast cancer could be demonstrated. Sato et al (15) obtained a pair of autologous specific CTL and target clone from the metastatic pleural effusion of a breast cancer patient. With cold inhibition assays the specificity of the clones could be shown. Nonspecific cytotoxicity against allogeneic targets and NK activity (see later) was not found. With monoclonal antibodies against T cell markers and HLA class I antigen it was demonstrated that the T cell antigen receptor (TiT3) on the clone and the specific antigen HMC8 on the cancer cell are involved in the killing. Kaieda (16) developed three T cell clones that lysed autologous breast cancer cells. Incubation with anti CD3 antibody decreased the cytotoxicity. Also the cytotoxic reaction was blocked by a mab against a specific antigen (ATM I) on the cell. This antigen ATM I was found in the sera of 8 of 12 breast cancer patients.

Natural killer cell activity

Natural killer (NK) cells are lymphoid cells, whose action on tumors is cytolytic. They are often discussed and a favoured object of studying the natural killing and protection against growth of tumor cells. Much is known about NK killing but the question of target recognition has not been uniformely resolved. The NK cells do not seem to be just one lineage within the hematopoetic lymphoid system rather natural killing is a function of different lymphoid subpopulations dependent upon the microenvironment. For their attack they do not require antibodies and unlike cytotoxic T cells they do not seem to have an immunological memory and MHC restriction. NK cells can lyse a wide variety of target cells, which can be allogeneic and autolog. The surface phenotyp of this population shows heterogeneity of the marker. They have receptors for Fc and some mediators as IFN and Il 2. These two mediators augment the lysis of target cells, while immune complexes and some metabolites may down regulate the effect. The cytotoxic reaction is mainly measured by testing the immune cells against NK sensitive cell lines, breast carcinoma lines included. The summary of several publications reveals a good cytotoxicity of NK cells in breast cancer patients up to stage II of the disease. Only some special results should be mentioned here. Blanchard et al (17) showed cytotoxic activity in a Cr 51 release assay in effusions from metastatic breast carcinoma after exposure to Il 2. The activity was found in cells carrying predominantly the phenotyps of CD 2 and CD 16, indicating natural killer/lymphokine activated cells. Bonilla (18) demonstrated NK activity in peripheral blood of breast cancer patients but not in regional lymphnodes. A. Hakim (19) divided PBMs in subpopulations by density gradient and panning. T helper cells and NK cells from stage IV breast cancer patients did not respond to PHA stimulation in comparison to those from stage I patients and healthy adults. Furthermore he found in the same patient group a less significant reaction of the NK cells to Il 2. Binding experiments with J 125-Il 2 revealed a loss of Il 2 receptor. An analysis of the enriched RNA profiles indicated a reduction of the mRNA fraction encoding the Il 2 in these cells.

Lymphokine activated killer cells

Recently lymphokine activated killer cells (LAK) are discussed very frequently, especially because they show functions in immunotherapy. LAK precursor seem to belong to NK cells as well as to T cells. An Il 2 activation is necessary for their production. In vitro tumor cells and supernatants from primary tumor cell cultures can inhibit their production. LAK activity is measured similarly to NK activity, however both - NK resistent and sensitive cell lines - are targets for the cytotoxic reaction. Bonilla (18) showed such LAK activity in regional lymphnodes of breast cancer patients after long term incubation (5 days) in vitro with Il 2, whereby the originally low number of cells with the NK marker Leu 11 (CD 16) and Leu 7 (CD 57) did not increase (see above).

Mediators (Lymphokines, Cytokines)

Immune cell derived mediators, which modify the function of other immune cells (as for example lymphocyte derived lymphokines), are important tools in the interaction of the different cells. They are used in the laboratory for testing all kinds of immune reactions. For a long time and even still to day leucocyte migration and leucocyte adhasion inhibition tests were used in immune monitoring of breast carcinoma. Their reaction is not identical but both measure the production of distinct mediators, at least from different cell populations. The leucocyte migration inhibition (LMI) test was regularly used by the Herberman group (12) and the antigen induced leucocyte adhasion inhibition (LAI) test was adapted to a so called tube test by Grosser et al (20). 47 breast cancer patients were compared in their LAI reaction to 32 controls. 40 patients showed significant adhasion inhibition, while no control was positive. From further 223 patients stage I and II breast cancer 85 % were positiv in this test, while only 45 % of 34 patients stage III and 29 % of 103 women with stage IV breast cancer gave positive results. A serum blocking factor is described that abrogates the LAI reactivity (21). Tsang et al (22) confirm these results and speak about an organ specific blocking factor, which masks the receptor on the effector cells. Fink et al (23) also found inhibition in the LAI test in 80 % of stage I and II breast cancer and 38 % of stage III and IV. Since the last authors used supernatant of breast cancer cell cultures as an antigen and since there was no inhibition, when other tissue cultures´ medium was used, an organ specific neo antigen is discussed as the source for the leucocyte sensitization. In general the LAI test had turned out to be handled with some difficulties and only skilled technical people were able to do it routinely.

Cellulare Immunity as a Prognostic Factor

The number of tumor cell positive lymphnodes and the size of the tumor at primary surgery are accepted clinical prognostic signs. Monitoring, which will follow changes in immunological parameters, can bring new prognostic criteria. Infiltration of the tumor with lymphocytes, discussed already above, is one of them. However criteria not dependent upon the biopsy are also needed. To illustrate this point some examples are given.

Black (24) showed by the skin window assay an in vivo reaction as prognostic favorable. This procedure involves the application of a coverslip, covered with the autologous tumor or with glycoprotein 55, to the scarified skin for approximately 30 hours. The coverslip is removed, stained and the extent of infiltrating cells is counted. From 267 postoperatively tested patients 80 developed metastasis in the time of 5 years. From these 80 only 17 showed a strong infiltration of immune cells on the coverslip, while from the 187 without metastasis 104 (56 %) were positive in this test.
Monitoring in vivo represents a burden to the patient, therefore it was looked for in vitro tests, which will employ peripheral blood lymphocytes (PBL). Cannon et al (25) published a comparison of the post surgery lymphoproliferative response of PBLs to autologous tumor extract (ATL) and allogeneic lymphocytes (MLC) with death after 10 years. The clinical risk factor of the patients revealed no evidence of metastasis beyond lymphnodes. Histological lymphnode positivity, a low ATL and high MLC corresponded to death in 73 %, while in the LN positive patient group with high ATL and low MLC no death occured (0/12 patients).

Changes in cellmediated immunity during and after therapy

In the years 1971-1976 900 Swedish breast cancer patients were divided into three equal groups: radiotherapy pre surgery, radiotherapy post surgery and surgery alone (26). These patients were initially tested for several immunological reactions, followed up and tested again in intervalls. After ten years 138 of these patients were examined for their lymphocyte and 107 also for their subpopulation count. The two radiotherapy groups were compared to the surgery alone group. It was shown that the two radiotherapy groups have still a

depression of the lymphocyte count. This was mainly attributed to a significant reduction of the helper T cells (p=0,005-0,001). Besides, lymphocytes from patients of this study were stimulated with PHA and Con A and in a mixed lymphocyte culture at diagnosis, within one month and 6-10 months after completion of radiation. For at least a decade the mitogen response was signifcantly lower in the irradiated compared to the unirradiated patient group. Mortality up to 8 years after irradiation was higher in the group with a low PHA response. The authors discuss that the irradiation induced decrease in mitogenic response is partly dependent upon an increase of lymphocyte with suppressor function since Con A inducible suppressor activity was found in the lymphocytes of irradiated breast cancer patients. The same authors also describe the possibility that the prostaglandin production by monocytes increases and causes so the immunosuppression (27).
Berger (28) analysed the alloantigen specific T lymphocyte precursor (CTLp) frequency in 10 patients with histological proven breast cancer, who received prophylactic radiotherapy. A 25 % decrease was seen immediately after irradiation. Values subsequently returned to pretreatment levels in the time of more than three months.

The effect of chemotherapy on the immune system must not always have a deteriorating effect. In some cases it even helps to activate the immune system. One example is cyclophosphamide, which can selectively damage T suppressor cells. This way positive anticancer response prevails. Most often however the chemotherapy harm the immune system. The NK activity of 83 breast cancer patients after chemotherapy in comparison to 24 healthy controls was measured by Bonilla (29). The NK activity was similar in both groups before chemotherapy of the patient group. Thereafter, inspide of no change in the cell count, the NK activity in the Cr 51 release assay went down (p=00,5) in the patients.

Tichatschek et al (30) shows a decrease of NK activity after 6 courses of CMF. In vitro stimulation with IFN and Il 2 did not convert the decrease. Also, the proliferative response to PHA and the production of sIl 2 receptor in response to this mitogen decreased in these patients.

Brenner (31) found low native and inducible natural killer activity of the peripheral blood lymphocytes in breast cancer patients after chemotherapy in comparison to nontreated patients. When the absolute number of the peripheral lymphocytes was depressed before therapy the decrease of the NK activity was even more pronounced.

Hormon therapy is mostly represented by the antiestrogen tamoxifen, which competes directly with estrogens for the receptor. There are some indications that such receptors are also on lymphocytes; so the interaction of this therapy with the immune system deserves some interest. Rotstein et al (32) found no changes in the cellular composition and amound of the immune cells in 23 patients after adjuvant tamoxifen. The proliferative response to Con A was high, while the NK activity against K562 was low. Scambia et al (33) found only a slight reduction of the CD4+/CD8+ ratio in 20 tamoxifen treated patients versus non treated persons. However during medroxyprogesteron acetate (MPA) treatment the decrease of the percentage of CD4+ cells was more pronounced. Also in this last patient group the response to PHA was reduced sharply. This inhibition of lymphocyte activation by PHA was restored, when Il 2 was added to the culture medium. The authors postulate an alteration of immuno competence by administration of high dose MPA. Valavaara (34) tested a new drug, toremefen, and found significant lower CD4+ cells, while the overall T cell count did not change. The mitogen stimulation of the patient´s lymphocytes increased in a follow up study during therapy, indicating a stimulatory effect of the drug on cell mediated immunity. Valavaara did not find any changes in NK cell cytotoxicity but Berry et al (35) showed an increase of the average NK cell activity of 17 patients during tamoxifen treatment. By others (36) such high NK cell activity was shown only in those patients, whose breast cancer had a high estrogen receptor content.

Immunotherapy

For some solid tumors as melanoma and renal cell carcinoma both types of immunotherapy - nonspecific and specific - show therapeutical success in a relative high percentage. Such results could not be expected in a tumor, histologically so heterogenous as breast carcinoma. Nevertheless combination of nonspecific immunostimulation with common therapy for breast cancer is an often used approach. A recent German publication (37) shows the use of a synthetic thymopentin (Timunox) in combination with chemotherapy. In comparison to patients receiving chemotherapy only those patients benefited by the approach, who had a limited spread of the disease. The benefit was seen in the clinical outcome. Treatment with another nonspecific stimulant, OK 432 (a lyophilized preparation from Streptococcus pyogenes, treated with penicillin G) also produces some objective positive results. In the here mentioned design (38) the treatment is combined with the transfer of autologous lymphokine activated lymphocytes. The aim was to treat liver metastasis of breast cancer. 9 of 14 patients responded with regression of the liver metastasis after intraarterial infusion. 4 patients had also regression of metastasis in other organs.

The in vitro stimulation of lymphocytes with Il 2 can be considered as a combination of nonspecific and specific. Il 2, mainly in high concentrations, stimulates lymphocytes with a broad spectrum of activity. However the already by the tumor prestimulated lymphocytes can have an increased concentration of Il 2 receptors and so respond better to stimulation. This presumption was used by Skornick et al (39) to stimulate lymphoid cells, infiltrating the tumor and from draining lymphnodes, because a higher proportion of tumor reactive lymphocytes can be here expected than in peripheral blood. From four breast cancer patients the in vitro properties of these cells revealed an increase in the amount of CD4+ cells over CD8+ cells in the time up to around 100 days. The early cultures demonstrated nonspecific cytotoxic activity against allogeneic tumor targets, while in one patient specific cytolytic activity occured after long time incubation (> 70 days). As mentioned above a preparation is possible of specific T cell clones against clones from single breast cancer cells. These clones were obtained with the help of low dose Il 2. The difficulty of immunotherapy in breast cancer is stressed by the fact that within a tumor cell clones exist with a different specificity. Therefore one case report should be mentioned (40). A patient with scirrhous breast cancer could not be treated with chemotherapy. An immunological approach was tried: PBLs were cocultivated with mitomycin treated autologous tumor and Il 2. The patient received cyclophosphamid to suppress the T suppressor cells prior to reinfusion of CTLs in intervalls of 1-2 weeks. The size of the tumor reduced.

Another approach of a specific immunotherapy is the immunization with tumorantigen(s) directly. Since the antigen(s) are ill defined in the case of breast cancer two possibilities are tested clinically. In Germany one trial uses Newcastle disease virus infected irradiated autologous tumor cells as a vaccine. There are several pilot studies only. The other possibility uses the fact that antiidiotype antibodies can represent an inner image of the tumor associated antigen. So these antibodies can be employed for vaccination. Such approach was tested in many experimental tumors and extensively by Koprowski (41) for colon carcinoma. To look for such possibility in breast cancer one should select patients with known autologous antibodies against their tumor. The feasibility of such approach was demonstrated in the rat model with mammary carcinoma (42).

References:

1. Black, M.M., Leis, H.P. N.Y. State J. Med. 70:2583, 1970
2. Foote, F.W., Stewart, F.W. Surgery 19:74, 1946
3. Moore, O.S., Foote, F.W. Cancer 2:635, 1949
4. Hamlin, J. Brit. J. Cancer 22:383, 1968
5. Black, M.M., Opler, S.R., Speer, F.D. Surg. Gynecol Obstet 100:543, 1955
6. Berg, J.W. Cancer 12:714, 1959
7. Whitford, P., Malcon, E.A., George, W.D. et al. Brit. J. Cancer 62:971, 1990
8. Bilik, R., Mor, C., Hazaz, B. et al. Cancer Immunol Immunother. 28:143, 1989
9. von Kleist, S., Berling, J., Bohle, W. et al. Int. J. Cancer 40:18, 1987
10. Shukla, H.S., Hughes, L.E., Whitehead, R.M. et al. Cancer Immunol. Immunother. 21:6, 1986
11. Koldovsky, U., Perschmann, U., Feldhammer, B. Aktuelle Onkologie 42:27, 1987

12. Dean, J.M., McCoy, J.L., Cannon, G.B. et al. J. Natl. Cancer Inst. 58:549, 1977
13. Jerrells, T., Dean, J., Herberman, R. Int. J. Cancer 21:282, 1978
14. Hoon, D., Korn, E., Chochran A. Cancer Research 47:1740, 1987
15. Sato, T., Sato, N., Takahashi, S. et al. Cancer Res. 46:4384, 1986
16. Kaieda, T., Imawari, M., Yamasaki, Z. et al. Cancer Res. 48:4848, 1988
17. Blanchard, D.K., Kavanagh, J.J., Sinkovics, J.G. Cancer Res. 48:6321, 1988
18. Bonilla, F., Alvarez-Mon, M., Merino, F. et al. Cancer 61:629, 1988
19. Hakim, A. Cancer 61:689, 1988
20. Grosser, N., Thomson, D.M.P. Cancer Res. 35:2571, 1975
21. Flores, M., Marti, J.H., Grosser, N. et al. Cancer 39:494, 1977
22. Tsang, P.H., Roboz, J.P., Holland, J.F. Immunol. Lett. 17:63, 1988
23. Fink, A., Shani, A., Feldman, B. Eur. J. Surg. Onkol. 15:17, 1989
24. Black, M., Zachrau, R., Hanky, B. et al. Cancer 62:72, 1988
25. Cannon, B.G., Pomeranz, R. Int. J. Cancer 44:995, 1989
26. Wasserman, J., Walegren, A., Blomgren, H. Cancer 58:348, 1986
27. Wasserman, J., Blomgren, H., Rotstein, S. et al. Bull. N.Y. Acad. Med. 65: 36, 1989
28. Berger, M., Irschick, E., Fritsch, E. et al. Immunobiology 180:261, 1990
29. Bonilla, F., Alvarez-Mon, M., Merino, F. Eur. J. Gynecol. Oncol. 11:103, 1990

30. Tichatschek, E., Zielinski, C.C., Müller, C.M. Cancer Immunol. Immunother. 27:278, 1988
31. Brenner, B.G., McGrea, E.L., Margolese, R.G. Anticancer Res. 8:653, 1988
32. Rotstein, S., Blomgren, A., Petrini, B. et al. Breast Cancer Res. Treat. 12:75, 1988
33. Scambia, G., Panici, P.B., Maccio, A. et al. Cancer 61:2214, 1988
34. Valavaara, R., Tuominen, J., Toivanen, A. Cancer Immunol. Immunother. 31:381, 1990
35. Berry, J., Green, B.J., Matheson, D. Eur. J. Cancer Clin. Oncol. 23:517, 1987
36. Zielinski., C.C., Tichatschek, E., Müller, C.H. et al. Cancer 63:1985, 1989
37. Mallmann, P., Krebs, D. Methods Final. Exp. Clin. Pharmacol. 12:333, 1990
38. Okino, T., Kann, N., Nakanishi, M. et al. J. Cancer Res. Clin. Oncol. 116:197, 1990
39. Skornick, Y., Topalian, S., Rosenberg, S. J. Biol. Response Mod. 9:431, 1990
40. Kitzukawa, K. Gan-To-Kagaku-Ryoho (English abstract) 16:1448, 1989
41. Koprowski, H., Herlyn, D., Lubeck, M. et al. Proc. Natl. Acad. Sci. 81:216, 1984
42. Smordinsky, N.I., Ghendler, Y., Bakima, R. et al. Eur. J. Immunol. 18:1713, 1988

NEW APPROACHES TO THE STUDY OF SELENIUM'S CHEMOPREVENTIVE PROPERTIES

D. MEDINA, R. MUKHOPADHYAY AND M. BANSAL

Department of Cell Biology, Baylor College of Medicine, Houston, Texas USA 77030

INTRODUCTION

Selenium (Se) compounds, both inorganic and organic, are potent inhibitors of mammary cancer in rodent model systems (1). The new organic compounds, such as selenobetaine and selenomethylseleno-cysteine are more effective than Na_2SeO_3 on a ppm basis (1,2). The salient features of selenium-mediated inhibition of mammary carcinogenesis appear to be the reversibility of the inhibition and the effectiveness of the compounds during either initiation or promotion stages (3). The reversibility of selenium's inhibitory effect is also observed during Se-mediated inhibition of mammary cell growth _in vitro_ (3). The basis of the inhibition of mammary carcinogenesis _in situ_ and cell growth _in vitro_ is not understood. Although several mechanisms of Se-mediated inhibition have been proposed, i.e., the modulation of DNA synthesis (4), RNA synthesis (5) and glutathione metabolism (6), the evidence of any of these having a central role is not extensive.

It is well-established that selenium binds and/or labels several cellular proteins (7). Other than glutathione peroxidase and Type 1 thyronine deiodinase, the nature and function of many of these proteins is unknown. In this review, two proteins which retain selenium avidly are discussed with respect to their characteristics and possible role in selenium-mediated inhibition of mammary carcinogenesis.

SELENOPROTEINS

Mammary cells grown in cell culture with medium containing ^{75}Se or organs collected from mice injected with ^{75}Se will contain a small number of proteins, 9-11, which avidly retain the selenium upon electrophoresis (8-10). Figure 1 illustrates the number and molecular weights of proteins in several organs collected from a mouse (8).

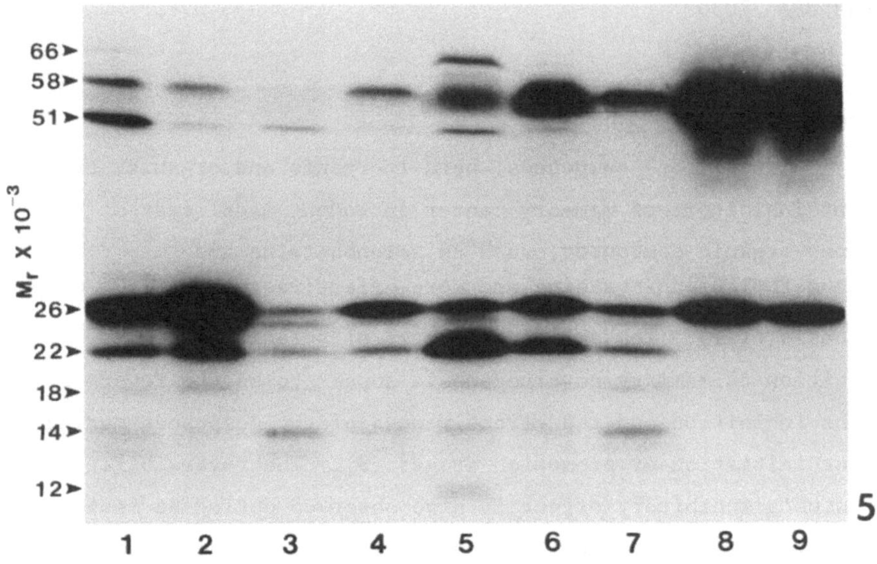

Figure 1. 1D-PAGE of selenoproteins from tissues labeled in vivo with $^{75}SeO_3$. One hundred μg of protein were loaded in each lane. Lanes 1, liver; 2, kidney; 3, pancreas; 4, stomach; 5, testis; 6, mammary gland; 7, mammary tumor; 8, plasma from a male; 9, plasma from a female.

The number and molecular weights of the proteins from the different organs is surprisingly similar. Several of the proteins, the 58 Kd, 26 Kd and 14 Kd are also observed in mammary epithelial cells grown in monolayer cell culture (8). Two of these proteins, the 58 Kd and 14 Kd, have been purified by a combination of gel filtration, ion-exchange, affinity chromatography and SDS-PAGE (11,

12). The characteristics of each of the two proteins is discussed in detail.

14,000 dalton selenium-labeled protein

A 14 Kd protein isolated from mouse liver was specific to liver. Polyclonal antibodies generated against purified 14 Kd protein recognized a protein only in liver and not in mammary gland or other organs, even though a selenium-labeled protein of 14 Kd is present in other organs (13). The explanation for this organ-specificity was obtained upon amino acid sequencing of the protein. The liver 14 Kd protein was identified as fatty acid binding protein (FABP), a family of proteins which includes liver, intestine, cardiac FABP'S, retinoic acid binding protein, myelin protein P2, adipocyte lipid binding protein, fibroblast growth regulator-soluble and mammary derived growth inhibitor (MDGI) (12). The two interesting features about this widespread family of proteins were the multiple ligand-binding properties of these molecules and the presence of at least 2 growth inhibitory molecules (i.e. MDGI, FGR-s). The MDGI was isolated from bovine and has only recently been shown to be present in mouse mammary gland (14, 15). It had previously been demonstrated that antibodies to liver FABP did not recognize other FABP's, whereas antibodies to cardiac FABP recognized proteins in mammary gland and adipocytes (16, 17). In recognition of the organ specificity of the liver protein, the 14 Kd proteins from virgin, pregnant and lactating rodent mammary glands were isolated, purified and sequenced at the amino acid level (18). The protein from virgin mouse mammary gland (which is 90% adipocyte cells) was 100% homologous along a 48 amino acid stretch to adipocyte lipid binding protein (ALBP). ALBP is roughly 65% homologous to rat cardiac FABP (19). The protein from lactating mouse mammary gland was 97% homologous to murine MDGI (15). The latter appears to be the major 14 Kd protein in the differentiated mouse mammary gland. Although murine MDGI is highly homologous to cardiac FABP (> 90%), there are at least 8 amino acid substitutions which distinguish between the two proteins. Interestingly, the protein isolated from pregnant rat mammary gland was 100% homologous to rat cardiac FABP over the

40 amino acid region that was sequenced. A similar finding was reported by Jones et al (16) who isolated the FABP for lactating rat mammary gland. The proteins from mammary gland bind long chain unsaturated fatty acids as well as selenium. It remains an unanswered question whether the 14 Kd protein from rat is the only species and if it is functionally homologous to MDGI. Also unanswered is the question if and how selenium interacts with the protein and interferes with its function. At this time, it is intriguing that selenium binds avidly to proteins which have growth inhibitory properties.

56,000 dalton selenium-labeled protein

The antiserum to the 56 Kd protein (originally described as 58 Kd in Figure 1) recognized a 56 Kd protein in liver, kidney, mammary gland, pancreas, testis and ovary but did not detect a protein signal in mouse muscle or plasma (13). The absence of the protein in muscle and plasma is intriguing since both body compartments accumulate high levels of selenium. In plasma, a 57 Kd protein (selenoprotein P) is present and easily identifiable as a selenium-binding protein (20). It is evident from the immunological and nucleotide sequencing data that the two proteins are distinct.

The cDNA which codes for the 56,000 Kd protein was cloned and sequenced for a λ/Zap mouse liver library (21). A significant portion of the protein (58%) was also sequenced at the amino acid level. The primary sequence has not been reported previously in any DNA data bank. Interestingly, the cDNA sequence did not contain an in-frame TGA codon that would code for selenocysteines, as occurs in prototypic selenoproteins. Hydropathy analysis suggested the protein was not a membrane spanning protein which was consistent with previous observations that the 56 Kd protein was a cytosolic protein(22). Inspection of the cDNA sequence revealed the presence of 9 potential phosphorylation sites on the molecule. As shown on Table 1 below, these sites include 3 protein kinase C sites, 5 casein kinase 2 sites and one tyrosine site.

Table 1. Predicted modification sites on the 56 Kd protein.

Amino Acid Number	Modification
132 -> 136	ASN-GLYCOSYLATION
87 -> 90	PKC-PHOSPHO-SITE
101 -> 104	PKC-PHOSPHO-SITE
295 -> 298	PKC-PHOSPHO-SITE
14 -> 18	CK2-PHOSPHO-SITE
36 -> 40	CK2-PHOSPHO-SITE
151 -> 155	CK2-PHOSPHO-SITE
316 -> 320	CK2-PHOSPHO-SITE
407 -> 411	CK2-PHOSPHO-SITE

The results so far indicate that SLP-56 is a unique protein, potentially phosphorylated, and represents a selenium-labeled protein distinct from GSH-Px with respect to the nature of selenium-binding.

The gene for 56 Kd is apparently well conserved in evolution since DNA regions amplified by PCR occur in genomic DNA of Aspergillus, Drosophila, Xenopus, rabbit, hamster and human (Mukhopadhyay and Medina, unpublished observations). Messenger RNA was readily detectable using a 0.9 Kb probe on Northern or slot blots in a variety of organs (Figure 2). The mRNA was detectable in liver, kidney, mammary gland (pregnant and lactating) and ovary, whereas only a very small amount was detected in muscle. The mRNA showed 2 message sizes in liver (1.6 Kb and the predicted 1.5 Kb) whereas only one (1.5 Kb) was detected in kidney, mammary gland and ovary.

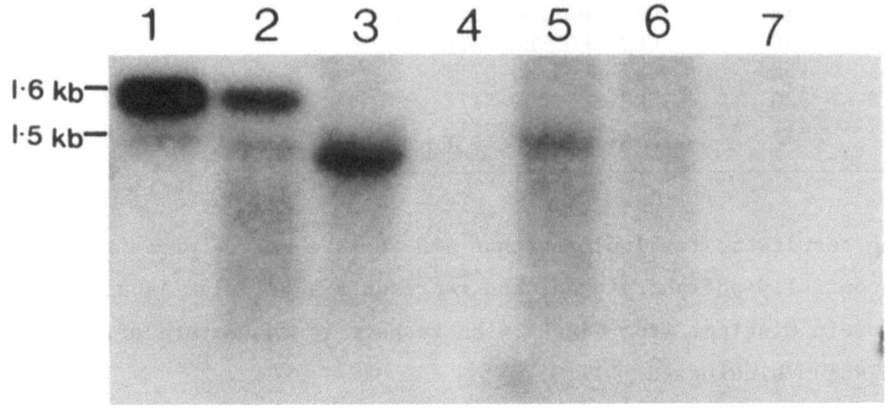

Figure 2. Northern blot analysis of RNA from mouse tissues. Two message size were observed (1.6 and 1.5 Kb). The lanes from left to right are liver (male), liver (female), kidney, heart, lung, small intestine and ovary.

CONCLUSIONS

There is a vast amount of convincing data on the chemopreventive efficacy of selenium compounds. The new generation of selenium compounds emphasize organic compounds which are more efficacious that Na_2SeO_3. The new organic compounds enter the same metabolic pathway of Na_2SeO_3 although at different entry points. Despite the relative good understanding of the metabolism of selenium compounds, the cellular events and macromolecules modified or influenced by selenium are relatively unknown. Although DNA synthesis appears to be one critical cellular events which is reversibly inhibited by selenium compounds, the molecular pathways between the introduction of selenium into the cell on one end and the inhibition of DNA synthesis on the other end remain a black box. The two proteins discussed here which avidly retain selenium have characteristics of proteins involved in growth regulatory processes. For this reason, they are of interest. The 14 Kd protein is a member of the FABF and recently has been identified as a growth inhibitor for the mammary gland. The 56 Kd protein is a novel protein with multiple phosphorylation sites. Phosphorylation of proteins and protein kinases play a pivotal role in signal transduction pathways as well as the pathways involved in DNA synthesis and mitosis (23, 24). In addition, the interactions between selenium and phosphorylated amino acids are deemed critical to selenium modification of amino acids (25). In the future, the central questions would appear to be if one or both proteins exhibit growth inhibitory (or stimulatory) effects on mammary cell growth and how selenium modulates the properties and functions of these proteins. In any event, the study of these two proteins (and other selenium-labeled proteins) offers a new and untraveled avenue in the study of selenium biology and function.

REFERENCES

1. Ip, C., Hayes, C., Budnick, R.M. and Ganther, H.E. Cancer Res. 51:595-600, 1991.
2. Ip, C. and Ganther, H. Cancer Res. 50:1206-1211, 1990.
3. Medina, D. and Morrison, D.G. Pathol. Immunopathol. Res. 7:187-199, 1988.
4. Medina, D. and Oborn, C.J. Cancer Res. 44:4361-4365, 1988.
5. Frenkel, G.D. and Falvey, D. Biochem. Pharmacol. 38:2176-2183, 1989.
6. LeBoeuf, R.A. and Hoekstra, W.G. J. Nut. 113:845-854, 1983.
7. Stadtman, T.C. Ann. Rev. Biochem. 59:111-127, 1990.
8. Danielson, K.G. and Medina, D. Cancer Res. 46:4582-4589, 1986.
9. Evenson, J.K. and Sunde, R.A. Proc. Soc. Expt. Biol. Med. 187:169-180, 1988.
10. Behne, D., Hilmert, H., Scheid, S., Gessna, H. and Elger, W. Biochem. Biophys. Acta 966:12-21, 1988.
11. Bansal, M.P., Oborn, C.J. Danielson, K.G. and Medina, D. Carcinogenesis 10:541-546, 1989.
12. Bansal, M.P., Cook, R.G., Danielson, K.G. and Medina, D. J. Biol. Chem. 264:13780-13784, 1989.
13. Morrison, D.G., Bansal, M.P., Kittrell, F. and Medina, D. In Vivo 3:167-172, 1989.
14. Kurtz, A., Vogel, F., Funa, K., Heldin, C-H. and Grosse, R. J. Cell Biol. 110:1779-1789, 1990.
15. Grosse, R. In: Breast Cancer: Cellular and Molecular Biology. R. Dickson and M. Lippman (eds), in press.

16. Jones, P.D., Carne, A., Bass, N.M. and Grigor, M.R. Biochem.. J. 251:919-925, 1988.

17. Bohmer, F.D., Sun, Q., Pepperle, M., Muller, T., Erikson, U., Wang, J.L. and Grosse, R. Biochem. Biophys. Res. Commun. 148:1425-1431, 1987.

18. Bansal, M.P., Oborn, C.J., Cook, R. and Medina, D. submitted for publication.

19. Matarese, V. and Bernlohr, D.A. J. Biol. Chem. 263:14544-14551, 1988.

20. Burk, R.F. J. Nutrition 119:1051-1054, 1989.

21. Bansal, M.P., Mukhopadhyay, R., Scott, J., Cook, R.G., Mukhopadhyay, R. and Medina, D. Carcinogenesis 11:2071-2073, 1990.

22. Morrison, D.G., Berdan, R.C., Pauly, D.F., Turner, D.S., Oborn, C.J. and Medina, D. Anticancer Res. 8:51-64, 1988.

23. Boulton, T.G. and Cobb, M.H. Cell Regulation 2:357-371, 1991.

24. Pines, J. Cell Growth Differentiation 2:305-310, 1991.

25. Lee, B.J., Worland, P.J., Davis, J.N., Stadtman, J.C. and Hatfield, D.L. J. Biol. Chem. 264:9724-9728, 1989.

SECTION VI

BIOLOGICAL FACTORS OF PROGNOSIS; THE METASTATIC PHENOTYPE

CELL KINETICS AS AN INDICATOR FOR PROGNOSIS AND THERAPY

R. SILVESTRINI

Oncologia Sperimentale C, Istituto Nazionale per lo Studio e la Cura dei Tumori, 20133 Milan, Italy.

The growing interest in breast cancer biology and the development of sophisticated technical approaches have contributed in the last few decades to a substantial increase in the knowledge at cellular and molecular levels of the different steps of disease progression. Several markers indicative of biologic aggressiveness have been identified (1), and some of them will pass as valid prognostic indicators from the laboratory bench to widespread clinical utilization.

In addition to the traditionally used pathologic prognostic factors, cellular markers peculiar for this malignancy, such as hormone receptors, or common to all neoplasms, such as rate of cell proliferation and DNA content abnormalities, were first proposed. More recently, molecular markers have been identified, such as qualitative and quantitative alterations in the expression of specific genes (HER-2/neu, p53, nm23) or proteins (cathepsin D, pS2, srp).

Most of these biologic markers are independent of the preclinical history of the tumor, in terms of local, regional and distant spread at the time of diagnosis. Conversely, most of them are related and their integration could provide a coherent picture of the successive steps of clinical progression of the malignancy.

Tumors that present at diagnosis with a rapid proliferative rate generally do not express hormone receptors and exhibit an aneuploid DNA content, which reflects considerable genomic alterations in terms of gene amplification or deletions. Conversely, present findings suggest the absence of a relation between most biologic factors and the expression of cathepsin D, a lysosomal protease which seems to be the most promising prognostic indicator among the molecular markers, as independently shown by recent, preliminary reports (2-4). If these results are confirmed and prospectively validated, the consideration of cathepsin D in addition to other markers already used in clinical practice, namely cell proliferative rate, hormone receptors and ploidy, could synergistically increase the prognostic power of biologic indicators.

Among the many biologic factors that have provided reliable information for breast cancer prognosis, cell kinetics has gained a prominent role. In fact, the availability of specific reagents and sophisticated methodologies and the promising results independently obtained in the early eighties by three laboratories on patients with early and advanced disease (5-7) have renewed interest and encouraged in the last decade speculative and applicative studies on cell proliferation. The many proliferation markers available are based on different rationales and are addressed mainly to detect cells synthesizing DNA, i.e., in the cell cycle S-phase, or generally cycling (8). However, such proliferation markers show different degrees of specificity and sensitivity for target cells, and for some of them further research is needed for a better comprehension of their functional role and of their actual relationship with biologic aggressiveness. Conversely, the proliferation indices traditionally used to detect the fraction of cells in S-phase by autoradiography (^{3}H-thymidine labeling index, ^{3}H-dT LI) or by flow-cytometry (FCM-S) have already completed or have been just submitted to the validation process for prognostic markers (9). Such methodologic validation foresees a definitive assessment on substantial series of patients submitted to local-regional treatment alone, to avoid any confounding factors due to the possible efficacy of systemic treatment.

In the last few years, efforts have been made to increase the reliability of FCM-S determination from DNA histograms and to overcome problems limiting its evaluability in aneuploid tumors, which represent the majority (70%) of breast cancers. However, present results do not unequivocally show a significant contribution of FCM-S to prediction of relapse for patients with stage I tumors (table 1). In fact, a review of the literature shows that FCM-S provides no prognostic contribution at all (10,11) or is directly related to the probability to develop a relapse only in diploid tumors (12), only in aneuploid tumors (13), or in both diploid and aneuploid tumors (14). In the latter study, however, about 20% of cases had been treated with adjuvant therapy, mostly hormonal, which could have benefited patients with slowly proliferating, estrogen-receptor-positive tumors, thereby reducing the risk of relapse and death.

Table 1. Clinical outcome related to FCM-S in patients with stage I breast cancer

Authors	Follow-up (years)	Survival (%) Relapse-free FCM-S Low	Inter-mediate	High	p	Overall FCM-S Low	Inter-mediate	High	p
Daidone et al.	3	77	-	77	ns				
Muss et al.	5	78		67	ns	87	-	70	0.04
Clark et al.[1]	5	90	-	70	<0.01	90	-	85	0.01
O'Reilly et al.[2]	5	78	-	52	0.006				
Sigurdsson et al.	4	89	81	69	<0.01	99	91	78	<0.01

[1]Diploid
[2]Aneuploid

On the whole, these controversial results emphasize the need for further studies focused on the optimization and standardization of modeling systems used to quantify FCM-S. In fact, results may be markedly affected by the mathematical approach used (planimetric or other complex mathematical functions) and by methodologic (presence of debris and doublets, recovery of cells from paraffin blocks or frozen specimens) or biologic conditions (multiclonality, presence of abnormal clones near the diploid region). The relative contribution of all these factors on the prognostic resolution should be carefully assessed before FCM-S is routinely introduced in clinical practice as a proliferation marker for prognosis.

In fact, an ideal marker should be feasible, biologically reliable, assessable on most tumors, reproducible and subjected to a quality control, which directs clinicians toward a network of credible laboratories that provide biologic data. These requirements are essential for the activation of multicentric clinical protocols, which prospectively select patients and treatments on the basis of biologic data.

Table 2. Clinical outcome related to ^{3}H-dT LI in patients with stage I breast cancer

Authors	Follow-up (years)	Survival (%) Relapse-free ^{3}H-dT LI Low	High	p	Overall ^{3}H-dT LI Low	High	p
Tubiana et al.[1]	15	75	43	<0.02	75	43	<0.02
Hery et al.	8	83	56	<0.02	100	36	<0.002
Silvestrini et al.	6	78	60	<0.0001	95	82	<0.0001
Meyer et al.	5	80	60	<0.001	89	65	<0.001

[1]Including patients with stage II and III cancers, given only local-regional therapy

Proliferative rate as measured by ^{3}H-dT LI has been found by several laboratories to be an important predictor of relapse and survival in stage I (table 2) and II tumors (15-19). In patients with early disease and/or subjected to only local-regional treatment, the probability to develop local-regional or distant metastases in all the published reports is about two-fold higher for patients with rapidly proliferating than for those with slowly proliferating tumors. ^{3}H-dT LI retains it predictive role even in the presence of the prognostic information obtained from tumor size, nodal involvement, histologic grade or hormone receptors. The prognostic contribution of proliferative activity could be further potentiated by considering it in association with other biologic aspects, such as hormone receptors or ploidy, or biologic factors independent of proliferative rate such as cathepsin D.

In view of the increasing interest in cell kinetics in clinical practice and of the activation of multicenter clinical protocols based or this biologic variable, we proposed to guarantee the past reproducibility of results by activating an inter- and intralaboratory quality control. This quality control is already operative for ^{3}H-dT LI and will begin shortly for FCM-S. The cross-blind evaluation has led to the demonstration of a high reproducibility among and within the different laboratories (20).

Once the validity of proliferation indices as markers to identify high-risk patients has been demonstrated, the subsequent step is to evaluate their usefulness to select tumors responsive to specific therapies or to recognize treatment modalities markedly effective on subsets of tumors differing for the proliferative pattern. No results are yet available from the recently begun clinical protocols prospectively designed on the basis of cell kinetics to assess the relation between proliferative rate and response to specific systemic treatments in breast cancer. Consequently, information can be derived only from retrospective analyses.

Indirect proof of the need for aggressive treatment for rapidly proliferating tumors has been observed in different clinical situations. In patients with node-negative estrogen-receptor-negative and rapidly proliferating tumors, an advantage in 7-year relapse-free survival was observed following treatment with surgery + adjuvant CMF over surgery alone (21). In patients with 1-3 node-positive, rapidly proliferating operable tumors, 5-year relapse-free survival was significantly higher following full CMF dose than lower dosages (22). Finally, in patients with stage II and III tumors (table 3), the objective clinical response was higher in rapidly proliferating cancers treated by polychemotherapy regimens including specific S-phase antimetabolites than two non-specific S-phase and cross-resistant drugs such as doxorubicin and vincristine (23-25).

As regards endocrine therapy, slowly proliferating indolent tumors appear to be the subset which maximally benefit (table 3). However, the finding of a higher response rate in advanced, slowly proliferating tumors than in rapidly proliferating tumors (26) cannot be ascribed only to the inverse relation between ER content and proliferative rate (27), since it was further confirmed in a larger subset of only ER+ tumors (28). Thus a high proliferative activity is responsible for failure to respond to endocrine therapy also in ER+ tumors.

Table 3. Objective clinical response[1] by cell kinetics

Authors	Stage	Treatment	Clinical response (%)		
			Proliferative rate[2]		
			Low	High	p
Silvestrini et al.	III	AV	50	50	ns
Sulkes et al.	IV	FAC±V	18	82	0.01
Remvikos et al.	II-III	FAC	46	89	0.004
Meyer et al.	IV	Hormonal	60	10	0.05
Paradiso et al.[3]	III-IV	Hormonal	88	46	0.05

[1] Tumor shrinkage >50%
[2] FCM-S for Sulkes, ^{3}H-dT LI for all the others
[3] Only ER^{+} tumors

The outcome of all the studies presently available in the literature is definitely in favor of a relevant role of cell kinetics, mainly confirmed for ^{3}H-dT LI, in the clinical management of breast cancer patients. Such evidence derives mostly from the validation process for prognosis, already completed for ^{3}H-dT LI, and in part from the emerging findings which indicate the rate of cell proliferation as a marker of differential response to different treatments. However, such encouraging findings should not be translated into a widespread use of any proliferative index proposed in the literature. All the recently proposed markers of proliferation should undergo the validation process already completed for ^{3}H-dT LI, which consists of biologic and methodologic assessments and optimization of cutoff values. This should be done by clinical validations with definitive studies on substantial and unselected case series and by reproducibility tests (9). In the absence of a clinical validation, new markers characterized by low cost, simplicity or rapidity could be introduced in clinical practice once they have shown a high agreement with other consolidated parameters such as ^{3}H-dT LI, which still represents the "gold standard" of clinically oriented proliferation studies.

Further efforts are needed to better define the cost-benefit ratio of the prospective use for breast cancer of the framework of biologic information which is integrating clinical and pathologic factors. However, available information supports the use of proliferation markers as a complement to traditional prognostic factors to identify high-risk patients and, possibly, to direct them to the most appropriate treatments.

REFERENCES

1. Merkel, D.E., Osborne, K. Hematol. Oncol. Clin. North. Am. 3:641-652, 1989.
2. Thorpe, S.M., Rochefort, H., Garcia, M., Freiss, G., Christensen, I.J., Khalaf, S., Paolucci, F., Pau, B., Rasmussen, B.B., Rose, C. Cancer Res. 49:6008-6014, 1989.
3. Spyratos, F., Brouillet, J.P., Defrenne, A., Hacene, K., Rouesse, J., Maudelonde, T., Brunet, M., Andrieu, C., Desplaces, A., Rochefort, H. Lancet 11:1115-1118, 1989.
4. Tandon, A.K., Clark, G.M., Chamness, G.C., Chirgwin, J.M., McGuire, W.L. New Engl. J. Med. 322:297-302, 1990.
5. Tubiana, M., Pejovic, M.H., Chavaudra, G., Contesso, G. and Malaise, E.P. Int. J. Cancer 33:441-445, 1984.
6. Gentili, C., Sanfilippo, O. and Silvestrini, R. Cancer 48:974-979, 1981.
7. Meyer, J.S., Friedman, E., McCrate, M.M. and Bauer, W.C. Cancer 51:1879-1886, 1983.
8. Quinn, C.M., Wright, N.A. J. Pathol. 160:93-102, 1990.
9. McGuire, W.L. J. Natl. Cancer. Inst. 83:154-155, 1991.
10. Daidone, M.G., Silvestrini, R., Del Bino, G., Di Fronzo, G. Proceedings of the American Society of Clinical Oncology 10:47,1991.
11. Muss, H., Kute, T.E., Case, L.D., Smith, L.R., Booher, C., Long, R., Kammire, L., Gregory, B., Brockschimidt, J.K. Cancer 64:1894-1900, 1989.
12. Clark, G.M., Dressler, L.G., Owens, M.A., Pounds, G., Oldaker, T., McGuire, W.L. New Engl. J. Med., 320:627-633, 1989.
13. O'Reilly, S.M., Camplejohn, R.S., Barnes, D.M., Millis, R.R., Rubens, R.D., Richards, M.A. J. Clin. Oncol. 8:2040-2046, 1990.
14. Sigurdsson, H., Baldetorp, B., Borg, A., Dalberg, M., Ferno, M., Killander, D., Olsson, H. New Engl. J. Med. 322:1045-1053, 1990.
15. Tubiana, M., Pejovic, M.H., Koscielny, S., Chavaudra, N., Malaise, E. Int. J. Cancer 44:17-22, 1989.

16. Hery, M., Gioanni, J., Lalanne, C.M., Namer, M., Courdi, A. Breast Cancer Res. Treat. 9:207-212, 1987.

17. Meyer, J.S., Province, M. Breast Cancer Res. Treat. 12:91-204, 1988.

18. Silvestrini, R., Daidone, M.G., Valagussa, P., Di Fronzo, G., Mezzanotte, G., Bonadonna, G. Eur. J. Cancer 25:1165-1171, 1989.

19. Silvestrini, R., Daidone, M.G., Valagussa, P., Di Fronzo, G., Mezzanotte, G., Mariani, L. and Bonadonna G. J. Clin. Oncol. 8:1321-1326, 1990.

20. Silvestrini, R. and the SICCAB group for quality control of cell kinetic determination. Cell Proliferation, in press.

21. Bonadonna, G., Valagussa, P., Moliterni, A., Buzzoni, R., Zambetti, M., Ferrari, L., Brambilla, C., Silvestrini, R., Veronesi, U. In: Adjuvant Therapy of Cancer VI (Ed. S.E. Salmon), 1988.

22. Daidone, M.G., Silvestrini, R., Canova, S., Valagussa, P., Bonadonna, G. Proceedings of the American Society of Clinical Oncology 8:24, 1989.

23. Silvestrini, R., Daidone, M.G., Valagussa, P., Salvadori, B., Rovini, D., Bonadonna, G. Cancer Treat. Rep. 71:375-379, 1987.

24. Sulkes, A., Livingston, R.B., Murphy, W.K. J. Natl. Cancer Inst. 62:513-515, 1979.

25. Remvikos, Y., Beuzeboc, P., Zajdela, A., Voillemot, N., Magdelenat, H., Pouillart, P. J. Natl. Cancer Inst. 81:1383-1387, 1989.

26. Meyer, J.S., Lee, J.Y. Cancer Res. 40:1890-1896, 1980.

27. Silvestrini, R., Daidone, M.G., Di Fronzo, G. Cancer 44:665-667, 1979.

28. Paradiso, A., Lorusso, V., Tommasi, S., Schitulli, F., Maiello, E., De Lena, M. Breast Cancer Res. Treat. 11:31-36, 1988.

CATHEPSIN D AND BREAST CANCER METASTASIS : BIOLOGICAL AND CLINICAL SIGNIFICANCE

Marcel GARCIA, Françoise CAPONY and Henri ROCHEFORT

Unité Hormones et Cancer (U 148) INSERM and Laboratoire de Biologie Cellulaire, Faculté de Médecine, 60 Rue de Navacelles, 34090 MONTPELLIER France

Most proteases that have been proposed to play a role in cancer metastasis are secreted and active at neutral pH. By contrast, cathepsins are ubiquitous proteinases that act at acidic pH (<5.5) and their major function is to degrade proteins in the lysosomes (1). Presently, 3 types of cathepsin (B, L and D) are shown to be over expressed and abnormally secreted in cancer cells and might be associated with metastatic potential. We mainly review the case of cathepsin D, whose gene expression is increased by estrogens and growth factors in breast cancer, and which has also been shown to be associated with increased risk of metastatic breast cancer in several independent clinical studies.

1. Cathepsin D gene expression is increased in breast cancer cells compared to normal mammary cells

While the amino acid structure of cathepsin D appears to be identical in breast cancer and normal mammary glands (2-3), its production is much higher in cancer cells which accumulate and secrete this protease more than normal mammary cells (4).

Using monoclonal antibodies and immunoperoxydase staining of frozen tissue sections, cathepsin D concentration was found to be much higher in most breast cancer tissues than in other tissues, including normal mammary cells (4-5). The staining was mostly located within breast cancer cells and not in the connecting tissue. Some macrophages were also stained occasionally. The higher cathepsin D production in cancer cells compared to normal mammary epithelial cells was confirmed at the protein level using immunoassay (4-5), and at the mRNA level by Northern blot analysis (6-7) and in situ hybridization of tumor sections (unpublished results). The 2.2 kb cathepsin D mRNA is induced by estrogen and growth factors in estrogen receptor positive breast cancers, whereas in estrogen receptor negative breast cancers there is a high or moderate constitutive level of this mRNA, which may explain the absence of correlation between cathepsin D and estrogen receptor status in breast cancer tissue (6-8). The mechanism of increased expression of cathepsin D gene by both estrogen receptor positive and negative breast cancer cells might prove to be very important in understanding mammary carcinogenesis.

2. Clinical prognostic value of cathepsin D in breast cancer

Most clinical studies have been performed on tumor cytosol collected at surgery and routinely prepared for steroid receptor assays to predict the aggressiveness of breast cancer and guide its therapy. Total cathepsin D concentration was assayed in cell extracts by solid-phase double-determinant immunoassay (ELISA or IRMA) using two monoclonal antibodies (D7E3, MIG8). These antibodies were prepared against the 52K-pro-cathepsin D of MCF7 cells, however they recognize different epitopes of the large chain (34K) of mature cathepsin D (9). These antibodies also recognize the same epitopes in the intermediate chain (48K) and the precursor form (52K) of the enzyme, thus total cathepsin D concentration can be assayed in cell extracts (10-11). The total cathepsin D assay is now commercialized by CIS International (ELSA-cath-D). Approximately 90% of cathepsin D is extracted by the homogenization procedure used in routine preparations of cytosol for estrogen and progesterone receptor assays (Tris EDTA buffer). Several independent clinical retrospective studies performed in several cancer centers have provided two sets of information. The most important concerns the prognostic value of high cathepsin D concentration for predicting relapse and metastasis according to the Cox multivariate model.

The first study in Copenhagen (12), the second in St-Cloud (11), indicated that cathepsin D has a high predictive value in both node negative and positive patients. Independently, McGuire's group, using polyclonal antibodies to cathepsin D and quantifying the 34K mature form of cathepsin D by immunoblotting, obtained predictive value only in node-negative patients (13). Subsequently, using the commercially available ELSA-cath D kit, other groups also found an inverse correlation between total cathepsin D levels and overall survival, with greater significance in some studies for node-positive patients (14,15). In all Cox-multivariate studies, cathepsin D was one of the top three significant prognostic markers. The cut-off level of total cathepsin D concentration, which helps to discriminate between breast cancers with good (low concentration) or bad (high concentration) prognosis, varied depending on the study but was generally close to the median value (40 to 60 pmoles/mg protein). The second set of information revealed that cathepsin D concentration and status is generally independent of classical prognostic markers such as nodes invasion, tumor size, receptors, Scarff and Bloom histological grade, age of patients (11,12,16), as well as more recently used markers such as neu-erb-B2 or int-2 oncogene amplification (17). There was a slight correlation between cathepsin D and estrogen receptor status in premenopausal patients (12), which is consistent with its constitutive high production in estrogen receptor negative cell lines. The predictive value of cathepsin D therefore supplements that of other markers and indicates that the overexpression of total cathepsin D in primary tumors is associated with the incidence of clinical metastasis occurring within the 5-6 years following surgery. This suggests that micrometastases are already present when primary tumors are removed. Moreover, cathepsin D might be very useful for determining which breast cancer patients would require adjuvant systemic therapy after surgery to retard or prevent early recurrence.

It is currently unknown whether secretion and altered processing of this protease also has some prognostic value but this can be investigated using antibodies specific to the proform (18).

The same antibodies can be used by immunoperoxidase staining of frozen sections to quantify cathepsin D or pro-cathepsin D in situ. A first study in benign breast disease indicated a correlation between ductal hyperplasia and cathepsin D staining (5). By contrast, one immunohistochemical study using different polyclonal antibodies reported that cathepsin D level was of favorable prognosis value (19). The reason for this discrepancy is currently unknown. However, we recently obtained a good correlation between cathepsin D level estimated by quantitative immunohistochemistry using the D7E3 antibody and computer-assisted image analyser and cathepsin D quantified by sandwich ELISA assay (Maudelonde et al., submitted for publication). It is therefore likely that both approaches for evaluating cathepsin D level will be able to provide the same prognostic information, as soon as immunohistochemistry staining can be objectively quantified in a sufficient number of cells.

3. A role of cathepsin D in metastasis ?

Two indirect lines of evidence suggest that the overexpression of cathepsin D in cancer cells may facilitate metastasis (20). First, when the enzyme is diverted from the lysosomal to the secretory pathway, it can degrade new substrates, such as basement membrane and growth factor receptors, and alter antigen processing. Second, as mentioned above, breast cancer patients whose tumors produce high levels of cathepsin D have a higher risk of developing clinical metastases.

To specifically test whether overexpression of cathepsin D promotes metastasis, we transfected a mammalian expression vector of human pro-cathepsin D, or the control vector alone, into a rat tumorigenic cell line 3Y1-Ad12 which secretes no cathepsin D in vitro. Stable transfectant clones which produced and secreted high levels of human cathepsin D were selected. These cells grew more rapidly in low serum concentrations than the control vector clones, displayed a more transformed phenotype and produced foci when cultured on plastic. Thus, cathepsin D transfection alone, appears sufficient to release 3Y1-Ad12 tumor cells from density-dependent growth arrest. In addition, when injected intravenously in athymic mice, their metastatic activity (mostly in liver) was significantly higher than that of control clones (21).

Taken together, these data suggest that cathepsin D may facilitate the growth of tumoral cells in distal tissues and thus accelerate the transformation of micrometastases into clinical metastases. However, the present data were obtained on the 3Y1-Ad12 rat tumor cell line and should be confirmed and extended by similar transfection studies in other cell types, such as breast-derived cell lines, to be closer to the clinical situation.

4. Mechanism of action of cathepsin D in metastasis

The mechanism by which cathepsin D facilitates metastasis is currently unknown and many hypotheses can be proposed to explain this effect. Cathepsin D transfection increases experimental metastases after i.v. injection of tumor cells, thus suggesting that it might facilitate distal steps of the metastatic process including invasion (resistance in the blood stream, extravasation) and subsequently survival and proliferation of tumor cells in the host organ.

Cathepsin D from normal or cancer cells contains both an aspartyl active site, responsible for proteolytic activity, and mannose-6-phosphate signals on its N-linked oligosaccharide chains, responsible for its interaction with mannose-6-phosphate/IGF-II receptor, internalization into cells and targetting to endosomes (22-23). These two structures might a priori be responsible for different biological mechanisms involved in metastasis.

a. The search for biological substrates of cathepsin D

A likely hypothesis is that cathepsin D, like other proteases, facilitates metastasis via its proteolytic activity. However, the biological substrate(s) responsible for breast cancer cell invasion and spread is currently unknown. Cathepsin D has a very wide specificity and can split most proteins at acidic pH. Therefore, there is an unlimited number of potential substrates which could be degraded or activated by high cathepsin D concentrations in breast cancer. No one has yet been demonstrated in vivo. A few possibilities are listed in Fig. 1.

POSSIBLE SUBSTRATES FOR CATHEPSIN D
IN BREAST CANCER METASTASIS

---

1. Extracellular matrix and proteoglycans
   → invasion, FGF release...
2. Triggering of a proteolytic cascade
   pro-cathepsin B/L → activated cathepsin B/L
3. Activation of growth factors
   - precursors ? (TGFβ, TGFα ...)
   - receptors (EGF-R etc...)
4. Others : adhesion proteins, proteases or growth inhibitors
   antigen processing etc...

Figure 1
While most of these hypotheses have been shown to be possible by in vitro experiments, there is presently no conclusive evidence to favor one particular mechanism occuring in vivo in breast cancer patients.

Both purified 52K pro-cathepsin D and conditioned media from estrogen-treated MCF7 cells can digest in vitro extracellular matrix synthesised by bovine corneal endothelial cells. However, optimal activity occurs at acidic pH (4 to 5). The degradation of extracellular matrix by secreted proteases present in conditioned media of breast cancer cells is mostly due to cathepsin D, since it is completely inhibited by pepstatin but not by other inhibitors. Several epithelial cancer cell lines have been found to secrete pepstatin-sensitive protease which correlates with cathepsin D antigen concentrations, as determined by ELISA (24). Thus, we could propose that the invasive property, associated with high concentrations of cathepsin D, is due to digestion of the basement membrane by the secreted and activated pro-enzyme. Autoactivation of secreted pro-cathepsin D in vivo seems to require an acidic micro-environment, which has currently only been demonstrated within the cells (endosomes, lysosomes). However, large acidic vesicles containing both mature cathepsin D and endocytosed extracellular matrix have been found more frequently in breast cancer cells than in normal mammary cells, suggesting that overproduction and derouting of cathepsin D may facilitate digestion of extracellular matrix following its internalisation by an endocytotic or phagocytotic process (25). In breast cancer cells, cathepsin D could thus potentially act in acidic intracellular compartments other than the lysosomes.

Cathepsin D may also behave as a processing protease that can be autoactivated at high concentrations and low pH. Moreover, it might process and activate other proteases, such as pro-cathepsin B, thus initiating a proteolytic cascade with latent plasminogen activators and collagenases also being activated to degrade extracellular matrix (Fig. 2) (26-31).

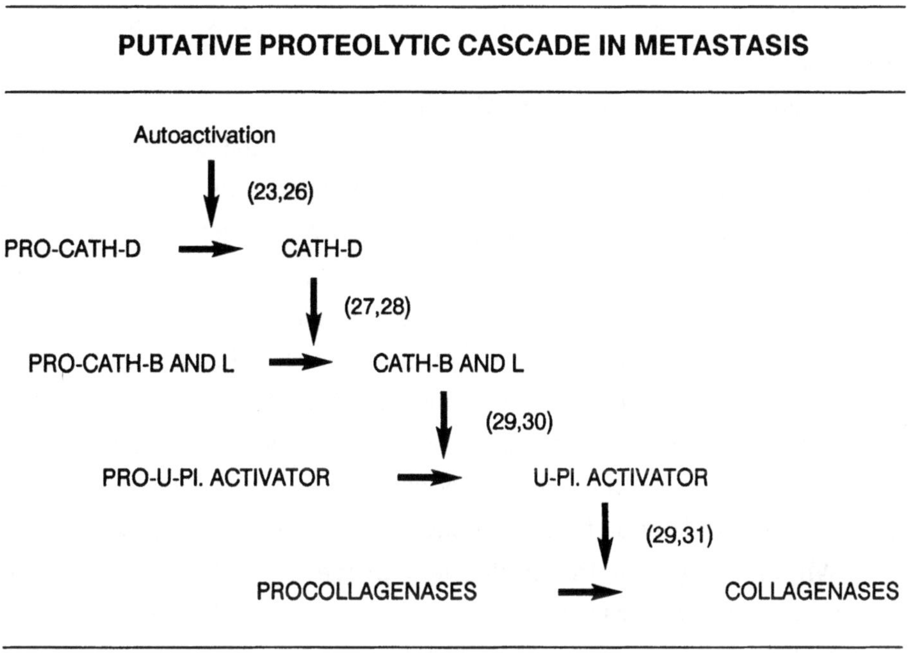

Figure 2
Putative proteolytic cascade in metastasis

Pro-cathepsin D might be decisive in triggering a proteolytic cascade, because of its unique property of autocatalytic activation at acidic pH. All of these proteases were shown to be produced in excess by malignant cells. Evidence demonstrating each activation step is described in the original references indicated in brackets.

Among these proteases, cathepsin D and urokinase (U-Pl.activator) have both been shown to be correlated with increased risk of metastases in breast cancer.

Both pro-cathepsin D and the mature enzyme have been shown to stimulate the growth of estrogen-deprived MCF7 cells (32). This autocrine mitogenic activity partially reproduces the effect of estrogens. By transfection of a cathepsin D cDNA expression vector, the cell proliferation of 3Y1-Ad12 cells was also increased in low serum culture conditions (21). The mechanism of this mitogenic activity of cathepsin D might involve the loss of density-dependent growth inhibition by degradation of some membrane components (adhesion proteins, proteoglycans...) as initially proposed for other proteases (33,34).

Like other proteases, cathepsin D may act indirectly by releasing growth factors from precursors or from extracellular matrix (FGFs family)

(35) and/or by activating growth factor receptors extracellularly or intracellularly.

b. Other questions and mechanisms

Cathepsin D, interacting with the mannose-6-phosphate/IGF-II receptor, like other lysosomal enzymes, might behave as a growth factor and stimulate cell proliferation by triggering this plasma membrane receptor which has been proposed to mediate the mitogenic activity of low concentrations of IGF-II (36). Crosslinking and binding experiments have shown that pure pro-cathepsin D from breast cancer cells directly interacts with this receptor. However, while cathepsin D is mitogenic when added alone to resting MCF7 cells, it was found to inhibit the mitogenic activity of low concentrations of IGF-II, thus suggesting that it behaves as a partial agonist-antagonist ligand of the mannose-6-phosphate/IGF-II receptor (37).

Which step(s) of the metastatic process is (are) affected by cathepsin D overexpression ? In the 3Y1-Ad12 cell line, cathepsin D significantly increased in vitro both cell density at confluence by cell-cell adhesion and the capacity to grow in low serum conditions or in an agar gel. These effects suggest that cathepsin D-producing cells acquired new properties to adhere, resist and divide under stronger environmental selection pressure. These properties are beneficial for metastatic cells to survive in successive steps of migration, invasion and proliferation in the host organ.

Is cathepsin D acting extracellularly or intracellularly ? In human breast cancer, overexpression of cathepsin D and down regulation of mannose-6-phosphate/IGF-II receptor by estrogens (38) results in saturation of receptors and derouting of the protease which is both secreted and increased in cellular compartments (endosomes) as a pro-enzyme. However, it is unknown whether cathepsin D is active in intracellular compartments or extracellularly or both. In resting MCF7 cells, the addition of cathepsin D in the culture medium increased cell proliferation either in its proform or processed form. Recently, when the 3Y1-Ad12 cathepsin D-transfected and control clones were cultured in adjacent compartments with communication between the two culture media, the cathepsin D-producing clone was unable to stimulate cell-cell aggregation that was responsible for higher saturation cell density in the control clones. This suggested that the increased aggregation of cathepsin D-producing clones might be due to intracellular cathepsin D and not to the secreted diffusing protease (M. Garcia and D. Derocq, unpublished results).

CONCLUSIONS AND PROSPECTS

A series of experimental data indicate that the overexpression of cathepsin D by cancer cells facilitates invasion and metastasis. According to clinical studies, high concentrations of cathepsin D in primary breast cancer are highly correlated with subsequent risk of developing metastasis. This increased accumulation of the protease is secondary to its increased gene expression in both hormone- dependent and independent tumors via a mechanism which is not yet understood but which could be studied at the gene level. Since we found no obvious alterations in the cathepsin D coding sequence, we are now looking for defects in its regulatory sequence (cis-regulatory elements) or in trans-acting factor(s) regulating cathepsin D gene expression in both estrogen receptor negative and positive breast cancers. Site-directed mutagenesis of amino acids engaged in cellular localization of this protease, its N-glycosylation and its proteolytic activity, might help to specify the mechanism by which cathepsin D stimulates in vivo experimental metastasis.

These results could be extended to other proteases which might act in concert with cathepsin D to stimulate metastasis (39). They should help to define new targets for breast cancer therapy aimed at inhibiting the critical steps of tumor growth and invasion.

ACKNOWLEDGEMENTS

We are grateful to all members of the INSERM laboratory who have contributed to these studies and are quoted in the original papers. We thank M. Egea for her skillful preparation of the manuscript, D. Derocq and C. Rougeot for their expert technical assistance. SANOFI and CIS Bio-International Laboratories and cancer centers in Copenhagen, Montpellier and St-Cloud (France) for clinical collaborative studies. We are grateful to Dr. Chambon and Dr. Rutter for gifts of biological material.

This work was supported by the "Institut National de la Santé et de la Recherche Médicale", the "Association pour la Recherche sur le Cancer", the University of Montpellier 1, the "Groupement des Entreprises Françaises dans la Lutte contre le Cancer", the "Fondation pour la Recherche Médicale" and the "Ligue Nationale Française contre le Cancer".

REFERENCES

1. Kirschke, H. and Barrett, A.K. In: Lysosomes : their role in protein breakdown (Eds. H. Glauman and F. Ballard), Academic Press, 1987, pp. 193-238.
2. Faust, P.L., Kornfeld, S., Chirgwin, J.M. Proc. Natl. Acad. Sci. USA 82:4910-4914, 1985.
3. Augereau, P., Garcia, M., Mattei, M.G., Cavaillès, V., Depadova, F., Derocq, D., Capony, F., Ferrara, P. and Rochefort, H. Mol. Endo. 2:186-192, 1988.
4. Capony, F., Rougeot, C., Montcourrier, P., Cavaillès, V., Salazar, G. and Rochefort, H. Cancer Res. 49:39O4-39O9, 1989.
5. Garcia, M., Salazar-Retana, G., Pagès, A., Richer, G., Domergue, J., Pagès, A.M., Cavalié, G., Martin, J.M., Lamarque, J.L., Pau, B., Pujol, H. and Rochefort, H. Cancer Res. 46:3734-3738, 1986.
6. Rochefort, H., Cavaillès, V., Augereau, P., Capony, F., Maudelonde, T., Touitou, I., Garcia, M. J. Steroid Biochem. 34:177-182, 1989.
7. Cavaillès, V., Augereau, P., Garcia, M. and Rochefort, H. Nucl. Acids Res. 16:19O3-1919, 1988.
8. Cavaillès, V., Garcia, M. and Rochefort, H. Mol. Endo. 3:552-558, 1989.
9. Garcia, M., Capony F., Derocq, D., Simon, D., Pau, B. and Rochefort H. Cancer Res. 45:709-716, 1985.
10. Rogier, H., Freiss, G., Besse, M.G., Cavalié-Barthez, G., Garcia M., Pau, B., Rochefort, H. and Paolucci, F. Clin. Chem. 35:81-85, 1989.
11. Spyratos, F., Maudelonde, T., Brouillet, J.P., Brunet, M., Defrenne, A., Andrieu, C., Hacene, K., Desplaces, A., Rouëssé, J., Rochefort, H. The Lancet ii:1115-1118, 1989.
12. Thorpe, S.M., Rochefort, H., Garcia, M., Freiss, G., Christensen, I.J., Khalaf, S., Paolucci, F., Pau, B., Rasmussen, B.B., Rose C. Cancer Res. 49:6OO8-6O14, 1989.
13. Tandon, A., Clark, G., Chirgwin, J., McGuire, W.L. New Engl. J. Med. 322:297-3O2, 199O.
14. Namer, M., Etienne, M.C., Fontana, X., Ramaioli, A., Lapalus, F., Héry, M. Breast Cancer Res. Treat. in press, 1991.
15. Romain, S., Muracciole, X., Varette, I., Bressac, C., Brandone, H., Martin, P.M. Bull. Cancer 77:439-447, 1990.
16. Maudelonde, T., Khalaf, S., Garcia, M., Freiss, G., Duporté, J., Benatia, M., Rogier, H., Paolucci, F., Simony, J., Pujol, H., Pau, B., Rochefort, H. Cancer Res. 48:462-466, 1988.
17. Brouillet, J.P., Theillet, C., Maudelonde, T., Defrenne, A., Simony-Lafontaine, J., Sertour, J., Pujol, H., Jeanteur, P., Rochefort, H. Eur. J. Cancer 26:437-441, 1990.
18. Freiss, G., Vignon, F., Pau, B., Paolucci, F., Rochefort, H. Clin. Chem. 35:234-237, 1989.
19. Henry, J.A., McCarthy, A.L., Angus, B., Westley, B.R., May, F.E.B., Nicholson, S., Cairns, J., Harris, A.L., Horne, C.H.W. Cancer 65:265-271, 199O.
20. Rochefort, H., Capony, F., Garcia, M., Cavaillès, V., Freiss, G., Chambon, M., Morisset, M., Vignon, F. J. Cell. Biochem. 35:17-29, 1987.
21. Garcia, M., Derocq, D., Pujol, P., Rochefort, H. Oncogene 5:1809-1814, 1990.
22. Von Figura, K., Hasilik, A. Ann. Rev. Biochem. 55:167-193, 1986.

23. Capony F., Morisset, M., Barret, A.J., Capony, J.P., Broquet, P., Vignon, F., Chambon, M, Louisot, P., Rochefort, H. J. Cell. Biol. 104:253-262, 1987.
24. Briozzo, P., Morisset, M., Capony, F., Rougeot, C., Rochefort, H. Cancer Res. 48:3688-3692, 1988.
25. Montcourrier, P., Mangeat, P., Salazar, G., Morisset, M., Sahuguet, A., Rochefort, H. Cancer Res. 50:6045-6054, 1990.
26. Hasilik, A., Von Figura, K., Conzerlmann, E., Nehrkorn, H., Sandhoff, K. Eur. J. Biochem. 125:317-321, 1982.
27. Nishimura, Y., Kawabata, T., Kato, K. Arch. Biochem. Biophys. 261:64-71, 1988.
28. Pagano, M., Capony, F., Rochefort, H. C.R. Acad. Sci. Paris 3O9:7-12, 1989.
29. Eeckhout, Y., Vaes, G. Biochem. J. 166:21-31, 1977.
30. Kobayashi, H., Schmitt M., Goretzki, L., Chucholowski, N., Calvete, J., Kramer, M., Gunzler, W.A., Janicke, F., Graef, H. J. Biol. Chem. 266:5147-5152, 1991.
31. Reich, R., Thompson, E.W., Iwamoto, Y., Martin, GR., Dreason, J.R., Fuller, G.C., Miskin, R. Cancer Res. 48:3307-3312, 1988.
32. Vignon, F., Chambon, M., Freiss, G., Garcia, M., Rochefort, H. Endocrinology 118:1537-1545,1986.
33. Sefton, B.M., Rubin, H., Nature. 227:843-845.
34. Carney, D.H., Cunningham, D.D., Nature. 268:602-606, 1977.
35. Briozzo, P., Badet, J., Capony, F., Pieri, I., Montcourrier, P., Barritault D., Rochefort, H. Exp. Cell. Res. in press 1991.
36. Morgan, D.O., Edman, J.C., Standring, D.N., Fried, V.A. Smith, M.C., Roth, R.A., Rutter, W.J. Nature 329:301-307,1987.
37. Mathieu, M., Rochefort, H., Barenton, B., Prébois, C., Vignon, F. Mol. Endo. 4:1327-1335, 1990.
38. Mathieu, M., Vignon, F., Capony F., Rochefort, H. Mol. Endo. in press 1991.
39. Goldfarb, R.H. In: Mechanisms of Cancer Metastasis (Eds. K.W. Honn, W.E. Powers, B.F. Sloane), Martinus Nijhoff Pub., Boston, 1986, pp. 341-375.

Diagnostic tools and prognostic factors in human breast cancer evaluated by morphological and immunohistochemical methods*)

A. Schauer[1), *D. Marx*[2), *I. Lipp*[2), *M. Schumacher*[2), *W. Sauerbrei*[3), *H. Rauschecker*[3) and *R. Sauer*[4)

With regard to the clinical management of breast cancer besides the radiological (mammography and magnetic resonance), ultrasound and galactographic image processing systems we need safe and fast-working, histopathological and immunohistochemical methods to make in uncertain cases the diagnosis sure and to obtain well defined informations with respect to the individual biological behaviour of every single cancer to be treated under optimal conditions according to the specific personal situation (Fig.1).

German Breast Cancer Study Group (GBCSG)

- Protocols -

1) Treatment of ductal carcinoma in situ (DCIS)

2) Treatment of small breast cancer ($pT_1N_0M_0$) with breast conserving surgery (start 1983)

3) Avoidance of radiation therapy in low risk cases

---

*) With Support of the German Ministry for Research and Technology and ICI-Pharma.
1) Dept. of Pathology, Göttingen, University, Germany.
2) Dept. of Statistics and Biometry, Freiburg, University, Germany.
3) Dept. of Surgery, Göttingen, University, Germany.
4) Dept. of Radiotherapy, Erlangen, University, Germany.

As a rule, experienced pathologists can give the clearcut diagnosis "breast cancer" using frozen sections already intraoperatively in a very high percentage of cases. Only seldom difficulties arise f.i. concerning the problems of

1. delineation of cancer from sclerosing adenosis,
2. delineation of small cell breast cancer f.i. "histiocytic type" from reactive or neoplastic histiocytic or lymphatic proliferation,
3. delineation of breast cancer – from epitheloid malignant hemangioendothelioma or similar special tumor lesions of the breast.

As already summarized in our earlier statements (*Schauer* et al. 1985, 1986, 1988) and further more by *Bussolati* 1985, and *Caselitz* et al. 1985), meanwhile, many immunohistochemical possibilities are available to obtain safe diagnosis.

The following principles can be summarized:

1. Ductal and lobular invasive cancers show identical cytokeratin pattern (*Moll* et al. 1982; *Schauer* et al. 1985). Furthermore it can not be discriminated between these two entities, based on only slightly variable cytokeratin patterns. In addition a small number of breast cancers according to the results of *Rilke* et al. 1990 and *Domagala* et al. 1990 show a simultaneous expression of cytokeratin and vimentin. According to statistical evaluated follow up investigations these tumors have a worse prognosis as compared to vimentin-negative breast cancers (*Domagala* et al. 1990). Furthermore, as lately pointed out by *Bässler* (1991) also S 100-protein is expressed too in some special cases. However these tumors are not positive for chromogranin, neuron-specific enolase (NSE) and synaptophysin like neuroendocrine tumors.
2. Lymphocytic or blastic reactive or neoplastic proliferations can be assured using antibodies directed to CLA (CD45) or by specific B- and T-cell markers such as 4KB5, L26 or UCHL 1 etc. (*Schauer* et al. 1985, 1988).
3. Histiocytic reactive or neoplastic lesions can be distinguished from "histiocytic type" of small cell lobular breast cancer using antibodies to lysozyme or alpha 1-antichymotrypsin or antibodies against macrophages (CD68) on the

one hand and pancytokeratin-antibodies on the other hand (*Schauer* et al. 1985, 1986, 1988).

4. Endothelial proliferations or neoplasias especially malignant hemangioendotheliomas are detectable and delineable by antibodies against factor VIII associated protein (*Schauer* et al. 1985, 1988).

Summarizing the efforts, how to exclude early stromal invasion in DCIS cases, antibodies to cytokeratins can be used, in order to detect single invasive cells in the stroma; on the other side defects of the basement membranes caused by early stromal invasion can be demonstrated using antilaminin or antikollagen type IV-antibodies (*Ekblom* et al. 1984; *Schauer* et al. 1985, 1986; *Remberger* and *Nerlich* 1985). However, we have to realize that in seldom cases f.i. tubular cancers can form basement membrane material. This is also a fact playing a role in low grade prostatic cancers (*Remberger* 1991). Concerning the lobular cancer in situ (LCIS) mostly without nuclear atypia, up till now, we have no possibilities to comment on the stage of carcinogenesis in facultative remaining foci of this often multifocal lesion, especially concerning the futural biological behaviour of rest-foci (*Rosen* 1978, 1980, 1981; *Schauer* 1985).

After discussion about how to make sure the diagnosis of invasive breast cancer and also the statements concerning early stromal invasion, we have to give an answer, about the risk for the patient, based on powerful prognostic factors.

Basically it is well known that tumor size and axillary nodal status are the most important factors and it is also well know that on the cellular level, the degree of malignancy, the proliferation activity, the proliferative compartment and the ploidy-status are also of importance.

With respect to these facts, we planned in our studies no further treatment of DCIS-cases after excision of this lesion only up to 2,5 cm after control of the margins in serial sections and gave up the claim of axillary revision. However, in cases with extension over 2,5 cm in which local invasion, increases to 46% retromamillary involvement to 25%, and axillary lymph node metastasis to approximately 8% (*Lagios* 1982; *Lagios* et al. 1989) axillary revision and radical subcutaneous mastectomy with histological control of the retromamillary ducts can not be avoided.

In our opinion special caution is necessary in cases with grade IIb and III tumor tissue (higher degrees of malignancy with c-erb B1 (EGFR) and or c-erb B2 positivity. In extensive lesions with these features in which early tumor invasion can not be excluded, with respect to nondetected early invasion, and therefore not excluded systemic spread, especially in pre- and perimenopausal cases, adjuvant chemotherapy should be taken into consideration to destroy early hematogenous systemic spread (*Schauer* et al. 1991).

Our experiences considering the worth of prognostic factors of invasive breast cancer for clinical decisions are based on our daily investigated routine material and also on data obtained from the First German Breast Cancer Study: Breast conserving surgery in pT1NOMO-cases, which started in 1983 (Reports see: *Schauer* et al. 1988, 1991). The investigations at our routine material showed that benign breast lesions as fibroadenomas showed no immunhistochemical membrane staining for p185-protein.
However, *Höfler* (1991) could demonstrate one case of fibroadenoma with clear p185-membrane-staining. Whether this case is one of the rare cases with initial step of malignant transformation or not is an open question.

The investigation of preneoplastic lesions showed positive reactions in a percentage rate of ~ 15% at dysplastic intraductal proliferations. In DCIS-cases especially the large cell high grade types, that means comedotypes, cribriform types with necrosis and large cell terminal lobular cancerization show positive reactions up to 60%, whereas the micropapillary small cell low grade types express the protein only in 10% (*Marx* et al. 1990; *Schauer* et al. 1990).

In DCIS-cases segmental atypical large cell proliferations showed intensive positive reactions for p185, whereas non proliferative small cell populations of the same duct in the neighbourhood were totally negative.

From these facts it can be followed that positive p185-membrane staining is already a significant signal for malignant transformation (Fig.2-6).

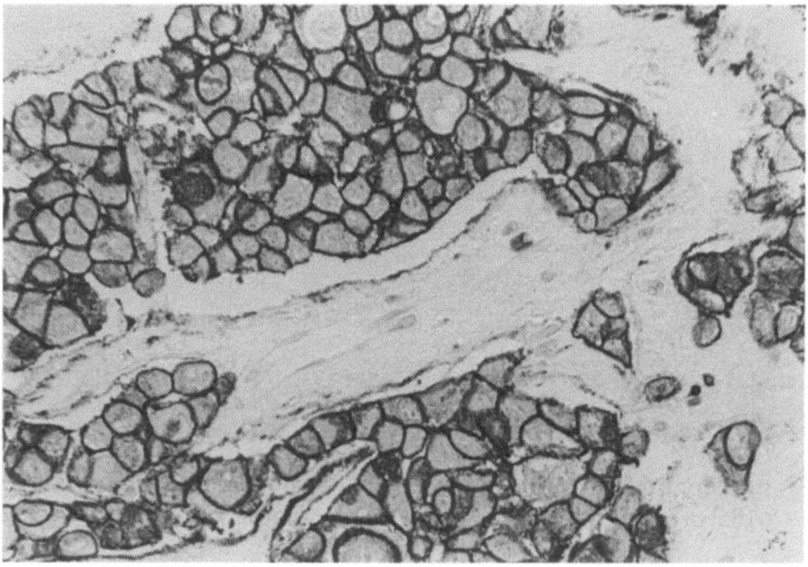

Fig 2: Invasive ductal breast cancer: Strongly positive immunohistological reaction for p185-protein at the tumor cell membranes

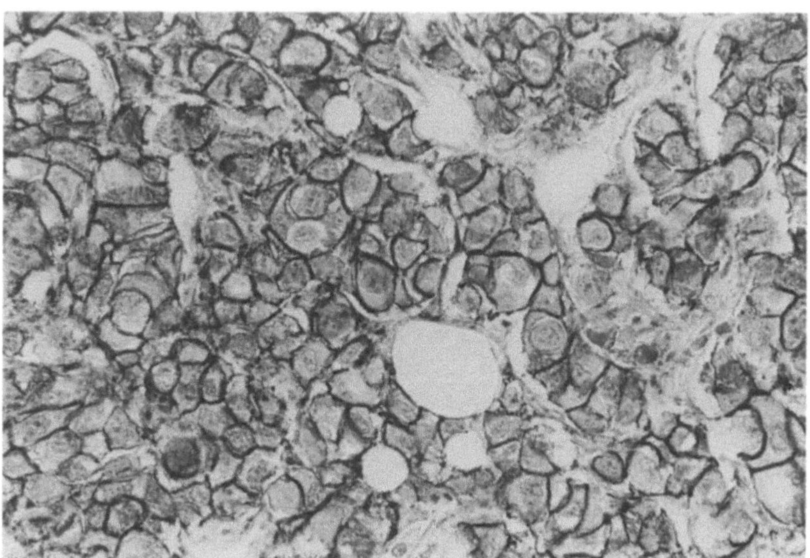

Fig 3: Invasive ductal breast cancer: Intensive homogenous immunohistochemical reaction for p185 transmembrane protein

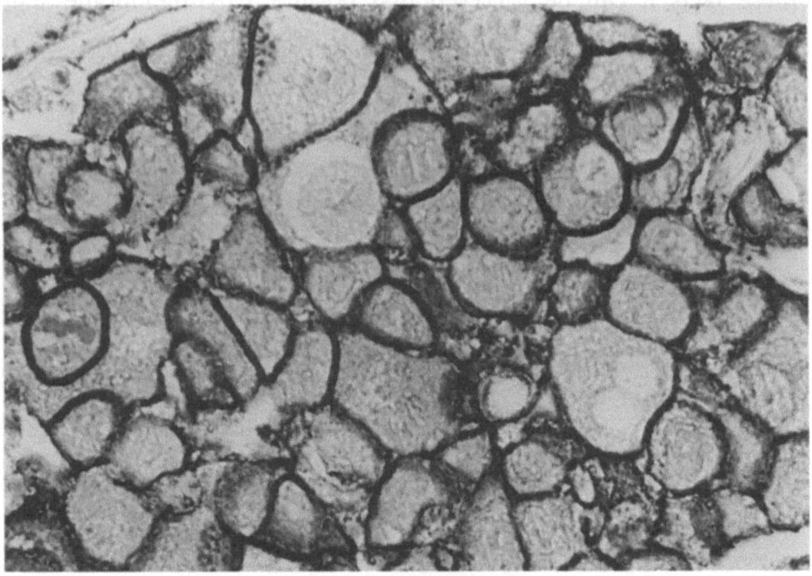

Fig 4: Invasive breast cancer: Strong immunohistochemical positive staining for p185 protein. Note the partly granular immunoprecipitate

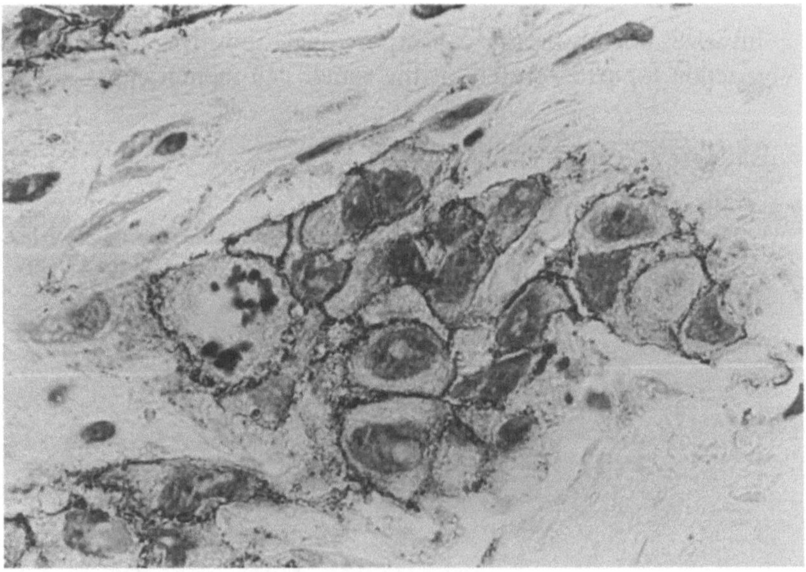

Fig 5: Large all high grade breast cancer positive for p185-protein. Note the positive reaction also during mitotic phase of the cell cycle

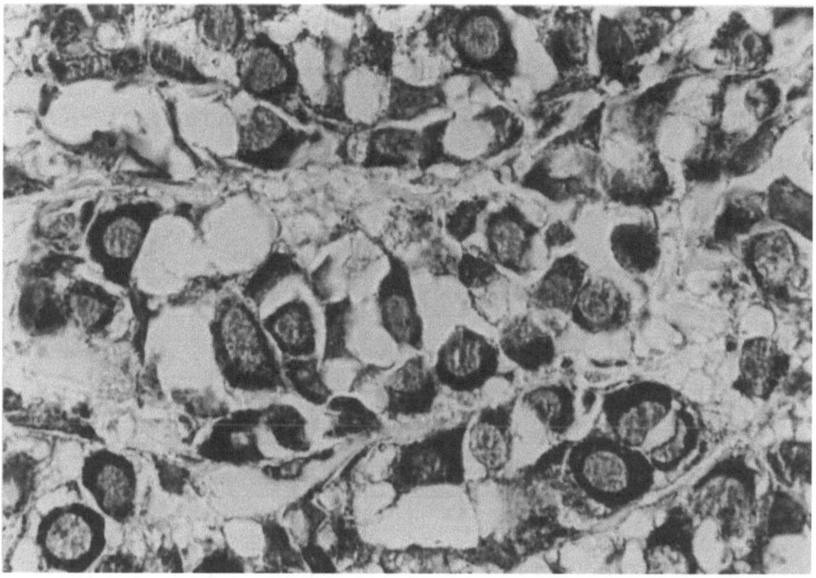

Fig 6: Invasive ductal breast cancer: False positive cytoplasmatic immunohistochemical reaction for p185. No positive membrane staining

In the cases with invasive cancer c-erb B2-oncogen-expression is related to the degree of malignancy and also to higher malignant subtypes. Whereas using native material Grade I-tumors in our series showed positive rates only in 4-6%, higher malignant tumors were positive up to approximately 30%. In comparison to these results *van de Vijver* found even no positive reactions in his Grade I-collectives (*van de Vijver* et al. 1991).

In our first preliminary series of 472 cases using paraffin-sections of our study the highly differentiated tubular cancers and also the differentiated low grade mucinous cancers showed only very seldom positive p185-reactions. Especially the dependence of p185 expression on the degree of malignancy and implicated proliferative activity are in contrast to the current opinion that c-erb B2-overexpression respectively amplification does not indicate worse prognosis in NO-cases (*Borg* et al. 1990, 1991) but only in cases with positive nodes (*Slamon* et al. 1987, 1989; *Zeilinger* et al. 1989; *Tandon* et al. 1989).

But this statement agrees with the fact that c-erb B2-positive cases show sometimes all investigated lymph nodes totally permeated by cancer cells. After our investigations at well defined routine cases, we looked for results, which could be obtained from the material of our study concerning pT1NOMO-cases coming from the National German Breast Cancer Study Group (Fig.7).

Univariate analyses of the effects of prognostic factors on disease-free survival

Variables		No. of pat. included	Estimated relative risk	Confidence interval	p-value (Logrank test)
Tumor size	< 10 mm	1033	1,00	-	0,024
	11-20 mm		1,68	[1,07/2,64]	
Estrogen receptor status	> 20 fmol/mg	829	1,00	-	0,36
	< 20 fmol/mg		1,20	[0,81/1,78]	
Progesterone receptor status	> 20 fmol/mg	810	1,00	-	0,1
	< 20 fmol/mg		1,40	[0,94/2,08]	
Tumor location	lateral	1030	1,00	-	0,65
	medial/central		0,92	[0,64/1,33]	
Tumor grading	I	1029	1,00	-	0,006
	II		1,58	[1,03/2,41]	
	III		2,36	[1,37/4,07]	
Degree of differentiation	> 75 %	1029	1,00	-	0,3
	10-75 %		1,23	[0,48/3,13]	
	< 10 %		1,59	[0,65/3,93]	
Pleomorphism	low	1029	1,00	-	0,031
	medium		1,99	[1,04/3,83]	
	high		2,64	[1,26/5,53]	
Mitotic index	< 1 mit/field	1027	1,00	-	0,034
	1-3 mit/field		1,52	[1,03/2,24]	
	> 3 mit/field		1,75	[1,01/3,03]	
Degree of dissociation	low	1029	1,00	-	0,18
	medium		1,39	[0,89/2,17]	
	high		1,59	[0,96/2,63]	
p-185	positive	425	1,00	-	0,001
	negative		0,28	[0,12/0,63]	
Myc	positive	425	1,00	-	0,42
	negative		1,31	[0,67/2,57]	

Fig 7

Of 1036 cases under long termed observation in this program, we could evaluate exact histopathological data. The mean valued follow up of 733 cases, treated by breast conservation with axilla revision and 303 cases treated by mastectomy also with axilla dissection is now three and a half years (Fig.8 and 9).

Recurrences in different treatment groups

	Mastectomy	Breast preservation	total
no recurrence	258 (85 %)	653 (89 %)	911
local	13 (4 %)	28 (4 %)	41
distant	14 (5 %)	32 (4 %)	46
second primary contralateral	5 (2 %)	5 (1 %)	10
regional or loco-regional or loco-regional and distant	4 (1 %)	7 (1 %)	11
death without recurrence	9 (3 %)	8 (1 %)	17
total	303 (100 %)	733 (100 %)	1036

Fig 8

Recurrence rates in correlation to tumor grading and different age groups:

Age		Degree of malignancy I + IIa	IIb	III	total	Recurrence rates n / %
<= 45	n	105	42	41	188	17
	% age group	55.8	22.3	21.8		9.0 %
	% Tu.-group	24.1	31.6	48.8		
46 - 60	n	152	57	31	240	20
	% age group	63.3	23.8	12.9		8.3 %
	% Tu.-group	35.0	42.9	36.9		
> 60	n	178	34	12	224	14
	% age group	79.5	15.2	5.4		6.2 %
	% Tu.-group	40.9	25.6	14.3		
Total:		435	133	84		652

Fig 9

In 23 of the 733 cases with breast conservation the tumorfree margins remained unceratin. In spite of homogenous local radiotherapy in these cases the locoregional recidive rate was very high, whereas when the tumorfree margins were measured, respectively controlled by histological examination the recidive rates did not depend significantly on the mm distance of the randominfiltrates of the primaries to the randoms of surgical excision. Furthermore the locoregional recurrence rates were quite similar in the group with breast conserving surgery and radiation therapy, as compared with the mastectomy-group (Fig.10)

Disease-free Survival-free margins

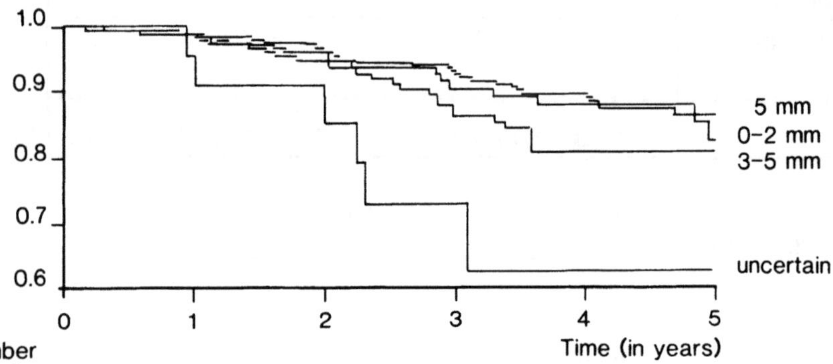

Number at risk	0	1	2	3	4	5
uncert	23	21	16	10	4	0
0-2	164	147	118	82	54	24
3-5	189	177	144	103	60	25
5	357	332	275	201	129	59
total	733					

Fig 10

From this follows that the recurrences mainly do not develop from intraductal atypical foci resistant against radiation therapy, but much more from extraductal tumor cell clusters surviving the procedures of both therapy regimens f.i. in lymphvessels of the subcutaneous tissue. In relation to this fact, the evaluation of lymph vessel invasion in the surrounding areas of the primaries seem to be very important.

In comparison to the prognostic factors evaluated in our pT1NOMO study: tumor size, degree of malignancy and also the c-erb B2-amplication measured by immunohistochemical demonstration of the p185-protein had the highest significance, as could be demonstrated by low p-values obtained in the logrank test (Fig.7).

While the locoregional recidive rates did not increase significantly in the breast conserved radiated group between 1 cm up to 2 cm tumors, the recidive rates increased three-fold in the mastectomy group, when the subgroups up to one centimeter in diameter and between one and two centimeters were compared. This is a very important point in working out plans for therapy regimens or study-programs concerned with the question. Can radiotherapy after wide excision be avoided in low risk cases. In this context it is also worth while to know that the recidive rate was approximately threefold in grade III-tumors as compared with the grade I-tumors (Fig.11). According to this fact one has to realize that the grading procedure needs optimal histological quality and great morphological experience as well as evaluation of the mitotic figures in at least 12 high power fields. In addition the outfit with the steroid receptor protein parallels positive to the grading system and the evaluations show that grade I and IIa tumors, that is up to 6 grading points in our grading scheme, show simular and higher positive rates than the grade IIb and grade III tumors.

Disease-free Survival by Tumor grading

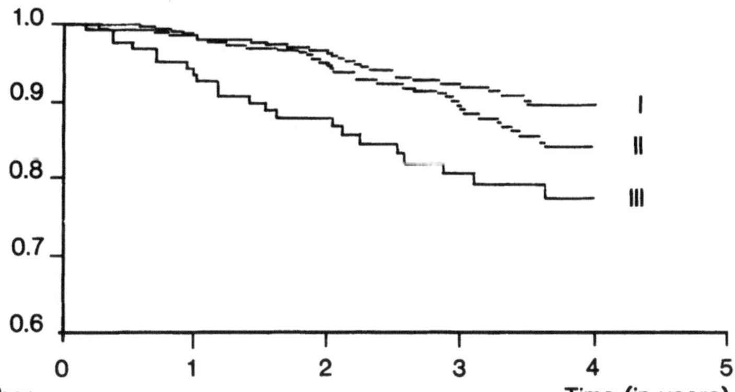

Number at risk

I	350	319	271	199	124	50
II	556	515	404	276	175	77
III	123	109	84	63	38	20

Fig 11

As a rule, the proliferation, measured by the antibody Ki67 (*Gerdes* et al. 1983, 1984) suitable for the visualization of the proliferation associated protein, is low with homologous and intensive staining (*Lellé* et al. 1985; *Schauer* et al. 1988; *Rothe* et al. 1989).

However, there are a few cases with high proliferation measured with the Ki67-antibody and intensively positive staining using ER und PR antibodies (Abbott). In so far especially in homogenous equipped tumors a down regulation of tumor growth can be expected by tamoxifen therapy for longer periods. This seems to be possible because late metastases sometimes show full equipment of the tumor cells with the receptor protein.

However this situation changes, when spontaneous or drug induced heterogeneity comes up. The heterogeneity of the receptor equipment can be measured by different sophisticated photometric systems (Zeiss, Becton and Dickinson) (*Harms* et al. 1986; *Adams* et al. 1988).

Besides the tumorgrading – as already pointed out the c-erb B2-amplification respectively over expression with p185-membrane staining was an important point, with respect to localregional recidives and distant metastasis, as could be found in our study. At first *Slamon* and coworkers found correlations between c-erb B2-over-expression respectively amplification and tumor progression. In the meantime many other groups confirmed this statement. However, there are also some other groups, who found no differences between p185-positive and negative collectives with respect to tumor progression. As already pointed out by *Slamon* an others, the progressive rate increases in p185 positive cases when more than three lymphnodes are involved. These data agree with older findings of *E. Fisher* and coworkers, who found very bad prognosis when more than three lymphnodes were involved with axillary macrometastases.
However, from the biological point of view this limited correlation seems not to be logical, because multiple metastases do not start immediately at the same point of time. Furthermore, the divergent results were obtained and can be explained by

1. looking for different only sometimes well defined collectives of patients
2. using different methods for the evaluation of c-erb B2 overexpression respectively amplification and
3. using different parameters with respect to tumor progression

In our still incomplete evaluation-using paraffinsections of the cases in our study in general, the rate of p185 negative cases without distant recurrence was significantly higher than the rate of p185 positive cases (Fig.12). With other words, the estimated relative risk was only 0,28 in negative cases as compared with 1,00 in p185 positive cases. The p-value of this composition according to the logrank test was 0,001. These data are in contrast to investigators who only found correlations to tumors progression in cases with more than three positive lymphnodes.

Disease-free Survival by p-185

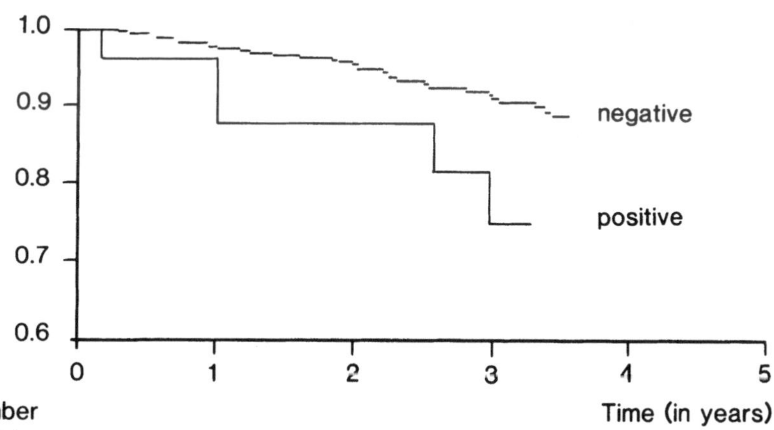

Number at risk						
pos	29	23	17	10	2	1
neg	396	365	290	186	89	26

Fig 12

Our data are supported by the results which demonstrate that in cases with locoregional recidives only 5% were positive for p185 protein, whereas in cases with systemic spread the five fold, namely 25% were positive. Furthermore in cases with early death with advanced breast cancer the p185 negative rate amounted to 17% whereas the positive rate to 57%. This is more than threefold (Fig.13).

c-erbB2- expression in relation to recurrences of 472 $pT_1N_0M_0$ cases used antibody (9G6) - [mean follow up 2.5 years]

	c-erbB2 (p 185+)	n	%
Recurrences	7	49	14
locoreg. Recurrence	1	21	5
others (systemic spread)	5	20	25
second primaries	1	8	13
dead with recurrences or systemic spread	4	11	36
11 cases died with breast cancer			
dead with progress of cancer	p 185 -	7 / 42	17
	p 185 +	4 / 7	57

Fig 13

If we take into consideration that the rate of p185 positive cases amounts to 25-30% in frozen sections and we have a loss of at least 10% in paraffinsections it makes more sense to look for the recidive and distant progression rates with and without p185 expression, than to evaluate the progressionrates based on the whole series.

Comparison with simultaneous or isolated EGFR expression gave no information about potentiating effects, but the death rate was three times higher in positive cases too (Fig.14-17).

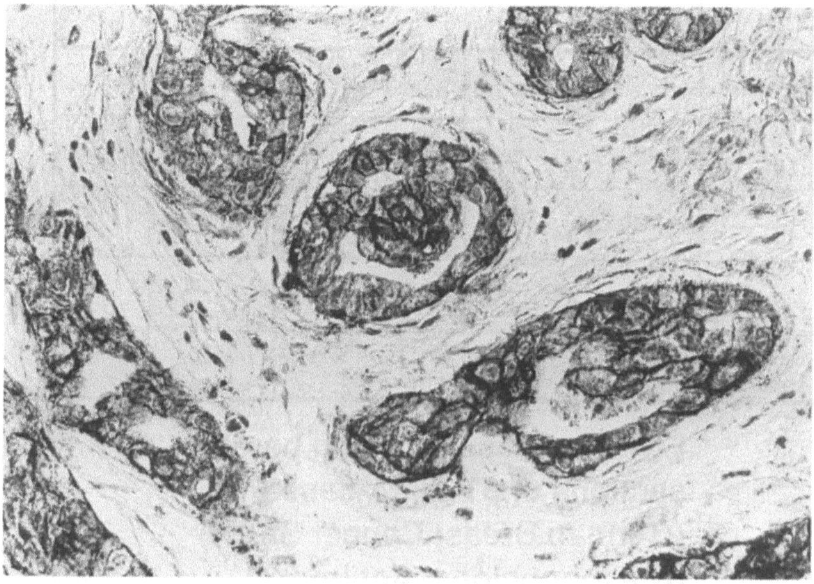

Fig 14: Predominantly intraductal tumor growth: Strongly positive reaction for EGFR at the tumor cell membranes

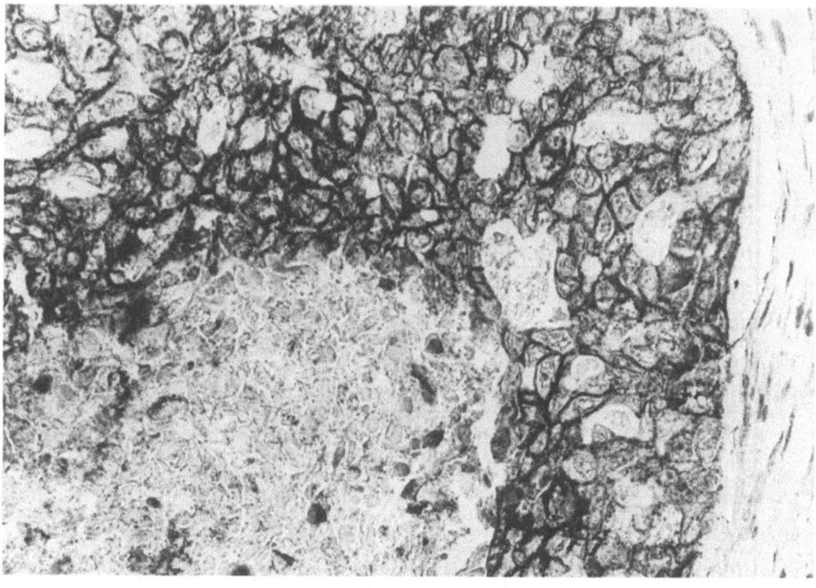

Fig 15: Positive EGFR-reaction at the tumor cell membranes. Antibody from Merck Company, FRG

EGFR / Grading at 363 cases

(German Breast Cancer Study)

	EGFR +	n	%
I	15	138	11
IIa	17	101	17
IIb	17	84	20
III	10	40	25
total	59	363	16

Fig 16

EGFR expression using paraffin sections of $pT_1 N_0 M_0$ cases (German Breast Cancer Study) by a monoclonal Antibody prepared by Merck Comp. and Correlation to recurrence rates.

	EGFR +	n	%
recurrences	8	38	22
locoregional recurrence	1	14	7
systemic spread	4	14	29
second primaries	2	5	40
combination	1	5	20
dead with recurrences or systemic spread	3	7	43
dead with progress of cancer	EGFR -	[4 / 30]	13
	EGFR +	[3 / 8]	38

Fig 17

The immunohistochemical evaluation of c-myc-protein expression product, localized in the tumor cell nuclei at the same collective of patients was not significantly correlated to the rates of disease free survial (Fig.18).

Disease-free Survival by c-myc

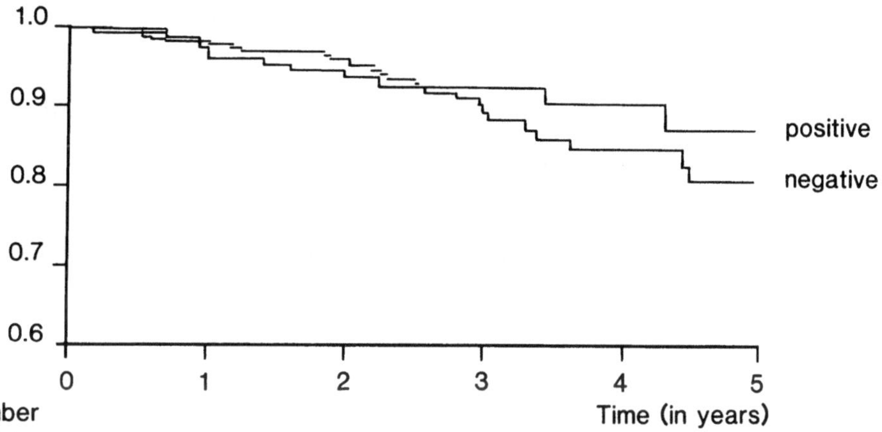

Number at risk						
pos	156	141	104	62	34	7
neg	269	247	203	134	57	20

Fig 18

In addition, there was no obvious correlation of the degree of tumor cell dissoziation to locoregional or distant recidive rates, whereas in our early investigations we found the rate of lymph node metastasis two fold higher in cases with a high degree of dissoziation as compared with cases with low degrees.

In conclusion:

Highgrade tumors i.e. Grade IIb or III tumors with p185 and/or EGFR expression must be treated very carfully.

Important open questions are:

1. significance of adjuvant chemotherapy in DCIS-cases high grade, oncogene positive c-erb B1 and/or B2 with or without minimal invasion
2. treatment of p185 and/or EGFR positive high grade tumors with EIC
3. Exclusion of these tumors in pT1NOMO study programs with the goal to avoid radiation therapy in low risk cases.

With view to futural individual therapy of breast cancer in our believe the time is comming that we have to overcome historical therapeutic methods in breast cancer treatment and, furthermore, "Simple thinking" in therapy study protocols which include over- and undertreatment in special cases and to open the doors for high qualified individual therapy on the basis of fast progredient knowledge based on molecular biology.

References

Adams, S., H. Harms, H.M. Aus, A. Schauer: Photometrische Steroidrezeptoranalyse des Mammacarcinoms. Verh. Dtsch. Ges. Path. 72: 391 (1988)

Bässler, R.: S 100-positive epithelial proliferations in small ducts and acinic cells of the breast not associated with initial carcinoid formation (to be published) (1991)

Borg, A., B. Baldetorp, M. Fernö, D. Killander, H. Olsson, H. and H. Sirgurdsson: Erb B2 amplification in breast cancer with a high rate of proliferation. Oncogene 6: 137–143 (1991)

Bussolati, G.: Markers of mammary cell types and their use in tumordiagnosis. In: Pathology of neoplastic and endocrine induced diseases of the breast. Ed. by Bässler, Gustav Fischer 1985, 184–190

Caselitz, Y., H.W. Stegner, M. Osborn, B. Walter and K. Weber: The Role of myoepithelial Cells in normal and neoplastic Mammary gland tissue. In: Pathology of neoplastic and endocrine induced diseases of the breast. Ed. by Bässler, Gustav Fischer 1985.

Domagala, W., Y. Lasota, A. Dukowicz, M. Markiewski, G. Striker, K. Weber and M. Osborn: Vimentin expression seems to be associated with poor prognosis in node negative ductal NOS-breast carcinoma. Am. J. of Pathol. 137: 1299–1304 (1990)

Ekblom, P., M. Miettinen, L. Forsman and L.C. Anderson: Basement membrane and apocrine epithelial antigens in differential diagnosis between tubular carcinoma and sclerosing adenosis of the breast. J. Clin. Path. 37: 357–363 (1984)

Gerdes, J., U. Schwab, H. Lemke, H. Stein: Production of a mouse monoclonal antibody reactive with a human nuclear antigen associated with cell proliferation. Int. J. Cancer 31: 13 (1983)

Gerdes, J., H. Lemke, H. Baisch, H.H. Wacker, U. Schwab, H. Stein: Cell cycle analysis of a cell proliferation associated human nuclear antigen defined by the monoclonal antibody Ki-67. J. Immunol. 133: 1710 (1984)

Harms, H., H.M. Aus, R. Schäffer, A. Schauer, R. Brehler, K. Hempel, O. Jacobi, H. Bloß, U. Gunzer: Tissue image segmentation with multicolor, multifocal algorithms. Nato Advanced Study Institute, Pattern Recognition Theory and Applications SPA. (1986)

Harms, H., H.M. Aus, A. Schauer and R. Brehler: Neue photometrische Bestimmungsmöglichkeiten der immunhistochemischen Rezeptoranalyse. In: Aktuelle Aspekte in der Diagnostik des Mammacarcinoms, Ferdinand Enke, Stuttgart 1989

Lagios, M.D.: Ductal Carcinoma in Situ: Relationship of extend of noninvasive disease to the frequency of occult invasion, multicentricity, lymphnode metastases, in short-term treatment failures. Cancer 50: 1309–1314 (1982)

Lagios, M.D., Fr. Margolin, P.R. Westdahl, M.R. Rose: Mammographically Detected Duct Carcinoma in Situ. Frequency of local recurrence following tylectomy and prognostic effect of nuclear grade on local recurrence. Cancer 63: 618–624 (1989)

Lellé, R.J., W. Heidenreich, G. Stauch, J. Gerdes, H.H. Peter: Determination of proliferative activity in carcinoma and benign changes of the breast by a monoclonal antibody. 11th World Congress of Gynecology and Obstetrics, Berlin, West Germany, Sept. 15–20, 1985. Arch. Gynecol. 237 (Suppl.), 1983

Marx, D., A. Schauer, Chr. Reiche, A. May, L. Ummenhofer, A. Reles, H. Rauschecker, R. Sauer, M. Schumacher: C erb B2 expression in correlation to other biological parameters of breast cancer. J. Cancer Res. Clin. Oncol. 116: 15–20 (1990)

Moll, R., W.W. Franke, D. Schiller, B. Geiger, R. Krepler: The catalogue of human cytokeratins: patterns of expression in normal epithelia, tumors and cultured cells. Cell Vol. 31: 11–24 (1982)

Moll, R. and W.W. Franke: Cytochemical celltyping of metastatic tumors according to their cytoskeletal proteins. Metastases Conference NIH March 1985 Proceedings

Osborn, M.: Vimentin expression in special cases of breast cancer (personal communication)

Remberger, K. and A. Nerlich: Diagnostic value of demonstration of basement membrane proteins in benign and malignant breast lesions. In: Pathology of Neoplastic and Endocrine Induced Diseases of the Breast. Ed. by R. Bässler, Gustav Fischer, 1986

Rilke, F.: Vimentin Intermediary filament expression in cases of breast cancer (personal communication)

Rosen, P.P., P.H. Liebermann, D.W. Braun, F.A. Kosloff: Lobular carcinoma in situ of the breast: Detailed analysis of 99 patients with average follow-up of 24 years. Am. J. Surg. Pathol. 2: 225–251 (1978)

Rosen, P.P., D.W. Braun, D.E. Kinne: The clinical significance of pre-invasive breast carcionoma. Cancer 46: 919–925 (1980)

Rosen, P.P., D.W. Braun, B. Lyngholm, J.A. Urban, D.W. Kinne: Lobular carciono-ma in situ of the breast: Preliminary results of treatment by ipsilateral mastectomy and contralateral breast biopsy. Cancer 47: 813–819 (1981)

Rothe, H., R. Brehler, I. Balzer und A. Schauer: Bestimmung des proliferationsaktiven Kompartments. Proliferationsaktivitäten in Mammacarcinomen. Aktuelle Aspekte in der Diagnostik des Mammacarcinoms. Hrsg. W. Jonat, Ferdinand Enke, Stuttgart 1989

Sauer, R., H. Rauschecker, A. Schauer, J. Dunst: Therapy of Early Breast Cancer. Preliminary Results of the German Breast Cancer Study. Recent Results Cancer Res. 115: 203–210

Schauer, A., R. Brehler, M. Bergholz: Immunhistochemische Brustkrebsdiagnostik. Verh. Dtsch. Ges. Path. 69: 171–186 (1985)

Schauer, A., R. Brehler, M. Bergholz: Immunohistochemically supported diagnosis of breast cancer. In: R. Bässler und K. Hübner (eds.): Patology of neoplastic and endocrine induced diseases of the breast. Fischer, Stuttgart-New York 1985, 191–205

Schauer, A., R. Brehler, M. Bergholz: Morphologische Kriterien für die brusterhaltende Chrirurgie. Langenbecks Arch. Chirurgie 369: 427–436 (1986)

Schauer, A., H. Rothe, I. Balzer, I. Fiebig, H. Rauschecker: Immunhistochemische Tumordiagnostik beim Mammacarcinom – Einsatz zur Evaluierung von Stadium und Biologie des sogenannten "Kleinen Mammakarzinoms". Röntgenblätter 41: 340–344 (1988)

Schauer, A., H. Rothe, I. Balzer, M. Bergholz, R. Brehler, I. Fiebig, H. Rauschecker, G. Nagel, H.C. Blossey, K. Weber, M. Osborn, aus HM, H. Harms, R. Sauer, H. Scheurlen, M. Schumacher: Monoclonal antibodies for improved avealuation of breast cancer prognosis. In: M. Rich, J. Hager, D. Lopez (eds.). Breast Cancer: Scientific and Clinical Progress. Kluwer, Boston 1988, 299–320

Schauer, A., D. Marx, L. Ummenhofer, H.F. Rauschecker, W. Gatzemeier, R. Sauer, M. Schumacher und W. Sauerbrei: Ref.-zentren Pathologie, Chirurgie (Univ. Göttingen), Strahlentherapie (Univ. Erlangen) und Statistik und Dokumentation (Univ. Freiburg): Die Multicenterstudie "Kleines Mammacarcinom" unterstützt durch das Bundesministerium für Forschung und Technologie. Deutsches Ärzteblatt 87, 3628–3638 (1990)

Slamon, D.J., G.M. Clark, S.G. Wong et al.: Human breast cancer: Correlation of relaps and survival with amplification for the HER-2/neu oncogene. Science 235: 177–182 (1987)

Slamon, D.J., W. Godolphin, L.A. Jones, J.A. Holtz, S.G. Wong, D.E. Keith, W.J. Levin, S.G. Stuart, J. Udore, A. Ullrich, M.F. Press: Studies of the HER-2/neu proto-oncogene in human breast and ovarian cancer. Science 244: 707–712 (1989)

Tandon, A.K., G.M. Clark, G.C. Chamness, A. Ullrich und W.L. McGuire: J. Clin. Oncol. 7: 1120–1128 (1989)

Van de Vijver: Grade I tumors of breast cancer are negative for p185. International Symposion on c-erbB_2 (neu) oncogen. 12. Januar 1991 in Hamburg. Springer in press.

Zeilinger, R., F. Kury, E.K. Czerwenka, G. Sliutz, W. Knogler, J. Huber, C. Zielinsky, G. Reiner, R. Jakesz, A. Staffen, A. Reiner, F. Wrba und J. Spona: Her-2-amplification, steroid receptors and epidermal growth factor receptor in primary breast cancer. Oncogene 4, 109-114 (1989)

SECTION VII

THERAPEUTIC STRATEGIES IN BREAST CANCER TREATMENT

OESTROGEN-DEPRIVATION IN BREAST CANCER: CLINICAL AND EXPERIMENTAL OBSERVATIONS

R.I. NICHOLSON and D.L. MANNING

Tenovus Institute for Cancer Research, University of Wales College of Medicine, Heath Park, Cardiff, CF4 4XX, U.K.

INTRODUCTION

Among the many malignancies of women, breast cancer falls into a fairly select category of tumour in that the requirement of the normal breast for oestrogens in relation to its growth, development and functions may, in some instances, be carried over into the malignant phenotype. This obviously offers opportunities for clinical exploitation which are based either on the removal of the source of oestrogens or their precursor molecules, or which interfere with oestrogen action at the tumour tissue level (1). Indeed, application of such therapies to patients with advanced breast cancer will bring about tumour remission, often lasting several years, in approximately 50% of women, and when applied to early disease can improve overall survival rates by about 20%. Significantly, oestrogens appear to be involved throughout the life history of breast cancer by virtue of their ability to stimulate, either directly or indirectly, the growth of the epithelial cell population (2). Thus, at puberty oestrogens stimulate ductal elongation and development, while in the mature gland they maintain aspects of the ductal lobular tree. This is widely envisaged as providing a permissive environment for tumour initiation to occur within the normal breast, and thereafter for oestrogens to be involved in both the promotion and progression of the disease, by providing a selective pressure for the growth of, in the first instance, abnormal lesions and ultimately the overt hormone-sensitive cancer. The magnitude of these associations is well illustrated by the epidemiological observation that oophorectomy prior to the age of 25 years, for reasons other than breast cancer, will reduce the lifetime incidence of the disease by 75%, and that significantly this is time-dependent factor, since delay of the operation towards the menopause diminishes its effectiveness (3).

These observations have led to two current trends in breast cancer therapy: firstly, to develop methods and drugs which will as efficiently as possible reduce the oestrogenic environment of the tumour, preferably through the use of antihormonal drugs rather than through ablative endocrine surgery, and, secondly, to apply the therapies as early as is feasible in the life history of the disease at a time of minimum tumour load and spread and when a more rigorous hormone sensitivity is envisaged. Indeed, it has recently been suggested that, if and when women at high risk of developing breast cancer can be accurately identified, some of the antihormonal treatments may be used prophylactically to prevent the development of the disease (1).

In recent years, the Breast Cancer Unit of the Tenovus Institute has maintained an interest in achieving these ends through the use of two distinct classes of pharmacological agents: luteinizing hormone releasing hormone (LHRH) agonists, as a means of suppressing ovarian activity, and antioestrogens, drugs which bind to breast tumour oestrogen receptors and block the effects of residual oestrogens. Our approach has included both experimental studies in tumour models, to establish the pharmacological properties of new or interesting drugs (4-8), and early clinical studies, to explore the efficacy of these preparations in patients with breast diseases, including the overt cancer (9-13).

In this light the current article briefly reviews our data on the endocrinological and clinical efficacy of combining Zoladex (ICI 118630; D-Ser(Bu^{t})^{6}Azgly^{10}HRH; goserelin) and Nolvadex (ICI 46474; trans-1-(4 dimethylaminoethoxyphenyl)1,2-diphenylbut-1-ene; tamoxifen) to produce an improved state of oestrogen deprivation in premenopausal women with advanced breast cancer, and on the biological and antitumour properties of the pure antioestrogen ICI 164384(N-n-butyl-N-methyl-1-(3,17 , dihydroxyoestra-1,3,5(10)-triene-7 -y 1) undecamide) as the ultimate means of depriving breast cancer cells of oestrogens (8,14).

LH-RH AGONIST AND ANTIOESTROGEN THERAPY IN BREAST CANCER

In addition to the use of LHRH agonists as single agents in premenopausal breast cancer patients (9,10,12,15) their use combined with other endocrine therapies are currently being evaluated. Emphasis is initially being placed on their actions in combination with the antioestrogen tamoxifen, since, although these compounds share a common line of action through their involvement with oestrogens, it is nevertheless envisaged that they have non-overlapping mechanisms of action. The studies are, therefore, based on the rationale that, while LHRH agonists reduce ovarian activity, they do not interfere with peripheral oestradiol production, a factor which is believed to play a major role in the promotion of hormone-sensitive breast cancer growth in postmenopausal women, and that the effects of this may be inhibited by the simultaneous administration of antioestrogens. Other arguments favouring combined therapies include the possibility that they may reduce the risk of early tumour flare and the time required to achieve a full suppression of ovarian activity. Significantly, our early endocrine studies in pre- and perimenopausal advanced breast cancer patients have not to date indicated any adverse interactions between the drugs (12,16). Indeed the combination of Zoladex (3.6mg depot/28 days) plus Nolvadex (20mg b.d.) results in a greater suppression of pituitary and ovarian function when compared to Zoladex alone. Moreover, in groups of women followed up for 1 year, the circulating concentrations of both follicle stimulating hormone (FSH) and oestradiol are significantly lower in patients using the combination. The clinical efficacy of combining Zoladex with Nolvadex is currently under evaluation in a multicentre trial (ICI study 2302/15). Early results in the Tenovus/Nottingham series have shown that 9/50 patients responded to the combination of drugs with a further 15 women showing stabilization of their disease. The rate of tumour remission is therefore similar to that elicited by Zoladex alone (approximately 45% (16). Comparison of the life-table curves for Zoladex-Nolvadex combination with Zoladex alone shows a significant advantage in terms of time to disease progression with median durations of remission of 29 months and 17 months respectively. Similarly, examination of the survival curves for these two groups demonstrates a clear benefit to women who respond to Zoladex plus Nolvadex, with only four deaths in 24 patients to date being recorded for this group (median survival time >60 months versus 43 months for Zoladex alone). Subdivision of the responding groups of patients according to the category of response shows that the combination of Zoladex and Nolvadex extends the time to disease progression (tdp) and survival (s) in women who experience both disease stabilization (Z + N tdp, 19 months and s, >60 months; Z, tdp, 11 months and s, 26 months) and a complete or partial response (Z + N, tdp 46 months and s, >60 months; Z, tdp, 20 months and s, 46 months). Tumour responsiveness to either Zoladex alone or Zoladex plus Nolvadex stems primarily from patients with ER positive disease. Examination of the time to disease progression curves for these women shows a more favourable outlook for patients with ER positive tumours. This is especially pronounced in the group of women receiving the combination of drugs. Evaluation of known prognostic markers for survival after the initiation of endocrine therapy (17), including sites of disease, histological grade of malignancy, ER and length of disease free interval, has failed to show an uneven distribution of the parameters between the group. The side effects of Zoladex therapy alone include cessation of menstruation, hot flushes, vaginal dryness and occasional nausea (9). In patients treated with Zoladex and Nolvadex similar side effects have been recorded (12).

These data provide considerable encouragement for the combined use of LH-RH agonists and antioestrogens in selected groups of primary and advanced breast cancer patients. Their superiority to single agent therapy, however, requires to be confirmed in prospective randomised trials. Such a trial is currently being analysed for Zoladex and Nolvadex (ICI study 2302/15).

ICI 164384, A NEW ANTIOESTROGEN LACKING OESTROGENIC ACTIVITY

A major difficulty associated with the use of the antioestrogens that are currently clinically available for oestrogen-deprivation studies is that, although their actions on the growth of hormone-sensitive breast tumours are predominantly inhibitory, they all possess a degree of oestrogen-like activity (18). This property is well illustrated in the rat, where the administration of Nolvadex to medically (19) or surgically ovariectomized(20) animals produces an increase in the weight of the uterus (agonism). The increase, however, is not as great as that provoked by oestradiol and, when administered concurrently with the steroid, will reduce the tissue response to oestradiol, to the level observed with Nolvadex alone (antagonism). The degree of agonism is dependent on the tissue examined, with Nolvadex stimulating a full oestrogenic response in the growth of the developing ductal system of the rat mammary gland and showing no antagonism within this tissue (20). Significantly, the oestrogen-like characteristics of Nolvadex have been linked to tumour flare and slow incomplete remissions in Nolvadex-treated patients (18). Moreover, it is the toxicological problems that are associated with the partial oestrogen-like activity of antioestrogens that has prevented their widespread use outside of breast cancer and their use in areas of benign conditions of the breast and high-risk states (21).

Antioestrogens now exist, however, that are biologically inert (22) and show no oestrogenicity in the above tests (23). Thus ICI 164384, when administered at identical doses to Nolvadex, does not induce an increase in uterine weight or mammary gland ductal development in ovariectomized rats and can antagonise the tissue actions of both oestradiol and Nolvadex (8). Indeed, our own data (8) have clearly shown that, when ICI

164384 is administered at high dose levels (0.35 mg/animal per day) in combination with Zoladex (1 mg depot) to mature non-castrated animals, the antioestrogen will significantly reduce uterine weights to values below those seen following castration. It appears, therefore, that the effects of these treatments are additive, with the LHRH agonist reducing the amount of ovarian oestrogens available to sensitive tissues, while the pure antioestrogen counteracts the effects of residual oestrogen production. Indeed, it is noteworthy that ICI 164384 at 1mg/day, when given in combination with Zoladex (0.5 mg depot) can completely block the maximum uterotrophic response to oestradiol (as the most potent oestrogen), to oestrone (as a less potent oestrogen that can be peripherally converted to oestradiol) and to androstene 3 ,17 -diol (as an adrenal androgen with weak oestrogenic activity) (23). The effects are not just restricted to whole tissue actions, with ICI 164384 antagonising the oestradiol stimulated increase in PgR levels in uteri to values below those seen in surgically or medically castrated animals.

An examination of the effects of the above treatments on the growth of hormone-sensitive dimethylbenzanthracene-induced mammary tumours has also shown that a combination of Zoladex and ICI 164384 is the most effective at promoting extensive tumour remissions (23). The rate of regression and the proportion of tumours responding to Zoladex and ICI 164384 are higher than those seen in Zoladex- and Zoladex plus Nolvadex-treated animals. The combination of LHRH agonist and pure antioestrogen is also more effective than the other treatments at preventing tumour regrowth on cessation of therapy and the development of new hormone-sensitive tumours. Indeed, while the tumours in Zoladex-treated animals regained their original mean size within 3 weeks following the cessation of Zoladex treatment with seven new hormone-sensitive tumours recorded in 12 animals, the corresponding figures for Zoladex plus ICI 164384-treated rats were 30% and three new tumours in 11 animals. These data suggest that the small amounts of oestrogens which remain in animals following castration are biologically important and that pure antioestrogens can prevent their cellular actions. It is also evident that in this model Nolvadex has substantial agonistic activity which decreases its effectiveness as an antitumour agent.

MCF-7 human breast cancer cells have also been used to study the antitumour properties of ICI 164384 (19,22). The data indicate that although MCF-7 cells grow well in an oestrogen depleted medium (phenol red free RPM1 medium supplement with 5% charcoal stripped serum), growth rates can be significantly increased by the addition of 10^{-10}M oestradiol. This results in an increase in the tumour cell growth fraction. Under these conditions ICI 164384 (10^{-7}M) is an excellent growth inhibitory agent, significantly preventing any oestradiol-induced growth and severely reducing tumour cell growth fraction (19). These results are paralleled by alterations in the PgR content of the cells, with oestradiol stimulating a very large increase in the proportion of MCF-7 cells expressing PgR, while ICI 164384 abolishes its expression. What is of particular significance, however, is that ICI 164384 ($>10^{-9}$M) is inhibitory to the growth of control cultures grown in the oestrogen-depleted media (no added oestrogens) and almost totally prevents increases in MCF-7 cell numbers. Indeed, ICI 164384 (10^{-7}M) down-regulates the already low PgR levels to values undetectable by immunocytochemistry and decreases the basal levels of expression of pLiv1 and 2 (pS2) and pSyd1-8, a series of oestrogen regulated genes isolated from c-DNA libraries of T-47-D and ZR-75-1 human breast cancer cells (23,24). An example of this is shown for pSyd 5 and 7 in Figure 1. The above actions of ICI 164384 on the growth of MCF-7 cells and on gene regulation appear specific since they are fully reversible by oestradiol (10^{-8}M) and are not observed in ER negative MDA-436 human breast cancer cells grown under identical conditions.

These data infer that even under culture conditions which severely reduce the amounts of oestrogens available to MCF-7 cells (phenol red free media, charcoal stripped serum), that sufficient biologically active steroid remains and is capable of

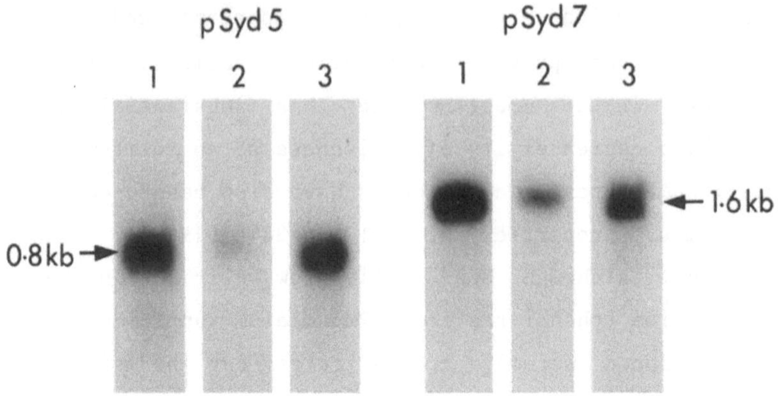

Fig. 1. Total RNA (10µg) isolated from T-47D cells grown for 7 days in the presence of 10^{-9}M oestradiol (lane 1) 10^{-7}M ICI 164384 (lane 2) or for 7 days with 10^{-7}M ICI 164384 resupplemented with oestrogen for 3 days (lane 3) was electrophoresed and transferred to nylon membranes. Hybridization to a ^{32}P-labelled cDNA probe for pSyd5 and pSyd 7 was performed and the membrane exposed to X-ray film.

The level of expression (as shown by hybridization signal intensity) for both pSyd 5 and 7 found in T-47D cells treated with oestrogen (lane 1) was markedly reduced by ICI 164384 treatment (lane 2) but reversed to the original value following oestrogen administration (lane 3).

maintaining basal levels of expression of a number of oestrogen regulated genes and aiding cell growth responses. Pure antioestrogens, however, when used at high concentrations can specifically inhibit the effects of residual oestrogens and prevent replicative events. Interestingly, recent cell biology experiments have shown that very small amounts of oestrogens can act in concert with growth factors, particularly those of the insulin-like growth factor family, to elicit the expression of oestrogen regulated genes and stimulate cell growth. Similar actions are also mediated by the concurrent administration of insulin-like growth factor I and hydroxytamoxifen, with the partial oestrogen-like activity of the drug apparently supplying a sufficient oestrogenic stimulus to maintain the responsiveness of the breast cancer cells to the mitogenic influence of growth factors (22). Pure antioestrogens cannot act in this manner due to their inert nature and therefore efficiently desensitise cells to growth factors (22). Interestingly, this desensitisation takes approximately 4 to 7 days to be established in the presence of added insulin, with cells responding normally to the protein hormone during this time (26). No further increases in cell number are observed after 7 days. It seems likely that the initial failure of ICI 164384 to block the mitogenic activity of insulin is due to residual oestrogens present in the MCF-7 cells, since the co-culture of insulin and ICI 164384 treated cells with oestradiol (10^{-9}M), which in itself is unable to reverse the growth inhibitory effect of ICI 164384, maintains the responsiveness of the cells to insulin (25). These data suggest that a relatively small oestrogenic stimulus to breast cancer cells in the presence of an alternative mitogenic supply may be sufficient to elicit a growth response and that this can be inhibited by pure antioestrogens.

Projection of this data and that derived from animal studies, to human breast cancer, suggests that since current clinical procedures uniformly fail to achieve total oestrogen deprivation and that the clinically available antioestrogenic drugs retain residual oestrogenic activity, that we may not as yet have achieved the maximum effects of endocrine therapy with respect to the rate of response, the duration of remission and the prevention of the development of hormone resistance. Pure antioestrogens which are able to bind to oestrogen receptors (14,26) and antagonise the cellular actions of oestrogens may, however, achieve this potential.

CONCLUSIONS

The studies outlined above indicate that progress is being made in both clinical and experimental areas to achieve oestrogen deprivation of sensitive tissues. We have established, in conjunction with our clinical colleagues, trials based on the use of the LHRH agonist Zoladex alone and in combination with the antioestrogen Nolvadex in advanced breast cancer patients. Through these studies we hope both to assess the efficacy of the preparations used and gain an understanding of their strengths and limitations in clinical practice. It is envisaged that this approach will be of value when high-risk states of breast cancer development are identified and interventive therapies are being planned. Indeed, experimental studies in animals have already been performed which support the view that early events in the development of cancer of the breast may be reversible by antihormone treatment and that this may be achieved through hormone-deprivation therapy (27). In this light, our current experimental results with pure antioestrogens are particularly encouraging and suggest that a state of total oestrogen deprivation produces a greater therapeutic response than does a medical castration with or without the partial antioestrogen Nolvadex. Since this state has probably never been clinically achieved due to the multiple sources of oestrogen (both endogenously produced and dietary in origin), we look forward to our forthcoming clinical involvement in this area.

RRFERENCES

1. Nicholson, R.I., Walker, K.J. and Davies, P. Cancer Surv. 5: 463-486, 1986.
2. Howell, A. Proc. R. Soc. Edin. 95B: 47-57, 1989.
3. Forrest, P. The last 30 years in the Proc. R. Soc. Edin. 95B: 1-10, 1989.
4. Nicholson, R.I. and Golder, M.P. Europ. J. Cancer 11: 571-579, 1975.
5. Maynard, P.V., Nicholson, R.I. Br. J. Cancer 39: 274-279, 1979.
6. Nicholson, R.I., Maynard, P.V. Brit. J. Cancer 39: 268-273, 1979.
7. Nicholson, R.I., Walker, K.J., Harper, M., Phillips, A.D., Furr, B.J.A. Rev. Endocr. Related Cancer 13: 55-62, 1983.
8. Nicholson, R.I., Gotting, K.E., Gee, J., Walker, K.J. J. Steroid Biochem. 30: 95-103, 1988.
9. Williams, M.R., Walker, K.J., Turkes, A., Elston, C.W., Blamey, R.W., Nicholson, R.I. Br. J. Cancer 53: 629-636, 1986.
10. Nicholson, R.I., Walker, K.J., Turkes, A. et al. In: Hormonal manipulation of breast cancer (eds. J.G.M. Klijn, R. Paridaens and J.A. Foekens), New York, Raven Press, 198, pp331-342.
11. Nicholson, R.I., Walker, K.J. Proc. R. Soc. Edin. 95B: 232-246, 1989.

12. Nicholson, R.I., Walker, K.J., McClelland, R.A., Dixon, A., Robertson, J.F.R. and Blamey, R.W. J. Steroid Biochem. Molec. Biol. 37: 983-987, 1990.
13. Dixon, A.R., Robertson, J.F.R., Nicholson, R.I., Walker, K.J., and Blamey, R.W. Br. J. Cancer. In Press.
14. Weatherill, P.J., Wilson, A.P.M., Nicholson, R.I., Davies, P. and Wakeling, A.E. J. Steroid Biochem. 30: 263-266, 1989.
15. Robertson, J.F.R., Walker, K.J., Nicholson, R.I. and Blamey, R.W. Brit. J. Cancer 76: 1262-1266, 1989
16. Walker, K.J., Walker, R.F., Turkes, A., Robertson, J.F.R., Blamey, R.W., Griffiths, K. and Nicholson, R.I. Europ. J. Cancer Clin. Oncol. 25, 651-654, 1989.
17. Williams, M.R., Todd, J.H., Nicholson, R.I., Elston, C.W., Blamey, R.W. and Griffiths, K. Brit. J. Surg. 73: 752-755, 1986.
18. Nicholson, R.I. In: Pharmacology and Clinical uses of Inhibitors of Hormone Secretion and Action. (Eds. B.J.A. Furr and A.E. Wakeling) London, Bailliere-Tindall 1987, pp68-86.
19. Nicholson, R.I., Walker, K.J., Bouzubar, N., Wills, R.J., Gee, J.M.W., Rushmere, N.K. and Davies, P. N.Y. Acad. Sci. 595: 316-327, 1990.
20. Diver, J.M.J., Jackson, I.M. and Fitzgerald, J.Z. Lancet 1986; March 24th: 733.
21. Wakeling, A.E. and Bowler, J. J. Steroid Biochem. 31: 645-653, 1988.
22. Wakeling, A.E., Newboult, E. and Peters, S.W. J. Mol. Endocrinol. 2: 1-10, 1989.
23. Manning, D.L., Daly, R.J., Lord, P.J., Kelly, K.F. and Green, C.D. Mol. Cell. Endocrin. 59: 205-212, 1988.
24. Manning, D.L., Archibald, L.H. and Ow, K.T. Cancer Res. 50: 4098-4104, 1990.
25. Dhoot, R. and Nicholson, R.I. Actions of pure antioestrogens and growth factors on the growth of human breast cancer cells. (Submitted).
26. Wilson, A.P.M., Weatherill, P.J., Nicholson, R.I., Davies, P. and Wakeling, A.E. J. Steroid Biochem. 35: 421-428, 1990.
27. Furr, B.J.A. and Nicholson, R.I. J. Reprod. Fertil. 64: 529-539, 1982.

POLYAMINES AND GROWTH FACTORS AS POSSIBLE TARGETS FOR ANTITUMOR THERAPY IN BREAST CANCER

Andrea Manni

Department of Medicine, Division of Endocrinology, Box 850, The Milton S. Hershey Medical Center, Hershey, PA, 17033, U.S.A.

INTRODUCTION

Recent evidence suggests an important role for autocrine/paracrine factors in the control of breast cancer cell proliferation. A variety of polypeptide growth factors are produced by breast cancer cells and, in hormone-dependent human breast cancer cell lines, their secretion has been shown to be hormonally regulated (1-4). In addition, breast cancer cells possess receptors for such growth factors and manifest a significant proliferative response when exposed to these peptides (1,5-7). Further support for the autocrine/paracrine theory of growth regulation is provided by the ability of antibodies directed against receptors of known growth factors such as IGF-I and EGF to inhibit breast cancer cell proliferation in vitro and in vivo (8-10).

Over the last several years, our laboratory has been interested in studying the role of polyamines (putrescine, spermidine and spermine) in breast cancer growth with specific emphasis on the interactions between the polyamine and autocrine/paracrine pathways. Initial studies performed in the NMU mammary tumor cultured in the soft agar clonogenic assay indicated that polyamines play a major role in the synthesis (11,12) and action (13,14) of hormonally regulated growth factors. Recent data indicate that, in this experimental system, NMU mammary tumor cells produce EGF/TGF-α-like peptides (15,16) and IGFs

(17) which appear to be critical mediators of hormonal effects. Studies conducted in the MCF-7 breast cancer cell line in liquid culture indicate that polyamines are involved in basal TGF-β secretion (18) but not in basal or estrogen stimulated IGF-I (19) and TGF-α (20) production. Polyamines, on the other hand, appear to be critical mediators of both IGF-I and TGF-α proliferative effects (19,20) although their involvement may be influenced by clonal variability and serum factors (20). Recently, we have provided evidence that polyamines may influence IGF action by effecting the secretion of IGFBP which are abundantly produced by breast cancer cells in culture (21).

Given the potentially important roles played by growth factors and polyamines in the control of breast cancer cell proliferation, it is conceivable that effective interference with these pathways may hold promise in the treatment of breast cancer. We will review here some of the experimental data providing support for this therapeutic approach.

Growth Factors as Targets for Antitumor Therapy.

Somatostatin Analogue Therapy. The development of long-acting somatostatin analogues has been a major advance in the treatment of several functioning endocrine tumors (22,23). These compounds could influence breast cancer growth indirectly by effecting the endocrine milieu of the host and directly at the tumor level. A possible mechanism of antitumor action involves inhibition of growth hormone and, under certain conditions, prolactin release (24-28). Consistent prolactin suppression can best be achieved by concomitant administration of dopaminergic drugs such as bromocriptine (29). Although human breast cancer is predominantly estrogen dependent there is evidence in the literature that growth hormone and prolactin, both lactogenic in women, could stimulate breast cancer growth (30-32). Suppression of circulating levels of IGF-I, the production of which is growth hormone dependent could also be instrumental in inducing tumor regression. Somatostatin analogues could also interfere with EGF/TGF-α stimulated breast cancer cell proliferation. Plasma concentrations of EGF have been found to be suppressed in patients treated with somatostatin analogue therapy (33). In addition, in different experimental systems, somatostatin has been shown to inhibit EGF action (34,35). Finally, somatostatin analogues could also exert a direct inhibitory effect on tumor growth as recently suggested in vitro in the MCF-7 breast cancer cell line (36). The presence of somatostatin receptors in a significant fraction of human breast cancer specimens (37) provides support for this potential mechanism of antitumor action.

Octreotide either alone or in combination with bromocriptine has been tested in few pilot clinical trials usually conducted in heavily pr/etreated women with advanced breast cancer (29, 38-40). Overall, these studies indicate that moderate suppression of growth hormone and somatomedin-C production can be achieved in most but not all patients. Additional efforts need to be placed in determining the optimal schedule of administration of the drug to maximize its endocrine effects. Occasional patients have been shown to experience objective tumor regression or disease stabilization. Due, however, to the heavy pretreatment in most patients, the therapeutic potential of this treatment cannot yet be adequately assessed. Larger clinical trials involving a more favorable category of patients are needed to establish the therapeutic efficacy of somatostatin analogues either alone or in combination with standard therapy in the treatment of metastatic breast cancer. It is encouraging that toxicity from octreotide is usually limited to mild and transient gastrointestinal symptoms consisting of abdominal pain, cramping, loose stools and steatorrhea. Glucose intolerance when present is mild and clinically insignificant. Perhaps of more concern is the development of cholelithiasis which has been reported by some investigators (41).

Anti-growth Factor Antibody Therapy.

The development of neutralizing antibodies directed against growth factors and/or their receptors offers potential for improved antitumor therapy in breast cancer. We have observed that administration of an anti-IGF-I antibody (α sm 1.20B) inhibited estradiol, progesterone and prolactin stimulated growth of NMU mammary tumors cultured in the soft agar clonogenic assay under serum-free media conditions (17). The same antibody, as well as an anti-IGF-I receptor antibody, inhibited estradiol and possibly progesterone stimulated MCF-7 breast cancer cell growth in the same culture system (42). In contrast to the NMU tumor, prolactin action was not inhibited in MCF-7 cells (42). We have also evaluated the effect of the anti-IGF-I antibody under conditions of anchorage dependent growth. We observed that addition of α sm 1.20B inhibited basal as well as estradiol-stimulated MCF-7 cell growth in liquid culture in the absence of serum (19). Overall, these data indicate that endogenously produced IGFs are major effectors of hormonally regulated growth of experimental and human breast cancer cells in culture. It should be noted that other investigators have failed to block estradiol stimulated growth of several human breast cancer cell lines including the MCF-7 with the administration of either an anti-IGF-I receptor antibody (8) or IGF-binding proteins (43). The reasons for these discrepant findings remain unclear.

Using an anti-TGF-α antibody, we have been able to block estrogen stimulation of NMU (16) and MCF-7 (44) breast cancer cell colonies in soft agar. Of most interest, in the same culture system we have been able to inhibit basal as well as E_2 stimulated growth of several primary human mammary tumors with the administration of an anti-EGF receptor antibody (16). These findings underscore the potential importance of TGF-α in hormonally regulated breast cancer growth as well as its candidacy as a target for antitumor therapy.

It is encouraging to observe that anti-growth factor antibody therapy is also effective in vivo in nude mice carrying human tumor xenographs (10,45). Finally, the feasibility of its application to humans has been suggested by recent Phase I clinical trials (46).

Polyamines as Possible Targets for Anti-Tumor Therapy.

We, as well as other investigators, have shown that polyamines are essential mediators of hormonal effects on experimental as well as human breast cancer cell proliferation in vitro (47-50). More recently, we have focused on the potential role of polyamines in breast cancer growth in vivo. We observed that administration of α-difluoromethylornithine (DFMO) an irreversible inhibitor of ornithine decarboxylase was able to completely abolish the stimulation of tumor growth induced by the administration of estradiol and perphenazine (to stimulate prolactin release) to ovariectomized NMU tumor bearing rats (51). The specificity of the DFMO effect through the polyamine pathway was supported by the ability of exogenous putrescine administration to reverse, at least in part, the antiproliferative action of DFMO. DFMO administration, on the other hand, failed to influence estradiol-stimulated progesterone receptor synthesis in the same tumors and uterine growth in the same animals (51). Taken together, these results emphasize the selectivity of polyamine involvement in hormonal action despite demonstration of hormonal control of polyamine synthesis in virtually every endocrine target tissue tested so far. Such selectivity if confined, indeed, to hormonal modulation of neoplastic cell growth could represent a major therapeutic advantage in the use of antipolyamine therapy in the treatment of human breast cancer.

In recent experiments, we have addressed the potential merit of combined hormone-depletion and antipolyamine therapy. Specifically, we focused on differential proliferative and morphometric responses of heterogeneous populations of breast cancer cells to modifications of the hormone and polyamine environment (52). In experiments conducted in the NMU mammary tumor, we observed that combined ovariectomy and DFMO induced a faster and greater suppression of the labeling indices of all cell types (glandular, myoepithelial and nonepithelial cells) than the individual treatments even though tumor regression was not superior to that produced by ovariectomy alone. Combination treatment also produced more profound morphologic changes consisting of a reduction in the fraction of glandular cells as well as a decrease in cell volume. It is conceivable that the lack of greater tumor regression observed with the combined treatment may simply be due to the short duration (7 days) of the experimental protocol. The ability, however, of combined manipulation of the hormone and polyamine pathway to rapidly influence tumor cell kinetics before inducing any major change in tumor volume may represent a significant step towards the implementation of kinetically targeted cytotoxic chemotherapy.

REFERENCES

1. Osborne, C.K., Coronado, E.B., Kitten, L.J., Arteaga, C.I., Fuqua, S.A.W., Ramasharma, K., Marshall, M., and Li, C.H. Molec. Endocrinol. 3:1701-1709, 1989.
2. Huff, K.K., Knabbe, C., Lindsey, R., Kaufman, D., Bronzert, D., Lippman, M.E., and Dickson, R.B. Molec. Endocrinol. 2:200-208, 1988.
3. Bates, S.E., Davidson, N.E., Valverius, E.M., Freter, C.E., Dickson, R.B., Tam, J.P., Kudlow, J.E., Lippman, M.E., and Salomon, D.S. Molec. Endocrinol. 2:543-555, 1988.
4. Knabbe, C., Lippman, M.E., Wakefield, L.M., Flanders, K.C., Kasid, A., Derynck, R., and Dickson, R.B. Cell 48:417-428, 1987.
5. Stewart, A.J., Johnson, M.D., May, F.E.B., and Westley, B.R. J. Biol. Chem. 265:21172-21178, 1990.
6. Osborne, C.K., Hamilton, B., and Nover, M. J. Clin. Endocrinol. Metab. 55:86-93, 1982.
7. Osborne, C.K., Hamilton, B., Titus, G., and Livingston, R.B. Cancer Res. 40:2361-2366, 1980.
8. Arteaga, C.L., and Osborne, C.K. Cancer Res. 49:6237-6241, 1989.
9. Ennis, B.W., Valverius, E.M., Bates, S.E., Lippman, M.E., Bellot, F., Kris, R., Schlessinger, J., Masui, H., Goldenberg, A., Mendelsohn, J., and Dickson, R.B. Molec. Endocrinol. 3:1830-1838, 1989.
10. Arteaga, C.L., Kitten, L.J., Coronado, E.B., Jacobs, S., Full, F.C., Allred, D.C., and Osborne, C.K. J. Clin. Invest. 84:1418-1423, 1989.

11. Manni, A., Wright, C., Luk, G.D., Davis, G., and Demers, L. Breast Cancer Res. Treat. 9:45-51, 1987.
12. Manni, A., Badger, B., Wright, C., Ahmed, S.R., Santner, S.J., and Luk, G. Breast Cancer Res. Treat. 10:191-196, 1987.
13. Manni, A., Wright, C., Feil, P., Baranao, L., Demers, L., Garcia, M., and Rochefort, H. Cancer Res. 46:1594-1598, 1986.
14. Manni, A., Wright, C., Hsu, C.-J., and Hammond, J.M. Endocrinology 119:2033-2037, 1986.
15. Manni, A., Wright, C., Badger, B., Bartholomew, M., Herlyn, M., Mendelsohn, J., Masui, H., and Demers, L. Breast Cancer Res. Treat. 15:73-83, 1990.
16. Ahmed, S.R., Badger, B., Wright, C., and Manni, A. J. Steroid Biochem. Molec. Biol., 1991 (in press).
17. Manni, A., Wright, C., Badger, B., Lynch, J., and Demers, L. Cancer Res. 50:7179-7183, 1990.
18. Cohen, F.J., Manni, A., Glikman, P., Bartholomew, M., and Demers, L. Eur. J. Cancer 26:603-608, 1990.
19. Glickman, P.L., Manni, A., Bartholomew, M., and Demers, L. J. Steroid Biochem. Molec. Biol 37:1-10, 1990.
20. Kim, I., Manni, A., Lynch, J., and Demers, L. Breast Cancer Res. Treat., 1990 (in press).
21. Kim, I., Manni, A., Lynch, J., and Hammond, J. Molec. Cellular Endocrinol. 1990 (in press).
22. Katz, M.D., and Erstad, B.L. Clin. Pharm. 8:255-273, 1989.
23. Gorden, P., Comi, R.J., Maton, P.N., and Go, V.L.W. Ann. Int. Med. 110:35-50, 1989.
24. Schally, A.V., Coy, D.H., and Meyers, C.A. Annu. Rev. Biochem. 47:89-128, 1978.
25. Schally, A.V., and Redding, T.W. Proc. Natl. Acad. Sci. USA 84:7275-7279, 1987.
26. Schally, A.V., Cai, R.Z., Torres-Aleman, I., Redding, T.W., Szoke, B., Fu, D., Hierowski, M.T., Colaluca, J., and Konturek, S. In: Neural and Endocrine Peptides and Receptors, (Eds. TW Moody), New York: Plenum Publishing Corp., 1986, pp. 73-83.
27. Schally, A.V., Redding, T.W., Cai, R.Z., Paz, J.I., Ben-David, M., and Comaru-Schally, A.M. In: International Symposium on Hormonal Manipulation of Cancer: Peptides, Growth Factors and New (anti) Steroidal Agents (Eds. JGM Klijn), New York: Raven Press, 1987, pp. 431-440.
28. Schally, A.V., Redding, T.W., Paz-Bouza, J.I., Comaru-Schally, A.M., and Mathe, G. In: Prostate Cancer, Part A. (Eds. GP Murphy, S. Khoury, R. Kuss, C. Chatelain, L. Denis), New York: Alan R. Liss, 1987, pp. 173-197.
29. Manni, A., Boucher, A.E., Demers, L.M., Harvey, H.A., Lipton, A., Simmonds, M.A., and Bartholomew, M. Breast Cancer Res. Treat. 14:289-298, 1989.

30. Manni, A., Wright, C., Davis, G., Glenn, J., Joehl, R., and Feil, P. Cancer Res. 46:1669-1672, 1986.
31. Malarkey, W.B., Kennedy, M., Allred, L.E., and Milo, G. J. Clin. Endocrinol. Metab. 56:673-677, 1983.
32. DeSouza, I., Morgan, L., Lewis, U.J., Raggatt, P.R., Salih, H., and Hobbs, J.R. The Lancet 2:182-184, I974.
33. Chirlanda, G., Uccioli, L., Perri, F., Altomonte, L., Bertoi, A., Manna, R., Frati, L., and Greco, A.U. Lancet 1983; i,65.
34. Viguerie, N., Tahiri-Jouti, N., Ayral, A.M., Cambillau, C., Scemama, J.L., Bastie, M.J., Knuhtsen, S., Esteve, J.P., Pradayrol, L., Susini, C., and Vaysse, N. Endocrinology 124:1017-1025, 1989.
35. Mascardo, R.N., and Sherline, P., Endocrinology 111:1394-1396, 1982.
36. Setyono-Han, B., Henkelman, M.S., Foekens, J.A., and Klijn, J.G.M. Cancer Res. 47:1566-1570, 1987.
37. Reubi, J.C., Waser, B., Foekens, J.A., Klijn, J.G.M., Lamberts, S.W.J., and Laissue, J. Int. J. Cancer 46:416-420, 1990.
38. Vennin, P.H., Peyrat, J. P., Bonneterre, J., Louchez, M.M., Harris, A.G., and Demaille, A. Anticancer Res. 9:153-156, 1989.
39. Pollak, M.N., Polychronakos, C., and Guyda, H. Anticancer Res. 9:889-892, 1989.
40. Stolfi, R., Parisi, A.M., Natoli, C., and Iacobelli, S. Anticancer Res. 10:203-204, 1990.
41. Ho, K.Y., Weissberger, A.J., Marbach, P., and Lazarus, L. Ann. Int. Med. 112:173-181, 1990.
42. Manni, A., Wright, C., and Buck, H. Role of insulin-like growth factors in the multihormonal control of MCF-7 breast cancer growth in soft agar. Program of the 82nd Annual Meeting of the American Association for Cancer Research, Houston, TX, May 15-18, 1991 (in press).
43. van der Burg, B., Isbrucker, L., van Selm-Miltenburg, A.J.P., de Laat, S.W., and van Zoelen, E.J.J. Cancer Res. 50:7770-7774, 1990.
44. Manni, A., Wright, C., Buck, H., and Heitjan, D. Role of transforming growth factors (TGF)-alpha and beta in the endocrine control of human breast cancer growth in soft agar. 73rd Annual Meeting of the Endocrine Society, Washington, DC., June 19-22, 1991 (in press).
45. Masui, H., Kawamoto, T., Sato, J.D., Wolf, B., Sato, G.H., and Mendelsohn, J. Cancer Res. 44:1002-1007, 1984.
46. Mendelsohn, J. J. Steroid Biochem. Molec. Biol. 37:889-892, 1990.
47. Manni, A., and Wright, C. J. Natl. Cancer Inst. 73:511-514, 1984.

48. Manni, A., and Wright, C. J. Natl. Cancer Inst. 74:941-944, 1985.
49. Lima, G., and Shiu, R.P.C. Cancer Res. 45:24662470, 1985.
50. Kendra, K.L., and Katzenellenbogen, B.S. J. Steroid Biochem. 28:123-128, 1987.
51. Manni, A., Badger, B., Lynch, J., and Demers, L. Breast Cancer Res. Treat. 17:187-196, 1990.
52. Manni, A., Lancaster, S., English, H., Badger, B., Lynch, J., and Demers, L. Breast Cancer Res. Treat. 17:179-186, 1990.

NEW DIAGNOSTIC METHODS AND TREATMENT MODALITIES IN BREAST CANCER

J.G.M. KLIJN, P.M.J.J. BERNS, M. BONTENBAL, J. ALEXIEVA-FIGUSCH and J.A. FOEKENS.

Division of Endocrine Oncology, The Dr. Daniel den Hoed Cancer Center, Rotterdam, The Netherlands

INTRODUCTION

Present research in the field of clinical breast cancer is focussed on new diagnostic methods and on the development of new treatment modalities. A number of modern cell biological parameters such as oncogenes, growth factors and secretory proteins, appear to be important prognostic factors because they strongly influence the behaviour of a tumor with respect to metastatic pattern, extent of cellular differentiation, growth rate and the development of therapy resistance. These factors are also relevant for the development of new treatment strategies. In this paper we will deal first with these new diagnostic methods and then we will summarize new developments in the treatment of breast cancer.

NEW DIAGNOSTIC METHODS

New diagnostic methods may more adequately select patients for certain treatment modalities. This can be reached by better characterization of individual tumors and by in vivo imaging of tumors by different techniques.

Tumor characterization and prognostic value

In the current discussion on application of systemic adjuvant therapy in primary breast cancer identification of high-risk and low risk patients is a major issue (1,2). Such identification is necessary in order to prevent overtreatment in low-risk patients and to apply intensive treatment in high-risk patients. A large series of classical and second-generation prognostic factors for human breast cancer has been reported (3). Patients characteristics are race, age, menopausal status, performance status and metabolic disease. Variables determined in blood are especially tumor marker levels (CEA, Ca15-3), alkaline phosphatase activity, liver function test and hormone levels. Most important are tumor characteristics. Stage, histological features such as differentiation grade and vascular invasion, and levels of steroid receptors (ER, PgR, AR, vit D-R) are well known prognostic parameters. Membrane receptors for hormones (LHRH, PRL, Somatostatin) and growth factors (EGF, IGF-1, TGF-β) are of increasing interest. Also enzymes, proteins and other cytoplasmatic factors are interesting, for instance cathepsin-D, pS2 protein, heat shock proteins, plasminogen activator expression, tyrosine kinase activities, growth factor content, aromatase activity, haptoglobin-related proteins, human milk fat globule antigens (HMFG-1), and prostaglandin levels. Chromosomal abnormalities in breast cancer have been demonstrated on chromosomes 1p, 1q,, 3p, 8q, 11p, 11q, 13q, 13p, 17q, 18q and 22. Aneuploidy occurs in more than half of all breast cancers and is related to poor prognosis. There are a lot of reports (3-14) on the prognostic value of amplification or (over)expression of various oncogenes (C-erbB-2, myc, int-2, bcl-1, hst-1). Amplification and overexpression of these oncogenes have been detected in a minority of patients (10-40%) and are frequently related to more agressive breast tumors and to poor prognosis. Also a high proliferative activity of tumors, measured by the thymidine labeling index, S-phase fraction, Ki67-index, and a short disease-free survival indicates poor prognosis. Finally, response to treatment is of course a very important factor especially with respect to patients with metastatic disease. For an extensive review on all of these prognostic factors I would like to refer to our paper in the Monographs of the European School of Oncology (3).

<u>Own results</u>

With respect to our own research efforts, we have investigated the incidence and prognostic value of a) some relevant oncogenes (HER2/neu, c-myc, int-2), b) hormone and growth factor receptors i.e. for estradiol (ER), progesterone (PgR), somatostatin (SS-R), insulin-like growth factor-1 (IGF-1-R) and epidermal growth factor (EGF-R), and c) estrogen regulated proteins as pS2 and cathepsin-D.

Oncogene copy numbers were studied by Southern analysis in DNA isolated from homogenates of 1052 human breast cancer samples collected both retrospectively from our tumor bank and in a prospective study (15-18). Oncogene amplification (>2 copies of the gene) was observed in 17.1% for c-myc, in 18.7% for HER2/neu and in 14.1% for int-2/bcl-1. The relationships between steroid receptor status and oncogene amplification are summarized in Table 1. HER2/neu amplification was more prevalent in both ER and PR-negative tumors. C-myc amplification was significantly related to PR-negative tumors, whereas amplification of int-2/bcl-1 was related to ER-positive tumors. A strong negative association between c-myc and HER2/neu amplification was found.

Table 1. Relation between oncogene amplification and steroid receptor status

	ER	PgR
HER-2/neu	$p < 0.0001$	$p < 0.0001$
C-myc	n.s.	$p < 0.05$
Int-2/bcl-1	$p < 0.001$	n.s.

Overall c-myc amplification appeared to be a much more powerful prognosticator than HER2/neu amplification (16,18). Amplification of c-myc was more frequently observed in larger tumors and in lymph node-positive patients, and strongly related with reduced relapse-free and overall survival. In multivariate analysis for relapse-free survival (RFS), c-myc amplification significantly added to the prognostic power of tumor size, lymph node status and ER-status with the highest relative failure rate (1.8) after lymph node status (2.2). C-myc amplification was predictive for outcome especially among patients with node-negative disease or steroid-receptor-positive tumors: 51 and 56% differences in actuarial five-year recurrence rates when compared to patients with tumors with normal C-myc gene copy numbers, respectively. HER2/neu amplification was not associated with RFS, but weakly with shorter overall survival in univariate analysis. Only in the relatively small subgroup of steroid-receptor-negative tumors, HER2/neu amplification may identify those patients with an increased risk of death.

C-myc and HER2/neu amplification appeared to be also of

value with respect to prediction of response to endocrine and chemotherapy in metastatic disease (16,18). HER2/neu amplified tumors showed a poor response to endocrine therapy but a good response to subsequent chemotherapy. On the other hand, C-myc amplified tumors showed a worse response to chemotherapy but not to endocrine therapy when compared to non-amplified tumors. Ultimately either for HER2/neu or C-myc, opposite effects on duration of response to endocrine and subsequent chemotherapy resulted in a lack of a significant association between gene amplification and overall postrelapse survival.

As demonstrated by many groups, we found a clear prognostic value with respect to ER and PgR levels measured by the dextran-coated charcoal assay (DCC-assay) (19,20). Recently we demonstrated that enzyme immuno-assays (EIA's) for determination of ER and PgR status in human breast tumor cytosols were equally suitable for predicting patient prognosis, but the optimal cut-points between receptor-positive and receptor-negative were slightly higher for the EIA (20). Since with immunocytochemical techniques an impression is obtained with respect to tumor heterogeneity of ER and PgR, combination of immunocytochemically assessed ER and PgR with biochemically obtained ER and PgR values may therefore be of additional value in the routine analysis of steroid receptors.

Somatostatin receptors (SS-R) have been demonstrated in 8-46% of primary breast cancers (21-23). A higher positivity rate (up to 46%) has been found in freshly prepared larger tumors (22). These SS-R positive tumors often contained neuroendocrine histological markers. In the first study (24, 25)on the relationship with survival, we demonstrated that patients with SS-R-positive tumors have a significantly better 5-year RFS than patients with SS-R negative tumors.

Receptors for IGF-1 were demonstrated by us (24, 26) and two other groups (27, 28) in 93%, 93% and 50-67% of primary breast cancers, respectively. Our study (24) on 214 patients showed no relationship between IGF-1-R and (relapse-free) survival, but recently Bonneterre et al (29) demonstrated in a study of 277 patients a longer RFS in a small subgroup of patients (± 15%) with very high levels of IGF-1-R than in those with lower levels.

Recently we reviewed a great number of papers on the clinical significance of EGF-R in human breast cancer (30). EGF-R positivity was shown to be present in 2500 (48%) of 5232 breast tumors of 40 different series of patients. The mean of the percentages of EGF-R positivity in the individual series is 45% (range 14-91%). Overall there are generally no clear differences between results obtained with different techniques although EGF-R positivity by immunological methods tends to be somewhat lower. A majority of the studies found a negative relationship between EGF-R and ER (28/31), PgR (11/18) and tumor grade (10/18), but only a minority found a significant relationship between EGF-R status and patient age (2/9), menopausal status (1/7), histologic type (3/7), tumor size (2/17), nodal status (5-9/20), ploidy (1/7) or proliferation indices (3/9). However taking the results of 5 studies together, we calculated a highly significant difference of EGF-R positivity between aneuploid and diploid tumors i.e. 38 and 15% respectively. With respect to prognosis Sainsbury et al (31) indicated that by multivariate analysis EGF-R status was the most important variable in predicting relapse-free and overall survival in lymph node-negative patients and the second most important variable in lymph node-positive patients. We found only a tendency (p=0.09) to a negative relationship between EGF-R and RFS (24). Reviewing the literature (30) 5 of 9 different groups of investigators showed significant prognostic value of EGF-R after short-term (1-4 year) follow-up indicating that patients with EGF-R-positive tumors have a poor prognosis. However, 3 of 5 groups with a maximal follow-up of at least 6 years found only a tendency to such relationship between EGF-R status and long-term outcome. With respect to metastatic disease EGF-R-positive tumors appeared to respond significantly worse to first-line endocrine treatment compared to EGF-R-negative tumors (32).

A new prognostic marker is the estrogen-regulated pS2 protein (pS2), which is a 84 amino-acid long protein with an as yet unknown function, and which is mainly expressed in ER-positive tumors. Using an optimal cut-off level of 11 ng/mg cytosol protein, we found a very strong prognostic value in both node-negative and node-positive patients, and in patients with ER-positive primary tumors (25, 33). Five-year overall survival was 97% in patients with ER+/PgR+/pS2+ tumors and only 54% in those with ER+/PgR+/pS2- tumors. In a preliminary study in 72 patients with advanced disease, Schwartz et al (34) showed that pS2 expression may define a subset of ER-positive patients that are more likely to respond to hormonal treatment. In a quite large serie of 289 patients, recently we did the same observation by quantitative assessment of pS2. In contrast to cathepsin D and independently, pS2-positive tumors responded better to endocrine therapy than pS2-negative tumors.

In vivo imaging

By using radiolabeled growth factors, hormones or radiolabeled monoclonal antibodies against receptors, tumors containing such receptors can be visualized in patients with primary or metastatic disease. Such techniques might influence treatment strategies, not only by detection of unexpected metastatic disease (35) but also by the development of new treatment modalities applying such techniques in the field of radiotherapy. For instance, the presence of SS-R and EGF-R in half of the patients with breast cancer makes such approach attractive.

NEW TREATMENT MODALITIES

Many steroid and peptide hormones, growth factors and other trophic substances are involved in the growth regulation of breast cancer. Most of these factors are derived from endocrine glands such as the pituitary, gonads and adrenals. Estradiol (E2) and IGF-1 are the most potent growth stimulatory factors. Endocrine treatment of breast cancer is designed to decrease plasma concentrations of one or more of these hormones and growth factors or to antagonize the biological effects of these trophic substances directly at the level of tumor cells. The involvement of so many hormones and other factors in the growth regulation of breast cancer offers many points of action for endocrine therapy, both directly and indirectly. Endocrine therapy of breast cancer consists of variety of both medical and surgical ablative treatment modalities but ablative therapy is increasingly replaced by medical therapy. Most endocrine therapies have more than one endocrine effect, frequently together with direct growth-inhibitory actions.

In the past decade the number of available endocrine agents has been drastically increased (36, 37). Novel approaches to the endocrine therapy of breast cancer are application of new antiestrogens, antiprogestins, new aromatase inhibitors, luteinizing hormone-releasing hormone analogues (LHRH-A), somatostatin analogues, inhibitors of prolactin secretion, and growth factor antagonists.

Tamoxifen is now the standard first-line therapy for postmenopausal metastatic breast cancer and is even accepted as an alternative to oophorectomy in premenopausal patients. However the stimulatory effect on the pituitary-ovarian function in the latter group with the occurrence of sometimes very high plasma estradiol levels is a point of concern and discussion (36). Therefore, it might be useful to add an LHRH analogue to this treatment to suppress estrogen secretion (38-41) and to reach "complete estrogen blockade", which subject is under investigation in several trials. At present, various new "pure" antiestrogens with less estrogen agonistic properties have been developed and are under investigation in experimental models and in the clinic (36, 37, 42). Interesting is the observation that some of these new antiestrogens have growth inhibitory effects on tumor cells being resistant for tamoxifen or even stimulated in growth by tamoxifen. In experimental models pure antiestrogens like ICI 164, 384 showed also a greater antitumor efficacy than tamoxifen in the absence of any (partial) estrogen agonistic actions.

Antiprogestins form a new category of antihormonal agents being of potential interest in the treatment of cancer. In vitro and in rats with mammary tumors clear growth inhibitory effects were demonstrated (43-45). Very interestingly, combination treatment with tamoxifen aiming blockade of both PgR and ER showed additive growth inhibitory effects (44). In a preliminary clinical study we demonstrated endocrine and clinical antiglucocorticoidal side-effects resulting in stimulation of pituitary-adrenal functions followed by increased plasma estradiol levels as a consequence of peripheral conversion of adrenal-derived androgens by aromatase activity (45). In spite of these unsuitable endocrine effects antitumor efficacy was observed, especially in patients with PgR-positive tumors indicating the presence of direct growth inhibitory action.

Aminoglutethimide is the only freely available aromatase inhibitor and as effective as other endocrine treatment modalities. Low dose aminoglutethimide (125-375 mg daily) is somewhat less toxic, but causes lower response rates (16-19%), while additional responses in 18-23% of patients have been shown after dose escalation to 750 or 1000 mg per day, especially when glucocorticoids are added (36, 37). The new very potent aromatase inhibitors need much lower dosages to reach similar reduction (50-80%) in plasma and urinary estrogen levels compared with aminoglutethimide. However, the antitumor efficacy seems not different from that caused by conventional aminoglutethimide treatment regimens, but the side effects might be less.

Apart from medical castration (36-41) treatment with LHRH analogues might have direct growth inhibitory effects in view of a) the presence of LHRH-like material in mammary tumor cells, b) the finding of specific LHRH binding sites in 52-67% of primary breast cancers and c) the observation of direct growth inhibitory effects on tumor cell lines in vitro (36, 39, 41). Such direct growth inhibitory effects might be responsible for the observed 10% response rate in postmenopausal women, but Dowsett et al (37) showed also decrease of postmenopausal ovarian androgen secretion and consequently a decrease of peripheral synthesis of estrogens, which endocrine effect might cause tumor remissions too.

In view of the observations that a) somatostatin analogues can decrease growth hormone and IGF-1 secretion (36, 46, 47) b) these analogues can inhibit growth of human tumor cells in vitro (48) and of mammary tumors in animal models (46), and c) somatostatin receptors have been demonstrated in about half of primary breast cancers (22), clinical treatment with somatostatin analogues might be worthwile. However, thusfar only a few results of treatment are available showing a low response rate in heavily pretreated patients (36). Studies on the efficacy of combination therapies with somatostatin analogues in previously untreated patients are needed.

We (49, 50) and others (36) showed that hormonal recruitment of tumor cells into S-phase increased the cytotoxicity of chemotherapy. However, in clinical studies the benefit from estrogen priming appeared to be modest (36, 51). New regimens have to be tested in randomized trials.

Therapy interfering with growth factor-mediated pathways such as with growth factor antagonists are promising in experimental models (52), but presently the lack of specific growth factor antagonists does restrict this type of therapy to only a few patient categories.

Apart from new developed agents with a new mechanism of action, especially combined therapies might be of value to improve treatment results in breast cancer. This concerns not only combinations of endocrine agents, but also combinations of endocrine-, chemo-, immuno- and radiotherapy. However, less is known on the interaction between hormones, growth factor antagonists, vitamins, interferons, interleukines, chemotherapeutic agents and irradiation. Therefore, in view of the fact that it is clearly impossible to test clinically all the possible combination therapies within reasonable time period, a better understanding of the biological principles involved and a rapid preclinical screening of potential powerful combination therapies are needed in order to improve the results of breast cancer therapy in the nineties.

REFERENCES

1. McGuire, W.L. N. Engl. J. Med. 320: 525-527, 1989.
2. O'Reilly, S.M. and Richards, M.A. Br. Med. J. 300: 346-348, 1990.
3. Klijn, J.G.M. and Foekens, J.A. In: Endocrine Therapy of Breast Cancer IV (Ed. A. Goldhirsch), Monographs European School of Oncology, Springer-Verlag, Berlin, 1990, pp.17-25.
4. Slamon, D.J., Clark, G.M., Wong, S.G., Levin, W.J., Ullrich, A. and McGuire, W.L. Science 235: 177-182, 1987.
5. MaGuire, H.C. and Greene, M.I. Seminars in Oncology 16: 148-155, 1989.
6. Gullick, W.J. Int. J. Cancer. Suppl., 5: 55-61, 1990.
7. Clark, G.M. and McGuire, W.L. Cancer Res. 51: 944-948, 1991.
8. Perren, T.J. Br. J. Cancer 63: 328-332, 1991.
9. Berns, P.M.J.J., Klijn, J.G.M., Van Staveren, I.L. and Foekens, J.A. In: Proceedings of International Symposium on the clinical and scientific relevance of HER2/neu/erbB2, Springer Verlag, Berlin, 1991, in press.
10. Berns, P.M.J.J., Klijn, J.G.M. and Foekens, J.A. Current Perspectivees on Molecular and Cellular Oncology, 1, 1991, in press.
11. Escot, C., Theillet, C., Lidereau, R., Spyratos, F., Champeme, M-H., Gest, J. and Callahan, R. Proc. Natl. Acad. Sci. USA. 83: 4834-4838, 1986.
12. Varley, J.M., Swallow, J.E., Brammar, W.J., Whittaker, J.L. and Walker, R.A. Oncogene 1: 423-430, 1987.
13. Roux-Bosseto, M. and Martin, P.M. Res. Virol. 140: 571-591, 1989.
14. Tsuda, H., Hirohashi, S., Shimosato, Y., Hirota, T., Tsugane, S., Yamamoto, H., Miyajima, N., Toyoshima, K., Yamamoto, T., Yokota, J., Yoshida, T., Sukamoto, H., Terada, M. and Sugimura, T. Cancer Res. 49: 3104-3108, 1989.
15. Berns, P.M.J.J., Klijn, J.G.M., Van Staveren, I.L., Portengen, H., Noordergraaf E. and Foekens, J.A. Proc. 82nd Annual Meeting AACR: 291, abstr. 1729, 1991.
16. Berns, P.M.J.J., Foekens, J.A., Van Staveren, I.L., Portengen, H., Van Putten, W.L.J., de Koning, H., Bontenbal, M., Alexieva-Figusch, J., Rodenburg C.J. and Klijn, J.G.M. 5th EORTC Breast Cancer Working Conference (Leuven, September 3-6), in press, 1991.
17. Berns, P.M.J.J., Klijn, J.G.M., Van Staveren, I.L., Portengen, H., Noordergraaf E. and Foekens, J.A. Eur. J. Cancer, in press 1991.
18. Berns, P.M.J.J., Foekens, J.A., Van Putten, W.L.J., Van Staveren, I.L., Portengen, H., de Koning, H. and Klijn, J.G.M. 4th Congress on Hormones and Cancer (Amsterdam, September 15-19), in press, 1991.
19. Alexieva-Figusch, J, Van Putten, W.L.J., Blankenstein, M.A., Blonk-van der Wijst, J. and Klijn, J.G.M. Cancer 61: 758-768, 1988.
20. Foekens, J.A., Portengen, H., Van Putten, W.L.J., Krijnen, H.L.J.M., Alexieva-Figusch, J. and Klijn, J.G.M. Cancer Res. 49: 5823-5828, 1989.

21. Reubi, J-C., Maurer, R., Von Werder, K., Torhorst, J., Klijn, J.G.M. and Lamberts, S.W.J. Cancer Res. 47: 551-558, 1987.
22. Reubi, J-C., Waser, B., Foekens, J.A., Klijn, J.G.M., Lamberts, S.W.J. and Laissue, J. Int. J. Cancer 46: 416-420, 1990.
23. Fekete, M., Wittliff, J.L. and Schally, A.V. J. Clin. Lab. Analysis 3: 137-141, 1989.
24. Foekens, J.A., Portengen, H., Van Putten, W.L.J., Reubi, J-C, Trapman, A.M.A.C., Alexieva-Figusch, J. and Klijn, J.G.M. Cancer Res. 49: 7002-7009, 1989.
25. Foekens, J.A., Van Putten W.L.J., Rodenburg, C.J., Reubi, J-C., Berns P.M.J.J., Henzen-Logmans, S.C., van der Burg, M.E.L., Alexieva-Figusch, J. and Klijn, J.G.M. J. Steroid Biochem. Molec. Biol. 37: 815-822, 1990.
26. Foekens, J.A., Portengen, H., Janssen, M. and Klijn, J.G.M. Cancer 63: 2139-2147, 1989.
27. Pekonen, F., Partanen, S., Mäkinen, T. and Rutanen, E-M. Cancer Res. 48:1343-1347, 1988.
28. Peyrat, J-P., Bonneterre, J., Beuscart, B., Djiane, J. and Demaille, A. Cancer Res. 48: 6429-6433, 1988.
29. Bonneterre, J., Peyrat, J-P., Beuscart, R. and Demaille A. Cancer Res. 50: 6931-6935, 1990.
30. Klijn, J.G.M., Berns, P.M.J.J. and Foekens, J.A. Submitted, 1991.
31. Sainsbury, J.R.C., Needham, G.K., Farndon, J.R., Malcolm, A.L. and Harris, A.L. Lancet i: 1398-1402, 1987.
32. Nicholson, S., Sainsbury, J.R.C., Halcrow, P., Chambers, P., Farndon, J.R. and Harris, A.L. Lancet i: 182-184, 1989.
33. Foekens, J.A., Rio, M-C., Seguin P., Van Putten, W.L.J., Faugue, J., Nap, M., Klijn, J.G.M. and Chambon, P. Cancer Res. 50: 3832-3837, 1990.
34. Schwartz, L.H., Koerner, F.C., Edgerton, S.M., Sawicka, J.M., Rio, M-C, Bellocq, J-P., Chambon, P. and Thor, A.D. Cancer Res. 51: 624-628, 1991.
35. Lamberts, S.W.J., Bakker, W.H., Reubi, J-C. and Krenning, E.P. N. Engl. J. Med. 323: 1246-1249, 1990.
36. Santen, R.J., Manni, A., Harvey, H. and Redmond, C. Endocr. Rev. 11: 221-265, 1990.
37. Dowsett, M. Eur. J. Cancer 26: 989-992, 1990.
38. Klijn, J.G.M. and de Jong, F.H. Lancet 1: 1213-1216, 1982.
39. Klijn, J.G.M., de Jong, F.H., Lamberts, S.W.J. and Blankenstein, M.A. J. Steroid. Biochem. 23: 867-873, 1985.
40. Klijn, J.G.M., van Geel, A.N., de Jong, F.H., Sandow J. and Krauss, B. Clin. Endocrinol. 34: 253-258, 1991.
41. Klijn, J.G.M. In: Peptides in Oncology: LH-RH Agonists and Antagonists (Ed. K. Höffken), Springer-Verlag, Heidelberg, in press, 1991.
42. Jordan, V.C. and Murphy, C.S. Endocr. Rev. 11: 578-610, 1990.
43. Bardon, S., Vignon, F., Montcourrier, P. and Rochefort, H. Cancer Res. 47: 1441-1448, 1987.
44. Bakker, G.H., Setyono-Han, B., Portengen, H., de Jong, F.H., Foekens, J.A. and Klijn, J.G.M. Endocrinol. 125:1593-1598, 1989.
45. Klijn, J.G.M., de Jong, F.H., Bakker, G.H., Lamberts, S.W.J., Rodenburg, C.J. and Alexieva-Figusch, J. Cancer Res. 49: 2851-2856, 1989.
46. Schally, A.V. Cancer Res. 48: 6977-6985, 1988.
47. Lamberts, S.W.J., Krenning, E.P., Klijn, J.G.M. and Reubi, J-C. Baillière's Clinical Endocrinology and Metabolism, Vol 3, pp: 29-49, 1990.
48. Setyono-Han, B., Henkelman, M.S., Foekens, J.A. and Klijn, J.G.M. Cancer Res. 47: 1566-1570.

49. Bontenbal, M., Sieuwerts, A.M., Klijn, J.G.M., Peters, H.A., Krijnen, H.L.J.M., Sonneveld, P. and Foekens, J.A. Br. J. Cancer 60: 688-692, 1989.
50. Bontenbal, M., Sieuwerts, A.M., Peters, H.A., Sonneveld, P., Foekens, J.A. and Klijn, J.G.M. J. Steroid Biochem. Molec. Biol. 37: 1097-1102, 1990.
51. Paridaens, R., Heuson, J.C., Julien, J.P., Veyret, C., van Zijl, J., Klijn, J.G.M., Sylvester, R., Mignolet, F. and EORTC Breast Cancer Cooperative Group. J. Steroid Biochem. Molec. Biol. 37: 1109-1115, 1990.
52. Klijn, J.G.M., Setyono-Han, B., Bakker, G.H., van der Burg, M.E.L., Bontenbal, M., Peters, H.A., Sieuwerts, A.M., Berns, E.M.J.J. and Foekens J.A. J. Steroid Biochem. Molec. Biol. 37: 1089-1096, 1990.

MIX
Papier aus verantwortungsvollen Quellen
Paper from responsible sources
FSC® C105338

If you have any concerns about our products, you can contact us on
ProductSafety@springernature.com

In case Publisher is established outside the EU, the EU authorized representative is:
Springer Nature Customer Service Center GmbH
Europaplatz 3, 69115 Heidelberg, Germany

Printed by Libri Plureos GmbH
in Hamburg, Germany